TRANSPLANT

TRANSPLANT

From Myth to Reality

Nicholas L. Tilney, M.D.

Yale University Press   New Haven and London

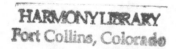

Published with assistance from the Mary Cady Tew
Memorial Fund.

Designed by James J. Johnson and set in Garamond types
by Keystone Typesetting, Inc.
Printed in the United States of America by R. R. Donnelley & Sons.

Library of Congress Cataloging-in-Publication Data
Tilney, Nicholas L.
Transplant: from myth to reality / Nicholas L. Tilney.
p. cm.
Includes bibliographical references and index.
ISBN: 0-300-09963-0 (alk. paper)
1. Transplantation of organs, tissues, etc.—History. I. Title.
[DNLM: 1. Organ Transplantation—history. 2. Transplantation—history. WO 11.1 T579b 2003]
RD120.6.T54 2003
617.9'5'09—dc21

                                                                            2003047966

A catalogue record for this book is available from the Library of Congress
and the British Library.

The paper in this book meets the guidelines for permanence and durability of the Committee
on Production Guidelines for Book Longevity of the Council on Library Resources.

10 9 8 7 6 5 4 3 2 1

For our patients, whose thirst for life,
steadfastness in facing an unknown future, and unflagging optimism
and support drive forward those of us who struggle
in this challenging field

Contents

Preface

Transplant: From Myth to Reality explores the parallel evolution of organ transplantation and transplantation biology, processes impelled by societal forces throughout much of their history. The theme of replacing diseased or deficient physical structures with the healthy tissues of others had its origins in myth and religion. The need for practical means of surgical reconstruction or repair even during the earliest stirrings of civilization led inexorably to the actual transplantation of a variety of body parts and then organs, particularly during recent decades. Unexpectedly, the remarkable success of this medical adventure has been tempered increasingly by an underlying atmosphere of competition, commerce, and exploitation—unwelcome signs, perhaps, that this hitherto limited and rather exotic specialty has reached maturity.

Having spent my entire professional career as a transplant surgeon and scientist in institutions from which important advances in patient care germinated and where lasting concepts in the biology of the subject were formed, I have experienced firsthand the joys and frustrations, adventures and misadventures, and triumphs and failures. My desire to tell the story of the evolution of organ transplantation stems from my continuing enthusiasm for this exciting and increasingly multifaceted undertaking.

Although the biomedical literature is replete with reports of discoveries, trends, results, and statistics, and some of the principal figures have described their own roles in their fields of interest, there have been few attempts to synthesize all aspects of the subject from its very beginnings. This account stems from an extensive review of published reports, grant applications, memoirs, and reminiscences, as well as a lifetime of experiences, communications, conversations, and discussions with friends and colleagues from many countries, who were and are involved in various aspects of the subject.

Transplant: From Myth to Reality is intended for a broad readership. My clinical and scientific peers may wish to refresh themselves in the history of their speciality. Our younger colleagues, trainees, students, and eventual successors often assimilate only snippets of prior events, hear the gossip and folklore surrounding parts of the subject, gape at the presence, stature, and eccentricities of the pioneers, and take for granted much of what has become routine treatment. They may learn from my accounts of the earlier struggles. My hope is that the book will also give perspective, knowledge, and confidence to patients with organ dysfunction and failure, with or without a transplant. Most especially, I seek to reach a general audience interested in the history of scientific ideas, desirous of understanding the translation of theoretical concepts into practical realities, and curious about the challenging search by those who strive to improve the lives of individuals encumbered with debilitating and often fatal illnesses. For ease of reference, a time line of pertinent discoveries and events is given at the back of the book.

The challenges implicit in wresting truths from Nature, and in particular in modulating or inhibiting bodily responses and systems that have evolved over millions of years, are familiar to scientists of every discipline. Equally difficult is the transformation of these truths and strategies into realistic means to combat or control human disease. The evolution of transplantation is a highly visible example of such a venture. Indeed, less than fifty years after the first successful kidney graft between identical twins, about forty thousand transplants of kidneys, hearts, livers, and other organs are performed each year by teams in hundreds of centers throughout the world. In many instances, these procedures have transformed the terminally ill into individuals of relative normalcy.

Many medical and scientific advances are deliberately designed and carried to fruition. Others arise purely by chance. Still others emerge as subtle clues from a mass of existing facts in relatively unrelated contexts that are identified, reinterpreted, and synthesized by alert investigators. Regardless of origin, the knowledge that has arisen is not only directly relevant to patient care, but has stimulated less obvious advances in bioengineering, pharmacology, immunology, genetics, and cellular and molecular biology. Driven forward on an international level by the constant sharing of information between those in the laboratory and those at the bedside, between universities and industry, between ethicists and policy makers, and—most important—by the patients themselves, organ transplantation has become one of the great success stories of twentieth-century biology and medicine.

Written in relatively general terms, this volume omits many specific descriptions of scientific and medical results. Relatively few individuals have been identified by name. This apparent lack of detail was deliberate, in an effort to make the text more readable. Those who were omitted, their supporters, and their colleagues know who they are and what they have accomplished, and I trust they will accept the spirit of this account.

I am extremely grateful for the interest and encouragement of those who read parts of the developing manuscript. They include Allan Mac-Donald of Dalhousie University in Halifax, Margaret Lock and Ronald Guttmann of McGill University, and Edgar Milford and Charles Carpenter of the Brigham and Women's Hospital and Harvard Medical School—all long-term colleagues who over the years have offered many points of information. Robert Sells of the University of Liverpool in particular spent a great deal of time and effort enhancing and improving two full drafts. His wisdom, common sense, and unflagging humor are greatly appreciated. Paul Terasaki at the University of California in Los Angeles kindly gave me permission to use several of his photographs from the early days of clinical transplantation, as did Hugues Joublin of Novartis Pharma France.

My surgical mentors, Joseph E. Murray and the late Francis D. Moore, involved me in the field as a young resident and have supported my efforts throughout my professional lifetime. My scientific teachers, especially Sir James Gowans of the University of Oxford, taught me much about the design of experiments to answer specific questions, and about accuracy and objectivity in interpreting laboratory data and reporting the results.

John Mannick and Michael Zinner, successive chiefs of surgery at the Brigham and Women's Hospital, the 1980 successor to the Peter Bent Brigham, provided the appropriate academic atmosphere and generously allowed me the time to complete this work. The resources of the Countway Library at Harvard Medical School are limitless; it is an unending pleasure to be able to find with ease books and articles ranging from those written early in the nineteenth century to current publications.

Special thanks go to Andrea Pribaz, who spent many hours editing, copying, and printing photographs as figures for this book; to Frances Tilney, for her organization and correction of the chapter references; and to Claire Martinez, who helped with permissions for photographs and, when desperately ill after her kidney transplant many years ago, taught us all what real courage means. Virginia LaPlante dragged readable and organized prose from my turgid first draft, teaching me much along the way. My agent, Kristen Wainwright, and her assistant, Heather Moehn, of the Boston Literary Group (housed unexpectedly across the Charles River in Cambridge) enthusiastically drove this venture to completion. Jean Thomson Black, Science Editor at Yale University Press, has been a tireless supporter and sensible advisor during the later evolution of this project. Her editing abilities seem infinite and her advice always sound. Vivian Wheeler expended vast effort on the final editing of the text. Brenda Hayslett uncomplainingly and cheerfully transcribed more drafts of chapters than I care to count. Her boundless enthusiasm, stamina, and organizational abilities are greatly appreciated.

Finally, the love and support of my wife, Mary, and our daughters, Rebecca, Louise, Victoria, and Frances, have been, as always, without parallel.

Legends, Possibilities, and Disasters

I

THE PHYSICIAN ASSURED AN OFFICIAL VOICE ON the other end of the telephone that he was indeed familiar with Joe Palazola, who had recently (in August 1964) been discharged from the Peter Bent Brigham Hospital in Boston following a successful kidney transplant. What was the call about? Palazola, the voice responded, had just been arrested as a suspected bank robber. A passing state trooper had spotted Palazola in his car, wearing a mask and a porkpie hat pulled low over his eyes. He had been forced to stop at the side of the road, then taken to the police station. Incredulous, the doctor retorted that the patient was receiving powerful immunosuppressive drugs to prevent rejection of his new organ; he had elected to wear a surgical mask outside the hospital as a rudimentary precaution against potential infection. Among those who had undergone this novel and hazardous procedure, Palazola was one of the few people to be released in reasonably good health and sustained by a functioning graft. Despite the explanation, the voice demanded that the patient's physicians come to the station to post bail. The following day, a picture of the suspect flanked by a burly policeman made its way into a local newspaper (Figure 1.1).

This awkward experience was emblematic of the opening phase of modern organ transplantation. At the time that Palazola received his graft, this innovative means of rescuing individuals with renal failure had been under way for only a brief time. Despite occasional favorable results, this period was known as "the black years" because of the consistently high failure rate of grafted kidneys and the inordinate

I

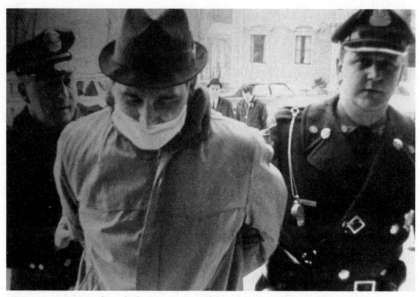

Figure 1.1 Joe Palazola being arrested by the Boston police

patient mortality. Doctors and patients alike were often frustrated and disappointed. Indeed, two thirds of the more than two hundred non-identical recipients transplanted by 1963 in all units in North America and Europe died within a few months of operation.[1] As soon as one set of complications of this radical treatment was recognized and treated, another arose.

Palazola illustrated both the positive and negative aspects of the emerging field. His newly placed kidney functioned promptly without significant rejection, transforming him from a person dying of irreversible end-stage disease into someone who was essentially healthy. The medical and surgical team was delighted. He and his family were thrilled. Unfortunately, sixteen months later he returned to the hospital with an enlarging mass involving the graft in his lower abdomen. Although the kidney donor was thought to have died from a brain tumor, in retrospect the cause was a brain metastasis from a lung cancer unrecognized at the time of organ removal.

The moment was dreadful for all involved. Immunosuppressive medications were abruptly withdrawn, in the hope that Palazola's immune system would recover and fight the new invader. As a result, he promptly rejected his kidney and returned to dialysis. When the organ was removed in an effort to control the cancer, the surgeons found an extensive and inoperable tumor surrounding it and incorporating many adjacent lymph nodes. To the collective amazement of all, and coincident with the return to normal of the patient's immune defenses, the tumor regressed and disappeared. But the operation itself produced complications, including the dramatic rupture of an artery that had been repaired upon removal of the graft; it had healed poorly because of the drugs he had taken. After six months of recuperation and considerable debate about the advisability of further attempts at transplantation, Palazola's mother donated a kidney. Despite the resumption of immunosuppression, Palazola remained cancer free until his death from unrelated causes twelve years later. He had been transplanted a third time and was awaiting his fourth organ.

I came to the Peter Bent Brigham Hospital as a resident at about the time Joe Palazola received his kidney. This was only ten years after the first successful transplant between identical twins and four years after chemical immunosuppression was initially administered to a kidney recipient. Following several years of general surgical training, I immersed myself at Oxford University in the burgeoning biology of the host responses to foreign tissues, spending the bulk of my career thereafter balancing clinical transplantation and relevant experimental studies. As these two subjects influenced each other so closely during their joint evolution, and as so many of the seminal events occurred during my professional lifetime, my goal here is to present their intertwining stories.

During the fifty years of its modern history, transplantation has mushroomed. The isolated, usually hopeless, early attempts of a few innovative surgeons to preserve by any means available an occasional patient dying from nonfunctioning kidneys have led to standardized and increasingly effective treatment for many individuals with failure of a variety of organs. From a clinical exercise of last resort, transplantation has become a vast, industry-driven enterprise involving the replacement of many vital body parts, whose relative scarcity is engendering increasingly fierce competition among transplant programs, among pharmaceutical companies, among physicians, and among the patients themselves. The result is an incredible chapter in humanity's ongoing effort to preserve life and improve the lot of the ill. Today we see "the largest entirely new field of medical care in this century . . . opening up a vast, previously unexplored territory of surgery and bio-medical science" and departing radically from established treatments.[2]

The expression of fantasy in literature and the arts has often ignited ideas that, while completely unrealistic at the time of their inception, later become applicable to the human condition. Although the modern history of transplantation is relatively short, the concept has been fueled richly throughout the ages by the vision of adding or substituting bodily features between humans or between humans and other species, a theme that has recurred since the beginning of time.[3] The ancient Egyptians and Phoenicians worshipped gods bearing the heads of animals. The Hindu deity Ganesha, the god of wisdom, bore an elephant's head put in place by another god, Shiva. In Greek mythology, creatures with attributes of both man and beast were plentiful: witness the centaurs who were half-man and half-horse, and the Minotaur with a human body and the head of a bull (Figure 1.2). Satyrs on their horse's legs raced after nymphs. Snakes coiled from Medusa's scalp; the unfortunate object of her glance was turned to stone. Homer sang of the sailors of Ulysses, who were changed into swine by the enchantress Circe. Indeed, Homer's Chimera—part goat, part lion, part serpent—has become the modern icon of transplantation (Figure 1.3). The most fearsome of all, perhaps, was the Sphinx, described by Sophocles as "the hooked, taloned maid." This monstrous creature with a woman's head and a lion's body guarded the gates of ancient Thebes, devouring anyone who failed to answer her riddles. Later in Rome, Virgil described a utopian Arcadia as a peaceful land in which dwelled the god Pan, half-goat and half-boy, Eurynome with a fish's tail, and Demeter with a horse's head.

   This motif continued throughout the Christian Middle Ages, fueled by the miracles of Jesus in reversing physical catastrophes that included blindness, disease, and even death. With supernatural aid, men were allegedly able to infuse life into inanimate forms. In the thirteenth century, the naturalist Albertus Magnus reputedly created the alchemist Cornelius Agrippa from brass. Paracelsus, a chemist and medical

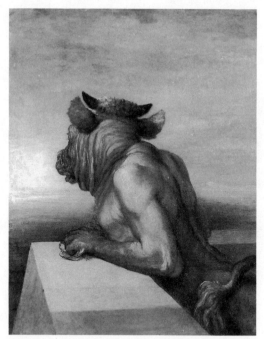

Figure 1.2 *The Minotaur*, by George Frederick Watts, 1877–1886 (© Tate, London, 2001)

thinker, described how to produce a homunculus from feces, semen, and blood.[4]

The early geographers were not immune from such influences. A fourteenth-century Benedictine monk and cartographer, Ranulf Higden, peopled his map of the mysterious continent of Africa with one-eyed denizons whose outsized feet covered their heads. In the next century, a geographic savant announced that Africans had one leg, three faces, and the head of a lion. The borders of illuminated manuscripts were replete with fantastic figures. Bestiaries of the time portrayed fanciful beings such as the manticore (lion's head, human body, scorpion's tail), the griffin (eagle's head and wings, lion's body), the hippocamp (head and forequarters of a horse, dolphin's tail), and the lemassu (part winged lion, part human). Mermaids with their women's bodies and fishes' tails swam the oceans. Hell was thought to contain bizarre beings, including humans with the heads, wings, or tails of birds. Some savants differentiated further between celestial angels who

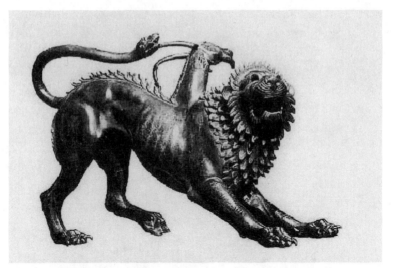

Figure 1.3 *Chimera*, Etruscan bronze sculpture, 5th–4th century B.C., in the Archeological Museum, Florence (A.K.G., London, with permission)

bore bird wings, and fallen angels from the underworld who sported those of bats. The Devil himself had horns and a tail. In the Renaissance, the Flemish painter Hieronymus Bosch portrayed the damned as anthropomorphic rats or with faces disfigured by beaks or animal features.

These themes abounded in literature, in the descriptions of the inhabitants of Heaven and Hell by Dante, Milton, and later by Blake, as well as in countless stories for both children and adults. Pinocchio's features were intermittently replaced with those of a donkey, depending on his ability to tell the truth. Mary Wollstonecroft Shelley's Frankenstein was a new being created by electrically vitalizing portions of the dead. Count Dracula could change both his personality and his physical appearance in the tradition of vampires or of reanimated corpses of werewolves. As the character of Oscar Wilde's Dorian Gray deteriorated, the face in his portrait became more bestial. Franz Kafka's commercial traveler Gregor Samsa changed overnight into a gigantic cockroach.

The transfer of body parts between living beings was only occasionally considered for therapeutic purposes. In China the surgeon

Tsin Yue-jen (407–310 B.C.), faced with two soldiers—one displaying a strong spirit but weak will, the other the reverse—allegedly anesthetized them both with wine, performed thoracotomies, and exchanged their hearts to cure the disequilibrium in their energies. The Old Testament prophet Ezekiel also suggested the replacement of organs, at least in a spiritual context: "A new heart also will I give you, and a new spirit will I put within you; and I will take away the stony heart out of flesh, and I will give you a heart of flesh."[5] In the West, pagans, infidels, and believers alike were adept at removing skin under torture, although there is no record of any suggestion that this tissue be used to cover diseased or open bodily areas. Raphael portrayed Mercury excising a sheet of skin from Marsyas. In *The Last Judgment* Michelangelo showed Saint Bartholomew, the patron saint of tanners and butchers, holding a flayed skin complete with the face of the artist—which he could reclaim on the Day of Judgment. In Renaissance anatomy texts, human figures were inevitably displayed with the skin removed; but that is as far as the technique went.

As long as believers considered illness or injury to be under divine control, replacement or repair of missing bodily characteristics remained a "supernatural" event. Christ directly restored the ear of a servant of the High Priest after an angry Simon Peter had cut it off with a sword. Saint Peter, who witnessed this accomplishment, was later able to replant the breasts of Saint Agatha after a Roman consul had removed them with tongs because she repulsed his advances (Figure 1.4). In the first century A.D., Saint Mark reattached a soldier's hand that had been lost in battle. Four centuries later, Pope Leo I amputated his own hand after becoming sexually aroused when a woman kissed it; the Virgin Mary restored it as a reward for resisting further temptation. In the twelfth century, Saint Anthony of Padua reimplanted a leg after a young boy had cut it off in a fit of remorse for kicking his mother.

Saints Cosmos and Damian carried out the most enduring example of tissue restoration by saintly surgery in the fourth century.[6] These Christian physicians traveled widely from Arabia through Syria, where they were called Anagyroi (silverless ones) for refusing payment for their medical skills. Out of fear that their good deeds might convert their patients and followers to Christianity, the Roman proconsul,

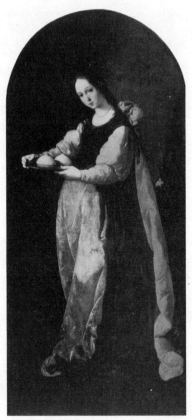

Figure 1.4 Saint Agatha holding
her amputated breasts, by Francisco de Zurburán (1537–1664),
© Musée Fabre, Montpellier
(Cliché Frédéric Jaulmes, with
permission)

Lycias, condemned the brothers to death in A.D. 303. The sentence
proved difficult to carry out. Stones bounced off the saints onto their
assailants; arrows reversed their flight in midair and killed the execu-
tioners; flames at the stake engulfed the spectators. When cast into the
sea, angels saved the two physicians. Although beheading finally completed their martyrdom, their healing powers persisted from the grave.
Prayers to them cured the faithful, including Emperor Justinian. The
brothers carried out their most famous surgical feat by reappearing in

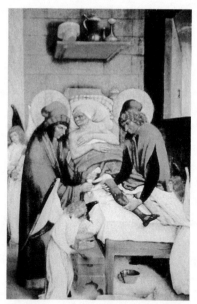

Figure 1.5 Saints Cosmos and Damian transplanting the leg of a dead moor to a bell-tower custodian. Detail of an altarpiece by an anonymous Swabian painter, about 1490 (Württenbergisches Landes Museum Stuttgart, with permission)

human form and substituting for the gangrenous, perhaps cancerous leg of the custodian of a Roman basilica the lower extremity of an Ethiopian gladiator recently buried in the church of Saint Peter in Chains (Figure 1.5). For this deed they are considered the patron saints of modern transplantation. That they also appeared to be identical twins was a remarkable harbinger of things to come.

The physician-priest François Rabelais provided a less sacred sixteenth-century example of direct tissue replacement in his book *Gargantua and Pantagruel.* After one of the characters, Epistemon, loses his head in a battle with giants, the author describes how Panurge manages to restore the head surgically: "He set it on very just, vein against vein, sinew against sinew and spondyl against spondyl, that he might not be wry necked . . . He gave it round some 15–16 stitches with a needle. . . . In this fashion, Epistemon finally healed, only that he had a dry cough of which he could not be rid, except by continual drinking."[7]

The reconstruction of injured or missing body parts with living tissue did not lie totally within the realm of legends, fantasies, and religious beliefs. It is likely, however, that these themes acted as triggers for novel approaches to the practical treatment of the afflicted. For they arose centuries before medical knowledge had accumulated to the extent that physicians could rescue individuals like Joe Palazola. Indeed, occasional early surgeons challenged established custom by devising unconventional and sometimes effective solutions to the problems of those seeking aid for their infirmities. Some of these innovators were criticized for deviating from accepted practice, while unrealistic enthusiasts grasped other ill-considered methods so firmly that many patients were substantially harmed.

Most techniques involved the repair of superficial abnormalities or injuries, particularly by covering denuded areas of skin or reconfiguring lost features. Tissue replacements included blood, whereas later departures, enhanced by the development of surgical asepsis and the boon of anesthesia, allowed the development of ever more complex operative procedures. These led ultimately to the transplantation of whole organs. While some of these advances remain part of routine care to this day, other less successful or even exotic practices (such as transplantation of teeth or of the sex glands) arose from a combination of misinterpretations of existing scientific knowledge, unrealistic hopes of the public, and professional illusions. These themes have resurfaced intermittently throughout the history of the field.

The earliest recorded attempts at surgical repair involved the face. Procedures devised in ancient India and later depicted in Egyptian papyri included the correction of nasal deformities. As in other cultures of the time, the Indians had a practice of cutting off the noses of wrongdoers and occasionally of prisoners of war. In his monumental treatise *Sushruta Samhita*, Sushruta, a surgeon of roughly 1000 B.C., described the transfer of skin flaps to cover the large and obvious area of tissue loss in such individuals. He first made a mold to size the nasal defect. With that as a pattern, he cut a corresponding skin flap from the

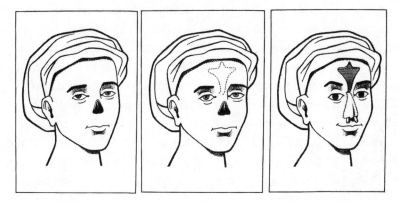

Figure 1.6 Reconstruction of the nose by Sushruta (G. Majno, *The Healing Hand*, Harvard University Press, Cambridge, Mass., 1979, with permission; originally in *Gentleman's Magazine*, London, 1794)

forehead, leaving it attached by a strip of skin between the eyebrows to maintain circulation. This was then turned and sutured to the edges of the missing tissue (Figure 1.6). Sometimes he used a flap from the cheek. The Sanskrit text explains the method: "Now I shall deal with the process of affixing an artificial nose. First the leaf of a creeper, long and broad enough to cover the whole of the severed [nose] is clipped off. Part should be gathered, and a patch of living flesh equal in dimension to the proceeding leaf should be sliced off [from down upward] from the region of the cheek and after scarifying it with a knife, swiftly adhered to the severed nose. Then the cool headed physician should steadily tie it up with a bandage decent to look at and perfectly sealed to the end for which it has been employed . . . The adhesioned part should be dusted with powders of Pattenya, Yashtimadhiekam and Rasannjana pulverized together and the nose should be enveloped in Karpase cotton and several times sprinkled with the refined oil of pure sesamum." Ears could be replaced in similar fashion: "A surgeon well-versed in the knowledge of surgery should slice off a patch of living flesh from the cheek. Then the part where the artificial ear lobe is to be made should be slightly scarified [with a knife] and the living flesh full of blood and sliced off as previously directed should be adhesioned to it [so as to resemble a natural ear lobe in shape]."[8]

These relatively sophisticated treatments were lost for centuries when medical learning shifted from centers in Egypt and Sumaria to those in other Mediterranean countries, to Asia Minor, and then to the rest of Europe. Throughout the Middle Ages, medical manuscripts in the great European libraries were often Latin translations of products of Arab writers. Contemporary teachings combined with the Arab commentaries or interpretations of Greek thinkers, particularly the physician-teachers Hippocrates and Galen, formed the basis for most scientific and medical knowledge of the time. A mixture of syllogistic precepts, Christian theology, and theoretical dialectic was involved. Surgery, so important to the ancient Greeks, was an object of disdain to the Arabs, who felt that touching the human body with the hands was unholy and unclean. Monastic and scholastic Christian minds furthered this theme, which culminated in the edict of the Council of Tours in 1163, "Ecclesia Abhorret a Sanguine." The result was a further separation of those who actually took care of physical problems by surgery and those who remained aloof from such matters. The field fell into disfavor and was relegated to barbers, sheep gelders, bath keepers, and itinerant journeymen.

Ancient surgical methods were reintroduced in Europe during the Renaissance, a period in which scholars began to broaden the interpretations of earlier Greek writings and to assimilate the exciting new discoveries in anatomy and physiology. Repair of damaged noses became important. Nasal amputation was a common result of swordplay and mutilating punishments during the period, and destruction of nasal cartilage was a frequent complication of syphilis, a disease that had become endemic in Europe. Many disfigured unfortunates lived in misery from the loss of this obvious facial feature. Gasparo Tagliacozzi, a professor of surgery in Bologna, embellished and refined Sushruta's operations. In 1557 he described his innovative methods of correcting abnormalities of the nose, lip, and ear in *De Cartorium chirurgia per insitionem*, the first book devoted to reconstructive surgery. Using a technique popularized by the Brancas, a Sicilian family of plastic surgeons, Tagliacozzi fashioned a flap of skin from the upper arm of the patient and attached it to the open site on the face, usually the nose (Figure 1.7). The immobilized arm, anchored to the patient's head with splints, allowed healing with restoration of the circulation

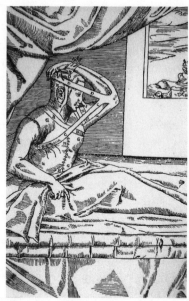

Figure 1.7 Gasparo Tagliacozzi's
method of rhinoplasty
(© Bettman/CORBIS)

between the skin flap and the afflicted area. He then detached the
lower segment of the flap from the arm and tailored the redundant but
living tissue into a shape appropriate to cover the defect.

Despite its practical success, the method came under criticism.
Some of his envious colleagues claimed that Tagliacozzi had used tissues from other people—a concept considered extreme—and ignored
his specific warning that "the power and force of individuality" would
prevent success of such grafts "because of the difficulty in getting a
permanent bond between grafted sites."[9] Important medical figures of
the time, such as the surgeon Ambrose Paré in France and the Paduan
anatomist Gabrielli Fallopius, reviled the procedure as too radical
a departure from established norms. The Church also became displeased, suggesting that such reconstructive operations (which later
included the repair of an area of bone loss in the cranium of a Russian
soldier with a piece of dog skull) violated canon law and interfered
with the will of God. After Tagliacozzi's death, those most offended
insisted that his remains be exhumed from his convent grave to be

reburied in unconsecrated ground. Removal of the healthy-appearing bone graft in the head of the Russian was also ordered.

Possibly as a result of these secular and ecclesiastical objections, nasal reconstruction became the subject of literary satire over the next century or more. Because of the high incidence of noses lost, the transfer of tissue from slave to master had reputedly become common. Although the grafts were said to heal successfully, the replanted noses were thought to survive only for the life of the donor and to slough off from the face of the recipient at death. One seventeenth-century account described this phenomenon, known as the sympathetic nose. "There was a certain Lorde or Nobleman of Italy that by chance lost his nose in a fight or combat, this party was counseled by his Physicians to take one of his slaves, to make a wound in his arme and immediately to join his wounded nose to the wounded arme of his slave and to bind it fast for a season, until the flesh of the one was united and assimilated unto the other. The noble gentleman got one of his slaves to consent, for large promise of liberty and reward; the double flesh was made all one, and a collop or gobbet of flesh was cut out of the slave's arme, and fashioned like a nose onto the Lorde, and so handled by his Chirugeon, that it served for a natural nose. The slave being healed and rewarded, was manumitted or set at liberty, and away he went to Naples. It happened the slave fell sicke and dyed, at which instance, the Lorde's nose did gangrenate and rot." Voltaire later perpetuated the myth of the sympathetic nose, as did Samuel Butler in *Hudibras*: "But when the date of Nock was out, off dropt the sympathetic Snout."[10]

The obvious effectiveness of vascularized skin flaps in facial reconstructions continued to stimulate interest among surgeons and patients alike. In the London of 1794, an anonymous writer in *Gentleman's Magazine* described the enduring practice in India in a case involving the repair of the missing nose of a bullock cart driver. The excitement produced in England by this and similar anecdotes was magnified by enthusiasm for Indian affairs during the consolidation of the empire. A surgeon-anatomist named J. C. Carpue became interested enough to practice the technique on cadavers while awaiting a live patient. In 1818 Captain Whitehouse of His Majesty's Regiment of Foot sought aid from Carpue about his nose, which had been destroyed by treatment with mercury for a nonvenereal condition. The success of the reconstruction further popularized the method of "Indian rhinoplasty."[11] That same year in Germany, Carl Ferdinand von Graefe in his book *Rhinoplastik* described "plastic" repairs of defects of nose, soft palate, and eyelids. It was the earliest application of the word, which connotes molding and shaping, in a surgical context.

The grafting of skin holds a critical place in the history of transplantation. The first formal descriptions of the rejection of foreign tissues appeared during World War II, and the individual performing the first successful kidney transplant in a human a decade later was a plastic surgeon concerned with skin coverage of severe burns.

The method was an ancient one. For millennia the Hindus had used free grafts to repair defects: "They chose a place on the buttock which they beat with hard blows from an old shoe until this repeated percussion had produced a suitable inflammation. They then cut from this inflamed part a piece of skin and cellular tissue (engorged with blood) in a triangular form which they transferred to the wound of the nose and to which they affixed with adhesive plaster. This living graft reunited marvelously." The possibilities of this transplantation technique later provoked interest among European natural philosophers and surgeons. In 1664, members of the Royal Society of London attempted to place free skin grafts on a dog, according to the society's minutes: "Dr. Charleton mentioned that the dog, a piece of whose skin had been cut off and sewed on again, had got it off; he decided to repeat the experiment at the next meeting, and think upon a way of securing the patch."[12] But the animal disrupted the planned experiment by running away. At the end of the century a Milanese surgeon, Giuseppe Baronio, initiated novel studies on the grafting of skin (Figure 1.8). Inspired by the ongoing political changes in his city as well as the new intellectual ideas of the Enlightenment, Baronio had become interested in subjects as diverse as infections, public health, poisons, electricity, chemistry, and the rights of prisoners. In his treatise *Degli innesti animali* (On grafting in animals), he noted that skin transferred between sites on a single host healed, but skin taken from other animals was inevitably destroyed, particularly if donor and recipient were of different species (say, a mare and a cow).

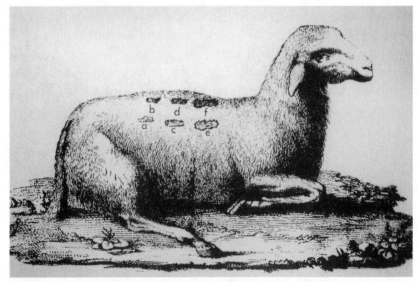

Figure 1.8 Giuseppe Baronio's experiment on skin grafting in a ram (1804 edition of G. Baronio, *Degli innesti animali*, Milan)

Despite only sporadic scientific reports on their efficacy, skin grafts were used increasingly in the nineteenth century to close skin defects in patients. The prominent London surgeon Astley Cooper successfully covered an open area on an individual's hand using his own skin. The record reads: "Hartfield, a young man admitted into Guy's Hospital (Cornelius Ward) April 9, 1817 with a diseased thumb: which Mr. Cooper, now Sir Astley, amputated between the phalanges on the 12th of July. He then cut off a healthy piece of integument from the amputated part and applied it to the face of the stump where he secured it by means of adhesive strips."[13] Over the next fifty years surgeons in France, Germany, and the United States transferred pieces of skin from the thigh or abdomen of patients to chronic superficial ulcers of their legs or to distant sites too large to be closed primarily or with a flap. With the advent of surgical asepsis and improving operative conditions, the transplantation of healthy skin to denuded or non-healing areas became the preferred treatment.

The basic doctrine of modern transplantation is that tissue moved between different areas on the same individual (an autograft) or between genetically identical twins (an isograft) will heal normally. In contrast, tissue from other members of the same species (an allograft) or from different species (a xenograft) will be destroyed or rejected promptly by the host. Differences in outcome for each type of skin graft, so clear in retrospect, puzzled earlier scientists and clinicians if, indeed, they considered them at all. The nineteenth-century German plastic surgeon Johann Dieffenbach, for instance, noted only that success of grafting was not inevitable. "We must admit that transplantation has frequently succeeded, why it has so often failed, we know not."[14]

To illustrate the not-infrequent parochialism of science, I should note that horticulturists had recognized for centuries the significance of a close relationship for successful grafting of trees or other plants, a subject probably initiated by the Egyptians and Hebrews and later described by Virgil. In seventeenth-century Florence, the Bizzaria orange, half orange and half grapefruit, was thought to have been developed through experiments carried out by a member of the Medici family. The wine industry in France was later rescued from destruction by the root louse *Phylloxeria vastatrix* by grafting French vines onto resistant California grape roots. Apple branches transplanted to pear trees or to other disparate species, in contrast, did not survive.

Even well into the twentieth century, only a few observant biologists appreciated the fact that autografts healed whereas grafts from other species did not. Based on extensive experiments on skin grafts carried out before the outbreak of fighting in World War I, German scientists recognized and explained allograft failure by evoking chemical and genetic differences between subjects. One clinical investigator covered a badly burned patient with small skin grafts from a large number of donors, including a brother. As the individual became extremely ill during the period of graft destruction, the clinician suggested that a systemic host response had developed against the foreign tissue. In 1924 Emile Holman, a surgeon working at the Peter Bent Brigham Hospital in Boston, grafted onto the extensive burns of several children pieces of their own skin and skin from their mothers. The destruction of the maternal skin but the healing of the autografts caused him to wonder about the relevance of individual differences in graft behavior. He also observed that a second crop of maternal skin was rejected more rapidly than the first grafts: "The destroying agency

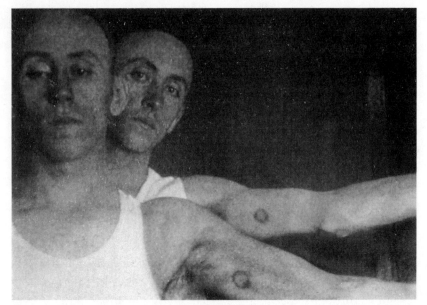

Figure 1.9 Healed skin grafts transplanted between identical twins (*Surgery*, with permission)

is specific for each set of grafts. It seems plausible to propose, thereafter, that each group of grafts develops its own antibody."[15]

James Barrett Brown, a Saint Louis plastic surgeon, confirmed Holman's opinion when he found that the skin from a given donor, transplanted after the rejection of a first set of allografts, was destroyed by the recipient more quickly and more intensely. He conjectured that the cause was some type of immune response: somehow the host, having already sloughed off the original donor tissue, produced a more powerful response against the repeat grafts. "If a second crop of homografts [a term later replaced by 'allografts'] from the same donor were applied to the patient . . . one would expect almost complete failure to take." He remained pessimistic about the chance of skin grafts surviving permanently in genetically dissimilar humans, despite acknowledging the success of isografts transplanted between genetically identical twins, including one of his own cases (Figure 1.9). His belief supported the pronouncements of an influential New York biologist of the time, Leo Loeb, that the prospects were hopeless. Indeed, in the early 1950s, Loeb declined to address the First International Conference on Transplantation, stating dogmatically that "the subject matter was a waste of time, the goal [of survival of foreign grafts] was impossible to attain."[16]

Ironically, when Brown was stationed in England during World War II, he suggested that a young Oxford zoologist interested in the problem, Peter Medawar, join Thomas Gibson, a plastic surgical colleague in Glasgow, to study skin grafts in humans. Building substantially on the previous anecdotal observations about the behavior of such grafts, their early studies on patients were to trigger Medawar's interest in the biology of rejection. This, in turn, launched the new field of transplantation biology.

The transfer of blood between individuals is a less obvious type of tissue transplantation than skin grafting, although it has become the most common and successful example. A renewable body product crucial to the viability of organisms, from the beginnings of history blood was endowed with mythic properties, probably because of the obvious association between its loss from the body and death. In ancient Rome, a ceremony called taurobolium, a symbol of spiritual rebirth, involved being soaked in and drinking the blood of a newly sacrificed bull. Encouraged perhaps by ancient traditions and by the emphasis of the Enlightenment on questioning authority, on observation of natural laws, and on development of experimental science, seventeenth-century Italian physicians were reputedly the first to attempt blood transfusions between animals and humans. The concept was an obvious extension of the long-term (but ill-considered) practice of phlebotomy or venesection—removal of blood from the ill by directly opening a superficial vessel or placing a hollow quill or metal tube within it.

After describing the circulation of the blood in 1657, William Harvey in England suggested injecting fluids into the bloodstream. A few years later, the architect Christopher Wren actually carried out intravenous injections in dogs. A not-atypical polymath of that productive age, Wren not only designed beautiful buildings, but was a mathematician and astronomer. He also dissected the brain, illustrated a neuroanatomical text, and was the first to note that an animal could survive without a spleen. Richard Lower, a failed scholar from the

University of Cambridge, then transferred blood directly from the carotid artery of one dog to the jugular vein of another, conjecturing that the blood of the first would mix freely with that of the second. In addition, he theorized that canine blood could be used "safely and advantageously" in patients who had lost blood by hemorrhage or venesection, as well as in lunatics or arthritics. During a period when bloodletting by phlebotomy was an all-too-common treatment for most diseases, Lower noted wisely that "perhaps as much benefit is to be expected from the infusion of fresh blood as from withdrawal of the old."[17] Indeed, he and a colleague transfused blood from a dog to a human late in 1667.

Others had the same idea. Satirical cartoons on the subject appeared (Figure 1.10). In November 1666 Samuel Pepys whimsically suggested in his *Diary* the transfusion of blood between humans: "At the meeting at Gresham College tonight . . . there was a pretty experiment of the blood of one dog let out until he died, into the body of another on one side while all his own ran out on the other side . . . This did occasion to many pretty wishes, as if the blood of a Quaker could be let into an Archbishop and such like." In 1667 Jean Denys, physician to Louis XIV, transfused sheep blood into a gravely ill 15-year-old boy. Six months later he administered the blood of a calf to a patient who died after the third treatment. In the ensuing legal action, the widow charged Denys with poisoning her husband, although some accused her of administering arsenic. Blood transfusions were then forbidden in France. No one attempted the technique again in England either, a decision perhaps reinforced by the first report of a fatal reaction in a dog receiving sheep blood: he "fell into a great disorder and agony and died . . . His heart was found full of coagulated blood, and the stomach black and bloody, and all his veins exceedingly distended."[18]

Transfer of blood between humans was not performed for more than a century. In 1818 an English obstetrician, James Blundell, having shown that dogs could survive blood replacement from other dogs but not from sheep, gave blood from several human donors to women dying of postpartum hemorrhage. He used a funnel and pump, then gravity, to infuse the blood into a peripheral vein. The subsequent invention of the hypodermic syringe and hollow needle enhanced this new treatment, later adopted by prominent surgeons in the United States.

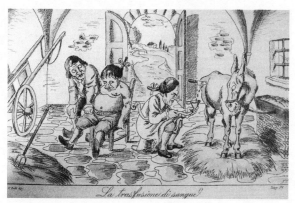

Figure 1.10 A 1628 blood transfusion between animal and man (Novartis, with permission)

The most critical factor—without which transfusion would often
be impossible—was the discovery in 1900 by Karl Landsteiner in
Vienna that serum from some individuals could cause the aggregation
or clumping of red blood cells of others when the two were combined
in a test tube. This observation led to the definition of the A, B, and O
major blood groups. The obvious importance of matching donor serum and recipient cells before the administration of blood emphasized
that, like skin-graft survival, individual differences between persons
and between species limited indiscriminant transfer. The subsequent
discovery that addition of small amounts of the anticoagulant sodium
citrate could prevent clotting outside the body opened the way for
modern blood banking and the use of stored blood in surgery or
trauma (particularly during World War II). The later introduction of
another anticoagulant, heparin, which could be given intravenously,
allowed routine performance of open-heart procedures, dialysis, vascular surgery, and organ transplantation.

Teeth also seemed an obvious superficial tissue to transplant, yet
like other innovations in the evolving field, the supposition was ill
founded. Hailed enthusiastically by the dental profession of the late
eighteenth century, actual transplantation of teeth had calamitous consequences. The Moorish surgeon Abul Cassis of Cordova had suggested the idea centuries before. John Hunter, one of the great figures

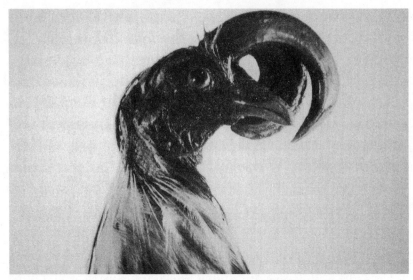

Figure 1.11 John Hunter's experiment in transplanting the spur of a cock to its comb (Royal College of Surgeons of England, with permission)

in experimental surgery, advanced it in more pragmatic terms. In 1748 Hunter became surgical consultant in London to a family of Scottish tooth-drawers and barbers, the Spences. Dentistry at the time was a primitive, dangerous, and painful field filled with eccentrics, quacks, and showmen; six hundred deaths per year in London alone were attributed to "teeth." Hunter first transferred the spur of a cockerel from its foot to the highly vascularized comb on its head (Figure 1.11). Emboldened by its growth, he transplanted a human tooth to the same area. Increasingly confident in the "disposition displayed by all living substances to unite when in contact with another substance" and impressed by the relative effectiveness of grafting between plants, he successfully replaced the first premolar of a patient several hours after it had been knocked from his jaw.[19]

Hunter's recommendations on the subject in his book, *The Natural History of Teeth*, were quickly taken up by contemporary dentists, who began to remove the teeth of the poor for a pittance and transplant them into the mouths of the rich. Their ardor, financial and otherwise, for the new technique—as well as the enthusiasm of their expectant patients—burgeoned despite undercurrents of criticism by more objective colleagues. Even individuals working in other fields began to ask questions. In his cartoon "Transplanting Teeth," the painter Thomas Rowlandson portrayed disdainfully the removal of teeth from poor children and their placement into the mouths of rich clients (Figure 1.12). The author Helenus Scott described this practice anonymously in her 1782 novel, *Adventures of a Rupee*: "The last of my master's customers was a chimney sweep about twelve years of age. My master observing that he had no teeth in the fore-part of his jaws, asked by what accident he had lost them. 'By no accident,' replied the sweep, 'my mother sold them when I was young, to a dentist, who transplanted them into the head of an old lady of quality . . . My sister . . . has had nothing but her naked jaw since she was nine years of age. It is but poor comfort to her that her teeth are at Court, while she lives at home on slops, without any hope of a husband.' "[20]

The use of teeth taken from corpses was even more common, despite the difficulties British dentists faced in collecting them (as did surgeons in obtaining intact cadavers for teaching, study, or experimentation). Today bodies are legally bequeathed to medical schools for anatomical dissection; in the 1700s they were procured by more nefarious means. The traffic in bodies by "resurrection men" was portrayed later by Robert Louis Stevenson in *The Body Snatchers*: in collusion with grave diggers, church sextants, and the like, these men pillaged cemeteries, stole corpses, and sold them to anatomical lecturers. The infamous team of Burke and Hare, who killed to provide bodies for the Edinburgh surgeon Robert Knox, was depicted in modern times by Dylan Thomas in his play *The Doctor and the Devils*.

In addition to these clandestine practices, passage of the Act of 1752 allowed the bodies of criminals executed in London and Middlesex to be legally conveyed to Surgeons' Hall for dissection. The new law led, after each hanging, to a scramble between the relatives and those wanting to profit from possession of the corpse. Even into the nineteenth century, scholars at the school of anatomy at Oxford were known to help themselves to a body from a passing funeral procession.

Considering that the deceased almost inevitably came from an urban underworld of poverty and disease, both the physicians dissecting them and the living patients they subsequently examined were at risk. The use of teeth from these corpses was equally hazardous. Hunter and others not only generated infections in the jaws of recipients, but

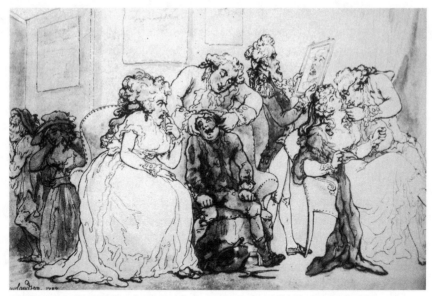

Figure 1.12 Transplanting teeth, engraving after Thomas Rowlandson (1756–1827) (*Lancet*, with permission)

often specifically inoculated the patients with syphilis. The result was sepsis, misery, and even death, as described in a 1785 report: "The transplanting . . . of teeth, has by some of our modern dentists been frequently attempted . . . A young unmarried gentlewoman had the misfortune of having one of the incisors of her upper jaw to become black and carious. This she determined to have removed and replaced by a found tooth . . . Things passed well but after a month her mouth became painful . . . The cheeks and throat, were corroded by large, deep, and foetid ulcers . . . Her strength gradually lessened, until death put an end to her sufferings . . . The progress of this putrid disease not being impeded by the most powerful antiseptics . . . cannot but suggest the taint was venereal." Indeed, after seeing the agony and death of tooth recipients, Hunter reconsidered the entire venture: "I may here remark that the experiment is not generally attended with success. I myself succeeded but once out of a great number of trials."[21]

The transplantation of skin and even teeth was possible for early surgeons; these procedures did not involve any vital internal organs and could be performed on patients who were awake. Similarly, blood could be transfused through a peripheral vein. By the middle of the nineteenth century, however, major advances broadened the scope of surgery and surgical care, setting the stage for the later development of organ transplantation. Control of sepsis was the first improvement stimulated by the scourge of puerperal fever, the often fatal infection of the uterus that could occur after childbirth. The concept that a third party such as a physician or nurse could spread this contamination and that simple hygiene could prevent it were revolutionary. In 1843 Oliver Wendell Holmes of Boston insisted that women in childbed should never be attended by doctors who had conducted postmortem examinations on individuals dying of the infection. At about the same time in Vienna, Philipp Semmelweis, horrified by the soaring obstetrical mortality rate in the city's premier hospital, the Allgemeines Krankenhaus, noted that the incidence of infection was highest in wards adjacent to the dissecting room and lowest in those where midwives trained under strict rules of personal cleanliness. After the initiation of hygienic measures that included the practice of washing hands between patient examinations, the mortality rate fell precipitously. Yet the tenor of the times was so conservative that Holmes faced prolonged and violent opposition from his colleagues. The hostility of the medical establishment drove Semmelweis to insanity and death.

Two decades later, a surgeon in Glasgow, Joseph Lister, put forth another critical improvement. Few patients were surviving an operation unscathed. Instruments were rarely cleaned between cases. Surgeons operated in pus- and blood-encrusted frock coats, with ligatures hanging from a buttonhole for use during the procedure. Under such conditions, operative sites often became septic and the sepsis led to death. The mortality rate of lower-extremity amputation, for instance, approached 50 percent, with most deaths occurring secondary to infection. Surgery was limited primarily to amputation of damaged limbs, removal of bladder stones, and minor superficial repairs. The chest was never entered; the abdomen, rarely. By chance, Lister had observed that one portion of the Clyde River, which received effluent from an adjacent chemical plant, was clear, whereas the remainder of the river was cloudy and polluted. He also learned that phenol wastes from the factory cleansed the water, and that Gypsies had used phenol-containing materials effectively for centuries to treat open wounds. After moving to London, he began to operate in a continuous spray of phenol-containing "carbolic acid," an antiseptic solution that enveloped surgeon, patient, and the surgical field alike. This radical departure from established tradition dramatically decreased the incidence of postoperative infection, but was accepted only after years of opprobrium from many in his profession both in Britain and in the United States.[22]

Anesthesia was an equally important development. Before it became available, operations were undertaken only as a last, dreaded resort. The operating theater was a torture chamber. Despite opiates such as laudanum, alcohol, and nostrums such as the Royal Navy's practice of beating a drum next to the victim's ears to take his mind off his pain, surgical procedures were carried out on screaming, struggling patients. Speed was essential. Robert Liston, a surgeon in London, for instance, could amputate a leg in a few seconds: "The gleam of his knife was followed so instantaneously by the sound of sawing as to make the two actions appear almost simultaneous." But according to a perhaps apocryphal story, in his hurry to perform a thigh amputation, Liston once "included two fingers of his assistant and both testes of his patient."[23]

Nitrous oxide, a gas, had been known since the end of the eighteenth century to produce pleasurable sensations, particularly laughter, among those who breathed it. Sometimes they became unconscious. Not until forty years later did the medical profession, particularly in the United States, consider seriously a remark that the material "seemed capable of destroying pain and might probably be used with advantage in surgical operations."[24] A Hartford dentist, Horace Wells, was the first to experience its anesthetic effects in 1844, having convinced a colleague to pull one of his molar teeth under its influence. His subsequent public demonstration was a failure; four years later, dispirited and derided, he committed suicide.

Almost simultaneously, a rural Georgia practitioner named Crawford Long noted that another gas, ether, dulled the pain of injury sometimes sustained by those who breathed it to unconsciousness during "ether frolics." Not one for publicity, Long was upstaged several years later, on October 16, 1846, at the Massachusetts General

Hospital by a young Boston dentist. William Morton used ether so convincingly that the surgeon John Collins Warren ligated a large vascular anomaly in the neck of one Edward Abbott calmly and without producing pain. Unhappily, the ensuing struggles for primacy and financial reward for the discovery led to lasting bitterness, even suicide, among those involved. British success with the use of chloroform for easing the agony of childbirth (including the parturition of Queen Victoria) and the first use of ether in Europe by Liston in 1846 cemented the acceptance of this new concept.

With the advances in asepsis and anesthesia allowing relatively safe surgical entrance into body cavities as the twentieth century opened, a few visionaries began to consider expanding the potential of organ grafting, particularly involving the kidney. However, increasing interest in the endocrine system, a group of "ductless glands" that secrete hormones into the bloodstream and specifically influence the function of other organs and tissues, caused the field to make an unexpected and short-lived detour. The existing data were intriguing. Removal of the thyroid produced death in dogs. Replacement with gland extract or even surgical implantation of pieces of thyroid in the muscles or under the skin could, at least temporarily, control the deficiency. Thyroid extract was even tried with some success in a few human patients with glandular insufficiency. Excision of the pancreas resulted in diabetes in dogs through loss of a factor secreted by the endocrine portion of that organ. Administration of a pancreatic extract later found to contain the hormone insulin prevented their inevitable deaths. However, it was possible manipulation of the sex glands that attracted the most attention.

Interest in these glands, particularly toward increasing their effects on energy and libido, was a universally popular subject. Throughout history, declining sexual prowess and vitality has been associated with growing old. The related concept that administration of tissues or their products from young and robust subjects could restore youth, revive the elderly, and delay aging has also been a constant theme. Much of this mystique has involved gonadal tissue—particularly the testes, long a symbol of vigor and bravery. In Greek legend Aeson, the father of Jason, for instance, was rejuvenated by Medea with a potion of organs of young crows and long-lived deer. Both the Greeks and the Romans took extracts of testes of goat or wolf (animals known for their sexual prowess) as a tonic. The emperor Caligula allegedly refreshed himself with such elixirs during his debaucheries. In the fifteenth century Pope Innocent VIII received blood from young boys as an antidote for the infirmities of advancing age. Ponce de Leon searched for the "fountain of youth" in the New World. Pharmacopoeias of the seventeenth century listed a multitude of substances made from the reproductive organs of several species. A century later in London, the ever-industrious John Hunter tested the concept by transplanting a cock's testes to a hen, but "without altering the disposition of the hen."[25] Reverse experiments transplanting an ovary into a rooster were also inconclusive. The enthusiasm of Asian cultures even to modern times for the aphrodisiac properties of their glands or other body parts has put the tiger, the rhinoceros, and other large animals increasingly at risk. Elderly Chinese take fetal tissues to enhance their vitality. In Western cultures too, the cosmetics industry touts various conditioning shampoos and creams containing extracts of human placentas to preserve youthfulness.

An eminent French neurologist of the late nineteenth century, Charles Edouard Brown-Séquard, did much to increase interest in the endocrine system. One of his important contributions, that adrenal function was necessary for life, was based on his finding that removal of these glands from animals was fatal. Subsequent highly publicized studies on rejuvenation also raised intriguing possibilities. Supported by the notion that celibates enjoy increased mental and physical energy, Brown-Séquard injected himself daily with seminal fluid, testicular blood, and gonadal extracts from animals. Summarizing the results of his experiments in 1889 in Paris, the 72-year-old scientist startled his audience with his conclusions that "everything I had not been able to do or had done badly for several years on account of my advanced age I am today able to perform most admirably." The "everything" he reported included increased strength and stamina, bladder control, and potency. Many of his colleagues were appalled by these pronouncements. "I consider the idea of injecting the seminal fluid of dogs and rabbits into human beings a disgusting one . . . It is time for the medical profession to repudiate it. Vivisection may be an open question, but self-abuse is not."[26] Despite the imprecations, within months of the report more than twelve thousand physicians in several countries began to treat patients with these fluids. Bolstered at least initially by the anecdotal information, the field of endocrinology, although referred to continuously in the media, remained relatively peripheral to much of established medicine until the discovery of insulin in 1921.

Uncritical practitioners became even more optimistic about the broader possibilities of glandular replacement through a series of widely read pseudoscientific books on the subject. The treatment also entered popular fiction: in one of Dorothy L. Sayers' well-known mystery stories, *The Unpleasantness at the Bellona Club*, the doctor commits murder to gain money for his research on endocrine glands. The subject even came up in the British music halls. One popular song ran:

Simpson was a clever man until the doctors treated him with thyroid glands—
He didn't have a monkey gland because they hadn't one;
He had it from a donkey, and as soon as it was done,
He tried to kick the surgeon, he nibbled bits of straw.
He tried to wag his rudder, and he shouted out "hee-haw!"[27]

Allusions to increased sexual prowess in the finale delighted a gullible public.

An exotic variation in manipulation of the endocrine system with gland extract was the growing interest in transplantation of portions or slices of the sex glands. This procedure was encouraged by the increasing breadth and scope of surgical operations; interest was stimulated further by the publicity surrounding sexual psychology as promoted by sexologist Havelock Ellis and the theories of Sigmund Freud about repressed sexuality and neuroses. Four years of destruction in World War I, the deaths of ten million young men, the wounding of thirty-six million others, and the loss of additional vast numbers from the subsequent flu pandemic sharpened these influences by causing the birth rate, already in decline in Europe, to diminish further. There was concern that the depopulated countries would lose their political power. At the same time, attention to eugenic improvement of the population was growing, possibly encouraged by the philosophy underlying the Russian Revolution and the new League of Nations that scientific principles could be applied to social organization.

Because of losing their "best" in the war, several societies not only exhorted their productive members to increase the number of children they produced, but passed draconian laws to limit the fertility of the "lower classes"—especially those who would be a potential drain on the existing social structure. "All eugenicists were agreed that manual workers were socially necessary. What they wanted was to improve the discipline, physique and intelligence of the working class by eradicating 'the lowest' elements of it. The eugenicists attempted to draw a line between socially useful and socially dangerous elements of lower orders."[28]

Britain targeted the mentally abnormal. In the United States, twenty-seven states passed laws calling for compulsory sterilization of the "unfit." In Virginia, for instance, 7,450 people were sterilized after a state eugenics law was passed in 1924, "in the name of purifying the white race." These included individuals with mental retardation, epilepsy, mental illness, alcoholism, criminal behavior, or immorality. In 1979 the law was finally repealed.[29] Germany would take this philosophy to extremes in the Third Reich, using language similar to that of the Virginia statute and evoking, in 1933, a law that ordered the forced sterilization of two million people. In his futuristic novel, *Brave New World*, Aldous Huxley also stimulated public consciousness with the concept of artificially engineering distinct classes of people; they were to range from leaders of imposing physical stature and high intellect (Alphas) to workers of small size and low mentation (Epsiloms).

As older males felt pressure to retain their youth, vitality, and potency, the prospect of rejuvenation by possible testes transplantation and other gonadal manipulation became increasingly attractive. In addition to the interest in Brown-Séquard's injections, a Viennese sexologist and hormone researcher, Eugen Steinach, stated that he had "discovered a charm to wean us from the vulgar habit of growing old." His highly publicized but untested claim stated that ligation of the secretory ducts of the testes would divert the flow of reproductive hormones into the bloodstream and thereby prevent the changes of senescence.[30]

Reports by surgeons in the United States also began to extol the efficacy of gland grafting in humans despite the lack of any supporting data. In 1916 Frank Lydston of Chicago described the results of a large series of slices of human testicles he had transplanted into the scrotum of patients, including his own: "I feel strengthened in my . . . impressions of the value of sex gland implantations, notably in the matter of increasing physical efficiency and especially physiosexual efficiency." In 1919 news from California claimed successful transplantation of pieces of the testes of an executed criminal, Thomas Bellon, into another inmate at San Quentin Prison. The prison surgeon, Leo Stanley, ultimately produced "an analysis of one thousand testicular substance implantations" in 656 prisoners, as well as describing the transplantation of testicular grafts from rams to five patients and the placement of minced testes from rams, goats, deer, and boars beneath the skin of others.[31] Physicians carried out similar rejuvenation procedures in other prisoners in the United States, particularly at Indiana State penitentiary, as did practitioners in Chicago and New York on their private patients.

During the 1920s in Kansas J. R. Brinkley was a prolific gland grafter as well as a radio station owner and a medical charlatan. Stimulated by the reports of Lydston and other Chicago surgeons, Brinkley started to transplant portions of the testes of goats, a species renowned for its sexual proclivities, to energize growing numbers of patients. A master of self-promotion, by 1930 he had reputedly collected fees of as much as $12 million from sixteen thousand gland recipients. The press finally investigated him, as he never published his results. He was eventually shut down by the Kansas State Board of Medicine for irregularities in his professional conduct and false claims of medical degrees. Despite it all, he narrowly lost a race for governor of the state.

Serge Voronoff, a Russian surgeon working in Paris, was the most visible proponent of this treatment in Europe. Eager to cap his career with an important and lucrative scientific contribution, he had already experimented with the transplantation of slices of testes from young rams or goats into the native organs of aging rams, alleging a marked increase in their energy and health. He established a sheep-grafting station in Algeria, intended to improve the industry with healthier, higher-wool-producing stock. At the same time, he emphasized the use of testicular transplants to restore potency in dogs, bulls, and stallions for breeding purposes. Claiming to have used monkey bone successfully in reconstructive operations on wounded soldiers during

World War I, he was ready to try endocrine-gland grafting in humans, an approach supported by many others in the medical establishment. Talented at keeping his name in the news, Voronoff was featured several times in the *New York Times*, which noted that he "cured a cretin by grafting the thyroid gland of a monkey to a child of 14. This resulted in immediate growth."[32] Beginning his clinical series in 1921, within five years he had transplanted slices of monkey testes into about a thousand patients, several of whom publicly extolled the virtues of the operation (Figure 1.13). To ensure a ready supply of appropriate donor organs, he developed a large monkey colony on the Riviera.

Both professional and public support of gland grafting in the United States and Europe remained high. Despite postwar disarray, the early 1920s were generally an optimistic period. The conflict had ceased, social mores were changing, science and technology held unlimited promise. Discoveries about the endocrine glands and clinical use of their products (insulin in diabetics, thyroid extract for children and adults with thyroid insufficiency) excited the imagination. Despite the extravagant but never-documented claims of the gland grafters and a spate of supportive publications, particularly by Voronoff, few voices of moderation emerged. Even the conservative *Boston Medical and Surgical Journal*, later to become the *New England Journal of Medicine*, gave the subject a cautious nod: "Like any new operations, testicular transplantation will have to pass first through a period in which it will be desired by the neurotic and the overstimulated. In many such cases, its results . . . can only be learned by experience . . . At any rate, a new chapter in surgery and physiology is being written. It will be surprising if, from this most interesting field of experimentation, something of value is not obtained for mankind."[33]

The tide of opinion turned when surgeons from Italy, Portugal, Brazil, England, and the United States began to question the entire venture. Not only were they appraising their own patients more carefully, but emerging scientific evidence was supporting a second look. In 1925, controlled studies showed that testicular transplantation was ineffectual in animals. A few years later, a leader in reproductive endocrinology, Carl Moore of Chicago, challenged the entire concept of transferring sex-gland material from human or animal. The first to

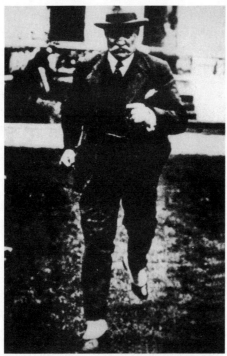

Figure 1.13 A monkey-gland recipient
showing off his new vitality (D. N. H.
Hamilton, *The Monkey Gland Affair*,
Chatto and Windus, London, 1986; with
permission)

develop dependable assays for detecting the presence of gonadal hormones in the blood, Moore was never able to demonstrate active secretion by any of the transplanted glands. Indeed, he later showed that
administration of testosterone, the major testicular hormone, to cas-
trated rats did nothing to reverse aging or enhance sexual activity. He
also concluded that "in the absence of functional incorporation of
living tissue . . . the transferred non-viable tissue . . . undergoes auto-
lysis and reabsorption, perhaps accompanied by inflammation, suppuration and sloughing."[34] In short, within days of their placement the
grafts were completely destroyed. An inspection on site by academic
veterinarians also cast doubt on the results of Voronoff's uncontrolled
sheep experiments in Algeria.

Finally, the rapid advances in steroid chemistry and increasing knowledge about the effects of hormone replacement obviated any lingering necessity for testicular transplantation. When the crash of the world's stock markets at the end of the decade ended the postwar gaiety and youth culture of the Jazz Age, common sense gradually replaced the unrealistic claims of the gland grafters. Few were ever heard from again.

New knowledge of the endocrine system and its products had stimulated the idea of testicular grafting. Like the transplantation of teeth more than a century before, uncritical science and excessive expectations and self-deceptions by public and physicians alike, fueled by the media, increased the popularity of these grafts. While Brinkley was a flamboyant entrepreneur without the scientific background, intellectual curiosity, or desire to evaluate his treatment, the same cannot be said of Voronoff. At least in the beginning, existing knowledge supported his concepts and the medical establishment accepted his reports. But as his clinical experience broadened, he became increasingly self-promoting and so conscious of his public persona that he deluded himself about his results. Unsubstantiated enthusiasm and subjective observations alone drove his claims of benefit in the animal trials, the value of which was cast into doubt because he had never included control groups.

This pattern of hope winning out over experience continues to arise intermittently in medicine and science. Doctors and scientists, like politicians, lawyers, stock brokers, and virtually everyone else, are vulnerable to the temptations of fame, adulation, and profit. During the 1950s, for example, physicians continued to inject endocrine cells to combat aging. Paul Niehans, a member of the Hohenzollern family, grandson of Frederick III of Prussia and director of Clinique la Prairie, a Swiss rejuvenation clinic for tissue therapy, exploited this technique with clients who were said to include Somerset Maugham, Aristotle Onassis, Bernard Baruch, Gloria Swanson, and the Duke and Duchess of Windsor. In 1953 he traveled to Rome to treat the ailing Pope Pius XII with tissues from pregnant ewes.

The revitalization of the elderly through grafting of animal tissues or cells involved even Christiaan Barnard, the surgeon who performed the first human heart transplant in 1967.[35] Years after this pioneering work, Barnard changed his career to become director of research at Clinique la Prairie, where by the 1980s more than sixty-five thousand patients had been treated with cells from fetal animals. Honing his not inconsequential entrepreneurial skills, he also promoted a cosmetic product that was reputed to reverse the effects of ultraviolet light on aging skin. Remarkably, the subject of gland grafting resurfaces to this day in sporadic reports of whole-testicle transplantation by joining the vessels of the donor gland directly to those of the recipient.

For nearly the first half of the twentieth century, the transplanting of tissue was limited to sporadic attempts. Although surgeons transferred skin to cover open sites on the same patient and occasionally transfused blood, they grafted only occasional organs, primarily in dogs. With the disastrous experiences of tooth transplantations and glandular grafts, reasonable expectations for eventual clinical use were few. However, with progressive refinements in surgical techniques, transplantation of vascularized organs such as the kidney suddenly became possible, causing both the public and its physicians to become aware of this new approach.

2

Attempts and Failures

A POLITICAL TRAGEDY IN 1894 TRIGGERED A
series of surgical contributions in two novel interrelated specialities,
vascular surgery and organ transplantation. After centuries of rudimentary attempts to control hemorrhage or prevent arterial rupture,
the development of methods to join or anastomose accurately two
vessels for repair, rerouting, or reconstruction was a crucial advance.
At the same time, application of the new techniques provoked investigations into the revascularization of solid organs after their trans-
position from their original location into another site in the same or a
different subject.

France at this time was in turmoil, with bombings, riots, and con-
frontations between police and workers angry at inadequate conditions, poverty, and social inequality. Even with these disruptions, the
still popular president, Sadi Carnot, continued to travel throughout
the country.[1] Upset with his lot, Santo Caserio, a baker's assistant
turned anarchist, bought a knife and took the train from his village to
the city of Lyon, which Carnot was then visiting. Pushing to the front
of the crowd surrounding the president's open carriage, he stabbed
him in the abdomen. Carnot bled massively and later died despite the
best efforts of the local surgeons. The liver had been perforated and the
great vein to that organ divided.

A young doctor at the Red Cross Hospital, Alexis Carrel, well
understood that expeditious repair of the severed portal vein could
have saved the president's life but that current knowledge and expertise were inadequate to the task. Indeed, the few times that operative

36

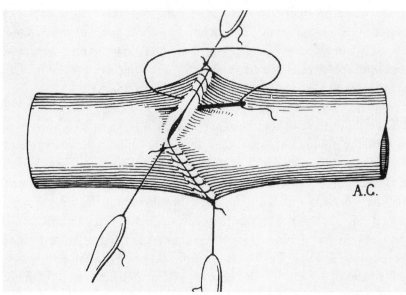

Figure 2.1 Alexis Carrel's method of vascular anastomosis (Novartis, with permission)

closure of open vessels had been attempted in patients, either bleeding continued or the surgically narrowed segment thrombosed. Stimulated by the circumstances surrounding Carnot's death, Carrel began to consider more effective means of vascular reconstruction, exploiting the availability of fine sutures of silk from his city (then the capitol of the thriving silkworm industry) and taking sewing lessons from an experienced embroideress, Mme Leroudier. He experimented on animals, attempting to devise methods to position the vessel ends accurately and to prevent clotting by presenting as little suture material as possible on the smooth vascular lining. In addition, he learned to separate the edges of the vessels to ensure perfect visualization and precise placement of the small oiled sutures on sharp needles (Figure 2.1).

Transplantation of organs was the next step. The kidney seemed an obvious choice; its blood supply usually consists of a single artery and vein, which allow it to be connected to appropriate vessels at several relatively accessible sites in the body. One of the paired kidneys could be removed surgically without disturbing the other, which could by itself sustain the subject normally. This fist-sized, bean-shaped organ filters waste products from the blood and controls fluid balance by excreting the appropriate amounts and concentration of urine. Once placed in a new location in the same individual or a new recipient, renal function could be assessed easily by following urine output. This organ seemed ideal for Carrel to try his new techniques.

The evolution of vascular surgery has been long, with a variety of methods to staunch bleeding described since ancient times. Sushruta first reported tying the umbilical cord at birth. Celsus, a Roman physician and man of letters, used the older descriptions of Galen to control hemorrhage in wounded gladiators. For first aid, the fingers were placed into the wound to compress the open vessel. For more definitive prevention of blood loss, the edges of the defect were twisted closed with a hook. Less consequential bleeding was stopped occasionally with "styptics," the best of which reputedly were made of frankincense, aloe, egg white, and clippings of the fur of a hare.[2]

Largely because the Islamic religion of the Arab physician-writers forbade the cutting of human flesh, hemorrhage was treated for centuries with red-hot cautery. Then the military surgeon Ambrose Paré and his Renaissance followers revived the use of ligation of the injured vessel with or without the addition of a compression tourniquet. The ends of the silk thread were left long, to facilitate removal when the wound underwent its almost inevitable suppuration and sepsis. Paré described his technique: "A gangreene happened to halfe of the legge of one named Nicholas Mesnager . . . Wee were constrained to cut off his legge to save his life . . . On the 16. Day of December 1583 . . . the blood was staunched by the ligature of the vessels, and he is at present cured and in health, walking with a wooden leg."[3]

Tying off the neck of an aneurysm (a dilated and weakened portion of an artery) to block blood flow through it and prevent its rupture was first chronicled in second-century Rome but was not taken up again until the early eighteenth century in France. John Hunter popularized the technique in England by ligating the femoral artery of a patient at midthigh to cause clotting of a large aneurysm behind the knee. His pupil, Astley Cooper, used the procedure successfully and unsuccessfully on aneurysms of other major vessels. America's first vascular surgeon, Valentine Mott of New York, himself a student of

Cooper, generated a large series of such cases. However, as many extremities became gangrenous beyond the site of occlusion, it was noted in Mott's 1865 obituary that he had also "amputed nearly 1000 limbs."[4] Despite these less than enviable results, the ligation method spread among practitioners during the remainder of the century, both in Europe and in North America.

The next conceptual advance in vascular surgery involved the repair of injured or severed vessels with sutures. In 1759 a Dr. Hallowell, a Yorkshire physician, closed a lacerated artery in the arm caused by a mismanaged attempt to bleed the patient by running a pin through the edges of the defect and tying a figure-eight ligature tightly around its ends.[5] A century later, a young Russian surgeon, Nicholai Eck, directly joined the ends of a divided artery with several sutures, then sewed two veins together. Others devised means to reconstitute partially divided arteries with multiple stitches or with a continuous suture method using fine lubricated needles. Placement of U-shaped sutures produced successful closure of large arteries in animals. On occasion, absorbable metal rings or cylinders were devised to join the ends of severed arteries, or the upstream proximal end of an artery was enclosed in the downstream distal end.

Shortly after the turn of the twentieth century, Emerich Ullmann of Vienna transferred a kidney from its normal location in the flank of a dog into its neck, using metal cylinders to join the vessels. The grafted organ produced "a liquid which resembled urine" for five days. Similar but unsuccessful experiments were performed by two of his colleagues, as well as by a Bucharest surgeon, Nicholas Floresco. This innovative individual previewed modern methods by using Carrel's vascular suture techniques to graft a canine kidney to the vessels in the lower abdomen, then joining the transplant ureter, the muscular tube that normally conveys urine from kidney to bladder, directly to the recipient bladder instead of leading it through the skin as his predecessors had done. Probably unaware of the activity in Central Europe, Carrel, who had "started research into the procedure of vascular anastomoses in order to be able to transplant several organs," reported the autotransplantation of a kidney to the neck of a dog. He noted enthusiastically that "organ transplantation, a simple surgical curiosity today, may one day have a definite practical value ... the replacement of the diseased organ by a healthy organ in order to treat, for example Bright's disease," an inflammatory condition of the kidneys that may cause their ultimate destruction.[6]

In 1904, unhappy about his chances for a career in experimental surgery in what he regarded as the provincial Lyonnaise surroundings (but more likely because he failed to achieve academic advancement), Carrel joined the physiologist Charles Guthrie in Chicago. The two investigators broadened the use of their techniques by transplanting blood vessels, thyroid and parathyroid glands, ovary, testes, kidney, and heart. Guthrie even transferred the entire head of one dog to the neck of another. They grafted two donor kidneys together into a cat, a refinement still used clinically in the placement of both kidneys from child donors into adult recipients.

With a growing reputation as a surgical investigator, Carrel moved to the Rockefeller Institute in New York in 1908. Guthrie, a self-effacing man, relocated to Saint Louis after a quarrel stemming from his colleague's ambition and vanity. "His [Carrel's] pre-eminence in publicity and personal promotion attributes have been widely internationally demonstrated."[7] Ironically, in 1912, the same year that Carrel won the Nobel Prize for Medicine and Physiology for his contributions to vascular surgery and transplantation, Guthrie published his important book *Blood Vessel Surgery and Its Application*. However, the reviews were unenthusiastic and the volume never gained the acceptance it deserved.

As Carrel's experiments in transplantation became known, interest in their potential application increased among his scientific peers and the public. For the first time, he examined changes in the function of a kidney transferred to a different location in the same animal. In one such study he removed an autografted kidney that had functioned successfully for three years, irrigated it with cold solution to protect the bloodless tissues, then retransplanted it into the same dog. She recovered and subsequently delivered two litters of healthy puppies, eleven in the first litter and three in the second, before dying of an unrelated complication. As the organ was normal at autopsy, Carrel concluded: "Such a transplantation did not interfere with the function of the kidney . . . Organ transplantation has become a reality." In his subsequent publications, he included whimsical photographs of dogs

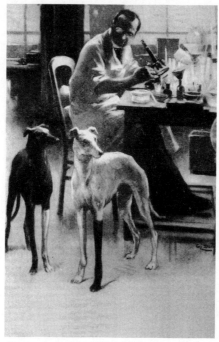

Figure 2.2 Alexis Carrel and recipients of limb transplants (Novartis,
with permission)

and cats that had received kidneys, as well as some with transplanted
legs (Figure 2.2). His growing enthusiasm produced further hyperbole: "A leg removed from a dog and replaced by the corresponding
leg of another dog was able to survive normally . . . This transplantation should be attempted in man with a limb derived from another
individual or from a cadaver dying from a violent death." The media
stirred public excitement further, the *New York Times* reporting inac-
curately that Carrel had "succeeded in transplanting the organs [kid-
neys and thyroids] in animals . . . grown them to monstrous size . . .
[and] used [them] with measurable success to replace diseased or worn
out tissue."[8] Human patients sought help. One asked him to replace an
arm; another desired a kidney from a cadaver or an executed criminal.

This initial enthusiasm did not survive the biologic reality. After
nine technically perfect kidney allografts in cats, Carrel sensed problems. Initial copious urine output from the transplanted organs ceased

after several days, function deteriorated, and the animals died. Examined under the microscope, the kidney was highly inflamed and many of its cells were dead. Carrel conjectured that such changes were caused by the absence of blood flow during the grafting procedure, or to the perfusion of the isolated organ before transplantation with cold salt solution. Agreeing with current knowledge about the behavior of transplanted skin and noting the increasing presence of white blood cells (leukocytes) in failing grafts, Carrel admitted to his colleagues that while autografts were almost invariably successful, allografts after "behaving satisfactorily over the first few days, almost inevitably failed." At about the same time, others described microscopic changes in slices of foreign kidneys transplanted to the ears of guinea pigs, with the addendum that after the ninth day "the actual destruction . . . seemed to be due to an invasion by [host] cells."[9]

Becoming increasingly involved in war-related activities, particularly the care of wounds, and sensing that undefined but inevitable host barriers precluded the success of transplants, Carrel left the field. He later turned his energies to the culture of cells and preservation of isolated tissues and organs outside the body.

The only attempt at renal transplantation between humans during the prewar period was undertaken in 1906 by Mathieu Jaboulay, Carrel's senior colleague in Lyon. Having perfected suture methods of vascular repair, he grafted donor kidneys to the arm vessels of two dying patients "to establish functional assistance for urine excretion by installing a foreign but healthy kidney to help the natural organ suffering from incurable diseases."[10] The kidneys failed. Eventually, all involved with this subject were forced to concede that although transplantation could be achieved by precise vascular anastomosis, and that the transfer of an organ to a distant site in the same animal did not appear to affect its function, kidneys—like skin grafts—survived only a few days when placed in a different individual.

The phenomenon of rejection, an invariable event that these early investigators were beginning to appreciate, has remained the principal enduring challenge to successful transplantation between genetically dissimilar individuals. The pattern of the acute process, regardless of type of tissue, is similar. The allografted organ acts normally after its placement into the recipient and resumption of its blood supply. But usually within days, function of the increasingly inflamed graft declines progressively before failing completely. Under the microscope, the graft substance is filled with host white blood cells, which mediate its progressive destruction.

The catastrophic effects of World War I evoked challenges more pressing than the continuing pursuit of this new subject. In postwar Germany the great medical clinics were in ruins. German scientists had become pariahs in the international community because of their support of the conflict and their role in the development of poison gas. The once-proud Viennese medical research establishment was virtually extinguished. The medical and social infrastructure of victorious France and Britain also lay exhausted and overwhelmed by the needs of the wounded, the bereaved, the unemployed, and the destitute. By contrast, in the increasingly powerful United States academic endeavors were stimulated by the philanthropic funding of libraries, research institutes, and laboratories. Carrel fueled the promise of science and technology by exhorting: "For the first time in the history of humanity, a crumbling civilization is capable of discerning the causes of its decay. For the first time, it has at its disposal the gigantic strength of science . . . It is our only hope of escaping the fate of all great civilizations of the past."[11]

Only rarely did surgeons and scientists involve themselves in transplantation during the years between the wars. Most recognized with Carrel that technical expertise alone could not assure survival of a new organ and that poorly understood host factors inevitably caused rapid destruction. Although the grafting of sex glands arose as an exotic and highly publicized interlude during the 1920s, research on renal transplantation almost ceased. Infrequent reports examined the benefits of cold preservation of isolated organs of dogs, the effects of drugs that could increase the urine flow of transplanted kidneys, and the relevance of genetic differences between canine donors and recipients. Clinical attempts were also scarce; the single instance, in America in 1923, was the unsuccessful placement of a lamb's kidney into a patient poisoned with mercury. Then in 1936, a surgeon working in relative isolation in a politically repressive society initiated a series of human-to-human renal transplants, a last-ditch treatment undertaken solely by Mathieu Jaboulay three decades before.

The unique experience of U. U. Voronoy, carried out in Russia and

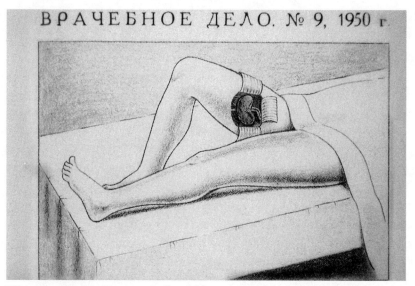

Figure 2.3 Yu Yu Voronoy's first kidney transplant (Novartis, with permission)

published in Russian, has only recently been appreciated in the West. Voronoy had previously investigated the use of cadaver blood for transfusion, using the new information on blood-group differences between donor and host. By 1929 he had detected complement in the serum of dogs grafted with slices of testes or receiving kidney transplants. Complement is a naturally occurring humoral substance, a major component of the host defenses via its ability to destroy foreign cells. Within a few years, Voronay encountered a 26-year-old woman who had developed renal failure after poisoning herself with "corrosive sublimate" (mercuric chloride). Convinced that a transplant was the only way to save her life, Voronoy grafted the right kidney of a 60-year-old male who had died from a skull fracture to vessels in her right groin. In the six-hour operation he covered the exposed organ with skin grafts (Figure 2.3). As the blood types of donor and host were different, he attempted a partial-exchange transfusion with donor blood. The patient put out small amounts of urine but died within a few days.[12]

Reporting in 1950 on his total experience with six human kidney transplants, Voronoy emphasized the benefit of using organs from cadavers. Clearly, his opinion was influenced by the climate in Russia at a time when the results of research had to agree with officially accepted dogma: in biology, the opinions of Trofirm Denisovich Lysenko strengthened the ideals of communism by repudiating the role of genetics and preaching that learned political beliefs could be inherited; in clinical medicine, the Stalin Prize winner V. P. Filov stated dogmatically that a variety of refrigerated tissues taken from a dead body formed "restorative biogenic stimulators" activated following reconstitution of their blood supply.[13] With this official imprimatur, Voronoy transplanted stored kidneys taken from cadaver donors nine to twenty days previously. As none of them functioned, he abandoned the approach. The remainder of his career was spent in the care of trauma patients and in investigating methods for blood transfusion. Isolated geographically and unrecognized by other workers until years after his death in 1961, Voronoy exemplifies a solitary investigator pursuing a novel scientific idea in an obscure area during an era not yet ready to accept it.

Although the initial experience with organ transplantation involved only a handful of surgeons interested primarily in its technical aspects, the field began to open up after World War II. The range of surgery widened into specialty areas as a result of lessons learned in combat. During World War I, surgical operations had been limited primarily to the repair of abdominal and head injuries, the debridement of contaminated or fragmented tissues, some plastic surgery, and wound care using antiseptic solutions designed and perfected by Carrel and his colleagues. More effective means of patient care during World War II and later during the Korean War included improved treatment of trauma and burns, repair of vascular injuries, management of fluid balance, blood banking, and the increasing availability of antibiotics.

Upon return to civilian life, surgeons became bolder and more expert in removing, restoring, and refashioning diseased, injured, or anomalous tissues. The thoracic cavity and its contents, anathema for centuries because operative invasion was considered a death sentence for the patient, were increasingly explored—first to remove pieces of shrapnel from around the heart and great vessels, then to eliminate portions of lungs destroyed by infection or involved with tumors. Operations on the heart itself also broadened in scope and complexity, particularly after the development of cardiopulmonary bypass techniques.

Stimulated by clinical advances and increasing biologic and medical knowledge, a few surgeons began to reconsider the feasibility of replacing diseased organs. Beyond its relative convenience for transplantation (which Carrel and earlier investigators had noted), the kidney lent itself well to the growing emphasis on physiology, diagnosis, and the relationship between the cause of a condition and its pathology. Although occasional individuals with kidney dysfunction secondary to anatomic abnormalities (such as localized obstruction of the ureter) or with systemic dysequilibrium (such as dehydration) could be salvaged by surgery, it was recognized increasingly that some chronic kidney diseases were genetically transmitted, other kidneys were destroyed by unremitting infection, and the cause of failure of the remainder was unknown.

Unfortunately, the picture of inexorable and progressive renal failure resulting from all these conditions was little different in 1950 than in 1836, when first described by the London physician Richard Bright. Although Hippocrates in ancient Greece had noted that cloudy and bubbly urine was a feature of some disease states, and fifteenth-century Italian observers had related scanty output to shrunken kidneys, Bright was the first to describe uremia, a condition where waste products excreted by normal kidneys collect in the blood when the kidneys function poorly or not at all. He also associated the symptoms and signs exhibited by uremic individuals with renal deterioration and failure. "The patient is usually subject to constant recurrence of his symptoms . . . He is suddenly seized with an acute attack of pericarditis [inflammation of the sac surrounding the heart], or with a still more acute attack of peritonitis [inflammation of the abdominal cavity], which, without any renewed warning, deprives him in 8–40 hours, of his life. Should he escape this danger . . . other perils await him; his headaches . . . become more frequent; his stomach more deranged; his vision indistinct; his hearing depraved; he is suddenly seized with a convulsive fit, and becomes blind. He struggles through the attack; but again and again it returns; and before a day or a week has elapsed, worn out by convulsions, or overwhelmed by coma, the painful history of his disease is closed."[14] This portrayal remains accurate today.

Regardless of differences in social philosophy and in the availability of medical resources in the postwar period, investigators in Paris and in

Boston initiated renal transplantation in an almost identical manner. Their increasing interest in the subject was galvanized in June 1950 when a Chicago surgeon, Richard Lawler, removed a kidney from an individual who had died of liver disease and placed it into his patient, Ruth Tucker. A 44-year-old woman of blood type similar to the donor, she had a hereditary condition that had gradually caused her kidneys to turn into ever-enlarging urine-filled, functionless cysts. Mrs. Tucker agreed to the transplant, as no alternative treatment was available to save her life. Lawler removed one huge polycystic kidney and replaced it with the normal donor organ before crowds of physicians and a camera crew in the operating room. News spread quickly, with the national press reporting hyperbolically that the operation was a first. *Newsweek* chimed in that "up to last week, no vital human organ had ever been moved from one person to another."[15] No one in the chauvinistic media troubled themselves to learn of the prior work in Europe or the more recent experience of Voronoy. For any American reporter to suggest that the Russians had performed anything first would have been anathema in that paranoid cold war era!

To everyone's surprise, the new kidney put out urine and Mrs. Tucker returned home (Figure 2.4). At fifty-three days the kidney's ability to excrete dye confirmed its continued function. At surgical exploration ten months later, however, it was found to be shrunken, discolored, and rejected. As the patient lived for five more years, her physicians came to believe that the grafted organ had survived as a bridge long enough to allow her remaining native kidney to recover partial function. Enduring both notoriety and sometimes vociferous censure by his peers, Lawler never performed another transplant.

Despite the relatively inconclusive results, this unique event served as a catalyst for surgeons in both France and the United States to pursue the subject in humans—or, as the French transplant pioneer René Küss pointed out, primarily in women (Figure 2.5). Küss, a distinguished Parisian urologist and one of the original group of transplanters, commented: "Lawler had an extraordinary impact on those of us in France who were doing experimental transplantation. He gave us the reason to believe that transplant surgery was possible in human beings . . . We were so anxious to apply the experience we gathered working on dogs to human beings that we used Lawler's success as an

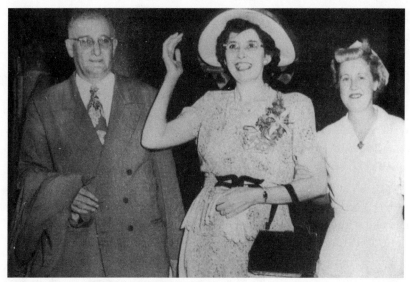

Figure 2.4 Ruth Tucker, discharged from the hospital in July 1950 after her kidney transplant (T. Stark, *Knife to the Heart*, London: Macmillan, 1996)

excuse to begin kidney transplants in man." Although doctors were enthusiastic, society generally did not accept the concept. The French public objected to the idea on ethical, philosophical, and pragmatic grounds. As Küss suggested, they "thought it was absolutely impossible to transcend the laws of nature by mixing two individuals, so public opinion was against this type of experimentation."[16] Even in the more laissez-faire United States, critics ranged from those who felt that removal of the kidney desecrated the body to those who questioned the justification for trying something so radical when all previous attempts had failed.

As a result of these pressures, appropriate organs were difficult to obtain. In France the first method considered was to recover organs from prisoners executed by the guillotine. In January 1951 two Parisian surgeons, Charles Dubost and Marcel Servelle, with the permission of the director, went to the Santé Prison and quickly removed the kidneys from a prisoner who had just been beheaded. Dubost and a colleague grafted one kidney to the pelvic vessels of a 42-year-old woman whose own organs had been destroyed by infection. The ure-

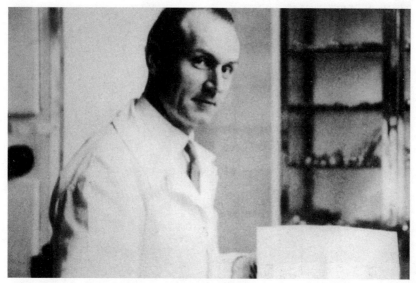

Figure 2.5 René Küss in the mid-1980s (Novartis, with permission)

ter was led through a defect in the skin, a technique they had previously perfected in dogs and which earlier surgeons had reported a
half century before. Despite initial function, rejection caused her death
on day 17. Servelle and his team placed the second kidney into a 22-
year-old female with a failing solitary kidney. While the transplant put
out abundant urine initially, on day 19 the patient suddenly died.[17]

Dubost and Servelle obtained the next few organs primarily from
living donors. These included single kidneys taken electively from
adults with irreversible abnormalities of the ureter, or from infants
with hydrocephalus whose retained ureter, after removal of the kidney,
could be used as a conduit to drain excess fluid from the brain into the
bladder via a plastic tube. Using an organ from a young woman with
an irreparably occluded ureter, the first from a living donor, Küss and
his group promptly performed the third transplant on a 44-year-old
female whose infected kidneys were filled with stones. They carried
out four more transplants in 1951, three from living adult and infant
donors and one from an executed criminal. Jean Hamburger and his
team at Hôpital Necker in Paris undertook the eighth transplant in
December 1952 on Marius Renard, a 16-year-old carpenter (Figure
2.6). A few days earlier Renard had ruptured his right kidney in a fall.

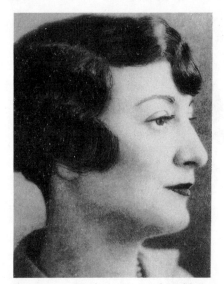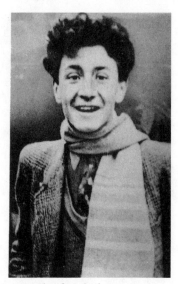

Figure 2.6 Madame Renard and her son, Marius, the first kidney transplant between relatives (Novartis, with permission)

The hemorrhaging organ had to be removed to save his life. As he put
out no urine at all postoperatively, it became apparent that he had been
born with only a single kidney (an occasional congenital anomaly). At
his mother's insistence, the surgeons transplanted her kidney into her
son on Christmas Eve in the first transplant between living relatives.
Despite immediate function and relief of uremia, rejection on day 21
led to Marius' death.[18] In short, no recipient survived in this disap-
pointing period, although over the next few years Küss reported that
occasional recipients of a transplant from a relative were supported by
their grafts for several months.

Boston was no more successful. An aging and rather drab city after the
war, its politics were insular and its finances insecure. Education, medicine, and science gave the city its lasting influence: it was replete
with universities, colleges, medical schools, hospitals, and laboratories,
many of which were benefiting from the postwar funding of research.
Kidney disease had been a long-standing interest of several physicians
in a small hospital on the west side of the city, the Peter Bent Brigham.
Conceived as a teaching hospital for the Harvard Medical School, it

welcomed its first patient in 1913. From the beginning, the atmosphere at "the Brigham" differed from its bigger, grander sister institution across the city, the Massachusetts General Hospital, founded in 1811. The former used each patient as a laboratory, gleaning as much physiological and pathological data as possible; the latter was more attuned to providing excellent care for large numbers of patients at the cost of a less investigative and inquiring spirit. Perhaps as a result, "Mass General" was heavily endowed through gifts from grateful patients, whereas the Brigham was financially less fortunate, with talk of closure during the 1930s and 1940s. The long, low brick-and-wood hospital of 250 beds was an unlikely site for innovation and originality. The physical plant was already outdated; it would take many decades before substantial rebuilding occurred. Yet the young institution had already established an international reputation in neurosurgery and was becoming known for its expertise in heart disease and the beginnings of cardiac surgery. Equally important, the staff was small in number and relatively few resident trainees were accepted into the highly competitive surgical and medical programs. All knew one another well and communication between the disciplines was open and easy.

In 1929 George Thorn, a medical student, invited a Brigham physician expert in renal disease to lecture at the University of Buffalo.[19] Stimulated by what he heard, Thorn applied for an internship at the hospital but was turned down. He would not return until 1942, when he was invited back as physician-in-chief. During his interim years at Johns Hopkins University, he became interested in the relationship between the kidney, the adrenal gland, and hypertension. High blood pressure could be produced in dogs by narrowing one of their renal arteries with a clamp. No one knew whether the condition was the result of factors circulating in the bloodstream or the direct influence of the nerves of the kidney itself.

That some mechanism other than an intact nerve supply was responsible was soon proven by Alfred Blalock, a young surgical investigator from Vanderbilt University, who showed that the elevated blood pressure of a dog did not fall following transfer to the neck of a kidney with a compromised artery from its native site in the flank.[20] Thorn related this experimental finding to the common syndrome of hypertension in patients with kidney disease. He theorized that the shrunken and scarred organs and their narrowed internal vasculature caused release of humoral substances into the circulation, thereby increasing blood pressure. He even predicted to his incredulous colleagues that hypertension could likely be cured by removal of both diseased kidneys.

One of Thorn's related interests was the influence on the blood pressure of at least some of the newly described steroid hormones. Compelling evidence for such a relationship was that the administration of cortisone or similar compounds could produce hypertension in individuals with Addison's disease, a state of adrenal insufficiency with diminished steroid production in which the patients ran strikingly low pressures.

The phenomenon of acute renal failure was now becoming recognized. English physicians first described this condition in civilians crushed by falling masonry and beams during the London "blitz" in World War II, who often went into hypotensive shock when dug from the rubble. Resuscitated by blood transfusions, their kidneys ceased to put out urine after several days—a phenomenon not previously appreciated, as such individuals usually died quickly from their other injuries. This condition of acute renal failure was also soon identified in patients experiencing hypotension from severe infection or hemorrhage. Examination of their organs under the microscope showed that the cells of the filtering portion of the kidneys, the tubules, were disrupted and dead from inadequate blood flow during the period of shock. Intrigued by these findings, Thorn showed that the tubular cells could regenerate and heal in animals and then in humans if the systemic salt and water abnormalities, and the buildup of toxic metabolites resulting from lack of urine production by the damaged kidneys, could be controlled long enough.[21] He and the relatively few others interested in the subject at that time began to understand a different aspect of the problem: that individuals whose kidneys had been irreversibly destroyed by disease were destined to die with progressive and irreversible uremia. Thus, the Brigham was gaining a reputation for expertise with patients suffering acute or chronic kidney failure. It was also becoming a center for the study of a new class of biological substances, the corticosteroids.

Two events in 1947 triggered what was to become an ongoing effort to extend the lives of individuals with end-stage renal disease: the introduction of the concept of hemodialysis, and transplantation of the kidney. Having heard that a Dutch physician, Willem Kolff, had been able to filter waste products from the blood of uremic patients via an external device called an artificial kidney, Thorn invited him to present his findings in Boston. Kolff had already donated his machines to hospitals in London, Cracow, Montreal, and New York. Most were unappreciated. In London, where there was professional antipathy toward the idea, one device was reputedly dismantled and its pieces used to improve the hospital's plumbing. Kolff later noted that the last "disappeared to Poland, behind the Iron Curtain and was never heard from since."[22] So he was able to offer only blueprints to the Brigham staff.

Thorn presciently asked two staff physicians to refine Kolff's apparatus—Carl Walter, an innovative surgeon and surgical engineer, and John Merrill, a newly graduated medical resident looking for a specialty. Working with a local engineering group, they redesigned and improved the prototype using nonwettable polyethylene tubing instead of rubber, and a rotation apparatus that could filter the blood effectively and gently without breaking the red cells. Walter's coincident invention of the plastic blood bag and other blood banking technologies, used to this day, allowed the sterile separation of whole blood into its red cell and plasma components.

Administration of the packed red cell fraction alone allowed many anemic dialysis patients to continue their treatments without the danger of receiving too much fluid. The success of the new machine was enhanced by the ability of a young surgeon, David Hume (Figure 2.7), to connect patients to it by inserting cannulae into their forearm vessels. The ability to dialyze a uremic individual more than once allowed time for the acutely damaged kidneys to recover. By 1950 Merrill and his team had carried out thirty-three dialysis procedures in twenty-six patients. And as Thorn later recalled, "The development of the artificial kidney was an integral part of a long range program leading to the transplantation of kidneys for irreversible renal failure or malignant hypertension."[23]

The second event in 1947 involved three surgeons at the Brigham

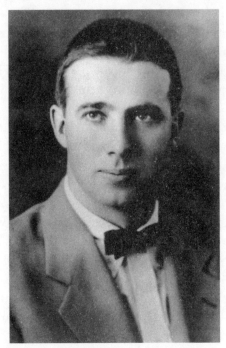

Figure 2.7 David Hume in 1949

faced with a patient dying of acute renal failure following a septic abortion and hemorrhage. The conundrum faced by staff surgeon Charles Hufnagel, chief resident in urology Ernest Landsteiner, and assistant surgical resident Hume was how to support the patient during the acute episode until her own kidneys could begin to function. Thorn, ever imaginative, suggested that a healthy kidney be used as a temporary bridge. Hume located a hospital employee who agreed to the removal of a kidney from a newly deceased relative. Under the light of two 60-watt bulbs in a side room near the ward, the surgeons isolated the major artery and vein at the patient's elbow and sewed the respective renal vessels of the donor kidney to them. Upon release of the vascular clamps, the organ became pink and began to excrete urine.

Hufnagel recounted the case in more detail:

In 1947 I had spent considerable time working with transplantation of the kidney [in dogs] . . . From time to time we had been on the lookout for a patient in whom a kidney transplant might be needed, as an urgent and desperate measure to save her life . . . In this case everyone was quite sure that the patient was not going to open up with urine output, and she was almost dead ... It was finally agreed that the patient should have a transplant from a cadaver to see if she could be tided over this problem long enough to get well ... Because the patient's condition appeared extremely critical, there was some administrative objection to bringing the patient to the operating room ... in the dark of night—about midnight. When the kidney had been obtained immediately after the death of the donor, our little group proceeded to do the transplant. The kidney itself with a short segment of the remaining ureter was wrapped in sterile sponges and covered with sterile rubber sheeting, leaving only the tip of the ureter exposed. An attempt to bury the kidney beneath the skin was made, but because of the position of the vessels a considerable part of the kidney was still uncovered ... Immediately the kidney began to secrete urine ... and by noon of the next day, the patient herself began to show marked improvement. She began to become more alert and by the following day was entirely clear in her mind. The day after the transplant the ureter began to show signs of swelling, and a portion of it was removed to allow for better drainage of the urine. By the following day the kidney was showing evidence of decreased output, and because of the great improvement in the patient, it was elected to remove it ... Two or three days after removal of the kidney, the patient began to enter a diuretic phase [putting out large amounts of urine] and her subsequent recovery was relatively uneventful.[24]

Unfortunately, she died several months later of hepatitis from a blood transfusion administered during her illness.

Interest in the possibilities of kidney transplantation with dialysis support as needed was encouraged by the Brigham's new surgeon-in-chief. Francis D. Moore had come from the Massachusetts General Hospital in 1948 at the age of 34, already distinguished in his scientific career. His enthusiasm, drive, and expertise in several fields, plus his close and enduring collaboration with Thorn, created a fertile ground for innovation (Figure 2.8). By chance, the first patient to receive dialysis prior to transplantation, a 37-year-old boiler repairman, was transferred from Springfield, Massachusetts, in March 1951. Ten days later, upon the patient's return to his home hospital, surgeon James Scola grafted a kidney removed from a living donor with cancer of the ureter, joining the renal artery to a large artery in the upper abdomen of the recipient. As the graft did not function initially, the patient again came to Boston for dialysis support before dying of rejection after five weeks.

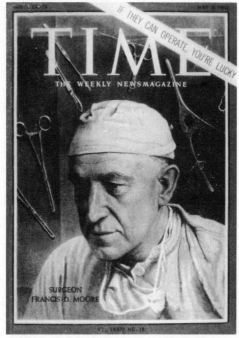

Figure 2.8 Francis D. Moore on the cover
of *Time*, May 2, 1963 (© 1963 Time Inc.,
with permission)

Because of the scarcity of available kidneys, those involved with
the new field realized that a supply of both cadaver and living-donor
organs would be necessary before a formal effort in transplantation
could be initiated. As an innovative surgical program to correct diseased heart valves was also beginning in the hospital at that time,
kidneys not infrequently became available following unsuccessful operations on the extremely ill cardiac patients. In addition, neurosurgeons were removing one kidney from children with hydrocephalus
on a relatively routine basis, to drain the fluid from their brains via the
native ureter.

After many discussions with Merrill, Thorn, and Moore, between
April 1951 and February 1953 Hume performed nine kidney transplants from such sources. Feeling that the patients were too ill to
withstand either a large intra-abdominal operation of the sort that had
been performed by Lawler and Scola, or placement of the kidney

behind the abdominal wall as described by Küss and his French colleagues, Hume devised an alternative approach by creating a skin flap
in the upper thigh, unknowingly using the same technique that Voronoy had.[25] When a kidney became available, its renal artery and vein
were anastomosed to the vessels in the recipient groin, and the skin
flap or a skin graft was used to cover the organ. The end of the ureter
was brought out through the skin of the thigh. Despite this less invasive operative approach performed under local anesthesia, plus the
availability of adjunctive dialysis, the first eight kidney recipients fared
no better than had the earlier patients.

The ninth recipient, however, reacted differently. A young physician from South America, Gregorio Woloshin, had developed chronic
renal failure years after a streptococcal infection. Hume placed his
kidney allograft, from a female patient of similar blood type who had
died following a heart operation, in Woloshin's right thigh. He surrounded the kidney with a thin plastic bag, thinking that this barrier
would prevent foreign proteins or antigens draining from the organ in
its lymph from stimulating the immune responses of the recipient.
After nineteen days of no output and a difficult postoperative course,
the patient began to excrete urine. By day 37 his renal function had
become normal. He was discharged on day 81, the first recipient in
that early period to be sustained fully by a functioning renal transplant. Although persistent hypertension remained his only problem
during the ensuing weeks, he died unexpectedly of kidney failure
about six months after the surgery. Microscopic examination of the
organ showed profound narrowing of its arteries, thought to be either
a result of high blood pressure or a recurrence of the original kidney
disease.

Two lessons seemed obvious. First, the failed native organs, considered to be the source of hypertension, should have been removed as
Thorn had originally suggested. Second, the relative success of this
transplant seemed to be inadvertently related to unrecognized similarities between the donor and the immunologically unmodified host.

The personnel involved in these early transplants changed quickly.
In 1953 Hume was called into the military during the Korean War. A
plastic surgeon, Joseph Murray, was appointed to the staff after experience in the army at a regional reconstruction and burn center in

Pennsylvania. He had grafted burned patients with autologous skin and had a developing interest in the potential use of skin from other donors. During his time in the military, Murray's chief was James Barrett Brown, previously chief consultant in plastic surgery for the U.S. Army Medical Corps. Brown had described differences in the behavior of skin isografts and allografts in humans, and while in England in the early years of the war had suggested that biologist Peter Medawar and surgeon Thomas Gibson collaborate in studies on rejection of skin grafts. His interest in transplantation undoubtedly influenced his younger colleague, Murray.

Caught up in the activity surrounding treatment of renal failure at the Brigham, Murray took over the laboratory experiments of Hufnagel and Hume, but transplanted the kidneys to the lower abdomen of the dogs (as Floresco had described a half century before) instead of to the neck. Based on this experience and on practice operations on cadavers, he used the same surgical approach in six patients in whom the kidney was protected by the abdominal muscles and the donor ureter implanted directly into the bladder. Like the majority of those previously transplanted, all died of rejection after several days.

Clinical attempts by other investigators followed. Gordon Murray, a surgeon at the University of Toronto, reported the engraftment of five recipients in 1954, one kidney transplanted to the arm and four to the lower abdomen.[26] One graft functioned for fifteen months, and the recipient returned to work as a stenographer. As with Lawler's patient, however, the actual contribution of the transplant was difficult to assess, as her retained native kidney still provided some function. One of the most imaginative and productive surgeon-scientists of the period was Michael Woodruff at the University of Edinburgh. He not only pioneered clinical transplantation, but also introduced several critical subjects into its biology. Others in Australia, England, and North America performed sporadic transplants as well.

It was clear by the mid-1950s that transplantation of a healthy donor kidney could effectively, though transiently, reverse renal failure. However, the complexities of the patients—which included the debilitating effects of uremia and an increased tendency toward infection, as well as the inevitable immunological destruction of the graft—contributed to the almost uniform failure of all attempts. Despite major experimental and clinical efforts by several teams, little optimism ensued. Küss summarized the state of the new subject: "The results from medical teams in France as well as the United States led us to believe that transplant surgery was impossible." Hume echoed these sentiments: "At the present state of knowledge renal homotransplantation does not appear to be justified in the treatment of renal disease."[27] Such opinions changed quickly, however, with the first human transplant between identical twins.

3

Hopes and Occasional Successes

WITH THE SINGLE EXCEPTION OF GREGORIO Woloshin, all the relatively small number of kidney transplants performed in a handful of centers during the early 1950s failed within a few days. The death of the recipients generated a difficult period for all concerned. Immunosuppression lay in the future. Dialysis backup was rare, and what was available was rudimentary. Hopes of success were remote. The new field was in sore need of a positive event to prevent its dissolution. Remarkably, such a situation surfaced and provided dramatic impetus.

Active and healthy at the age of 23, Richard Herrick developed high blood pressure, swelling of his legs, and protein in his urine—all serious signs of renal dysfunction. Over the next year, with worsening kidney failure he began to experience all the symptoms that Richard Bright had described a century before. Fatigue increased, his energy diminished, and weakness became pronounced. Loss of appetite and an unpleasant, persistent metallic taste progressed to nausea and vomiting. His weight dropped alarmingly. His hands trembled. He developed severe headaches. His vision blurred. His skin turned a bronze color and his body gave off an ammoniacal odor. The volume of urine lessened. Toward the end of 1954 he entered a local hospital, lethargic, hypertensive, and having sustained several seizures. He was difficult to control because of paranoid delusions. His physician restricted salt and fluid intake and transferred the desperately ill patient to the Brigham for dialysis. At the same time, he astutely broached the possibilities of kidney transplantation to John Merrill, having discovered that Richard had an identical twin, Ronald.

The team of surgeons and physicians, now including the urologist Hartwell Harrison, considered the precedents for such a novel step. They knew that skin had been successfully transplanted between at least three sets of identical twins. Joseph Murray had already performed a large number of renal autografts in dogs after removal of the other native kidney, designing "a transplant operation which, in the absence of an immunological barrier, could produce normal renal function indefinitely."[1] With the organ placed in the abdomen of the recipient, its vessels attached to one of the large arteries and veins in the pelvis, and the transplant ureter sewn directly to the bladder, several animals remained healthy for as long as two years. These successful results conflicted strikingly with those of earlier investigators; they had ascribed the progressive functional abnormalities after a kidney had been transferred to a different site in the same animal to interruption of lymphatics, division of nerves, changes in temperature during placement, and other variables. More likely, the technique of draining the ureter externally through the skin allowed infection to travel up the exposed conduit and gradually destroy the organ.

As Richard's condition improved and stabilized with dialysis treatment, the clinicians had first to prove that he and his brother were truly identical, sharing all of their genetic material. A check of their birth records confirmed a common placenta, almost invariable with these types of twins. All known blood groups were similar and differed from those of their two other siblings. Eye color, pigment patterns, and structure of the iris were the same. Most conclusively, exchanged skin grafts healed normally and exhibited similar gross and microscopic features. As final proof, documentation that the fingerprint patterns of the brothers were identical was confirmed at a police laboratory. A news reporter assigned to the police station realized the potential significance of these goings-on, and by that evening the newspapers were trumpeting, "Brigham doctors plan daring operation."[2] From then on, as Herrick and his twin awaited the transplant, local and national news continuously carried the developing story.

Like Carrel and Lawler before him, Murray was ill prepared for the media attention. "It was both an education and a shock to discover how sustained and widespread public interest in organ transplantation was." Some of his more skeptical colleagues were outspoken against the chances of success, advising the young surgeon that he was jeopardizing his career by embarking on such a risky venture. In spite of these warnings, Murray performed the operation on December 23, 1954. He used the lower abdominal retroperitoneal operative approach that he had refined from the technique described by Küss and his colleagues. Even as Murray was isolating Richard's vessels for anastomosis with those of the kidney, in the next operating room Harrison was removing a kidney from Ronald. To gain adequate length of renal artery, he clamped it at its origin on the aorta before dividing it. While the attention of those present focused on the recipient operation, the vascular clamp on the short arterial stump of the donor suddenly slipped off. Fortunately, Harrison was able to control the dramatic bleeding deep in the incision. Despite that near-catastrophe, the kidney was transplanted uneventfully, with both patients tolerating their surgeries well. The revascularized organ produced urine immediately.[3]

Herrick improved quickly. Murray contrasted the immediate success of the isograft with reversal of uremia and striking improvement of the twin recipient, "exceeding our highest hopes," with the earlier more somber experiences of those who had received cadaver kidneys. "In those patients, renal function was always delayed, poor in quantity and short in duration. The . . . operation performed on Richard Herrick has been the prototype for human renal transplantation ever since." Within a few days, however, he developed increasing hypertension. Realizing that the failed native organs could be responsible for these changes and encouraged by Thorn, Murray removed them sequentially. Following the second nephrectomy, the blood pressure stabilized, confirming Thorn's prediction. The unexpectedly rapid transformation of a terminally ill individual to one who had completely recovered was striking (Figure 3.1). Herrick married his nurse and fathered two children, emphasizing by his return to a normal life that any long-term effects, psychological or otherwise, stemming from receiving an organ from another could be overcome by the organ's continuing function. In his understated follow-up summary of this seminal case, Merrill wrote: "This report documents the successful transplantation of a human kidney from one identical twin to another. The

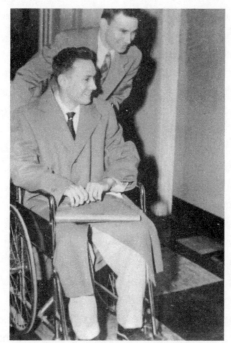

Figure 3.1 Richard and Ronald Herrick as they were discharged from the hospital in February 1955 (with permission)

function of the homograft [he uses the wrong term] remains excellent 12 months after the operative procedure."[4]

Over the next few years, more identical twins received successful kidney isografts at the Brigham. Similar surgeries were carried out in Portland (Oregon), Montreal, and Paris. By the mid-1970s, the overall experience with thirty-five twin transplants had created a unique resource for those treating patients with renal failure, leading to improved dialytic preparation and refinements in anesthesia and surgical management.[5] The responsible doctors formulated firm criteria for acceptance of donors and recipients and explained fully to all involved the adverse aspects and possible complications of the procedure. In addition, a complete evaluation confirmed the health of the donors, including the presence of two normal uninfected kidneys and a functioning bladder. The anatomy of the aorta and renal arteries was ascertained preoperatively by intra-arterial dye injection. (A technical failure of revascularization with loss of the organ had occurred when a kidney was unexpectedly found at operation to have two small unreconstructable arteries instead of the usual single vessel.) Conversely, only potential recipients with irreversible renal disease were considered for transplantation. Control of urinary tract infections and correction of any anatomical causes became routine. The primary disease process that had destroyed the native organs had to be quiescent before grafting could take place—a lesson learned when the original condition, glomerulonephritis, unexpectedly recurred and destroyed several of the new transplants.

The identical twin experience yielded significant physiological dividends. Disruption of the nerve supply of kidneys and ureters was found not to affect their performance. Isolated kidneys withstood relatively short periods of time without blood flow and upon revascularization resumed urine output immediately. Bladder function improved with reversal of the uremic state. Several recipients of successful transplants experienced uneventful pregnancies and delivered normal babies. Children whose growth had been stunted by renal disease grew quickly after restoration of function. Above all, this unique clinical experiment showed unequivocally that patients dying of uremia could be restored to full health with a successful graft (Figure 3.2).

The ethical grounds for saving one individual by removing a normal kidney from another by means of a major operation that in no way contributed to that person's welfare were unexplored at the time of the Herrick case. The obvious question of whether it was justifiable to place a potential donor at risk to secure a vital organ for use in a relatively untested and hitherto unsuccessful treatment was difficult. To prevent future recriminations, it was particularly necessary that the donor understand the ramifications of the sacrifice. Ronald Herrick was never urged to donate; every possible ethical, philosophical, and medical issue was raised to stress his freedom of choice. His reaction on a preoperative visit by the Brigham team cleared the way for the remainder of the identical twin experience. Although highly motivated, knowledgeable, and committed to his brother, Ronald questioned whether the physicians would guarantee treatment for any future health needs resulting from his surgery. Harrison, who was to

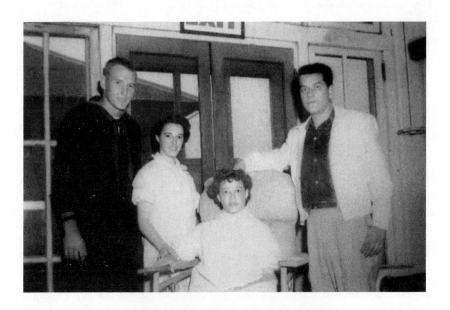

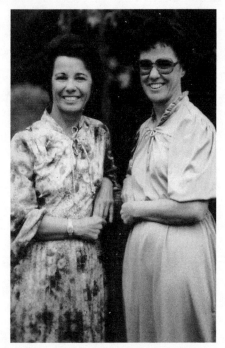

Figure 3.2 A, Edith Helm, her sister Wanda, and their husbands before their transplant in 1955; B, the sisters twenty-five years later (with permission)

remove the kidney, countered: "Do you think that any of us doctors here in the room would ever, at any time, refuse to help you to the best of our abilities?" The donor quickly realized that both his and his twin's future rested on professional integrity and sense of responsibility, rather than on legalities.[6]

A judicial judgment regarding the special circumstances surrounding the transplantation of identical twins under legal age was first tested in the Massachusetts courts in 1957, in connection with a 13-year-old donor-recipient pair. During the following year, in which the moral and legal aspects of using an organ from a minor were studied and discussed, the affected twin slid inexorably into kidney failure. It was arranged that the family would bring the case at once before the Supreme Judicial Court for permission to allow the operation to proceed. Parental consent was obviously necessary for medical treatment of minors even though such treatment benefited the child. A transplant would certainly help the recipient, yet removal of a kidney from the healthy twin had questionable justification, as such a loss could potentially endanger the child in later life.[7] Psychiatric interviews of both twins concluded that, because of their special relationship, the healthy individual could potentially suffer severe emotional upset if the sick twin died. Thus, the court ruled that the operation was necessary for the patient's survival and that the well twin's fully informed consent was valid.

In another instance, a 7-year-old identical twin donor continued to exhibit, thirty-two months after the kidney operation, "persistent concern about injury to her body." She was, however, comforted by the thought that since her sister, the recipient, also had only one functioning kidney, for them as twins "it was like having two kidneys." In her fantasy life, she could retain both kidneys through her twinning relationship. The court agreed.[8] These positive early decisions, as well as the continuing effectiveness of the transplant procedure, laid a stable foundation for more general use of living donors.

The success of the transplant between Ronald and Richard Herrick, set against the almost universal failures of the past, was a critical event in the history of the field, stimulating its ultimate acceptance into medical practice.[9] The decision to proceed was encouraged by the Brigham's long-standing interest in kidney disease, in conjunction with the availability of dialysis as a backup if initial graft function was poor or absent. Another impetus was the interactive spirit of that small institution, with a staff and administration that generally supported this unprecedented surgical procedure.

The transplant between the Herrick twins, although a medical curiosity, evoked new thinking about the potential of such treatment for kidney failure. The obvious next step for Murray was "to broaden the use of renal transplantation in humans beyond that of identical twins. So we, and everybody in world, were trying to break down the immune barrier. The most apt protocol seemed to be total-body irradiation followed by bone marrow infusion. Chemical immune suppression was just a will o' the wisp at that time."[10]

When they found that radiated rabbits produced fewer antibodies against foreign proteins than normal animals, German scientists had recognized at the beginning of the twentieth century that massive doses of radiation could inhibit host immunity.[11] Antibody responses to sheep red blood cells were then shown to be markedly depressed in rats whose circulating lymphocytes had been destroyed by repeated doses of x-ray. The investigation concluded that such cells—the bone marrow, spleen, lymph nodes, and other lymphoid tissues that were substantially affected by this modality—were the sites of antibody formation. In 1930, Swedish workers successfully transferred leukemia to immunologically compromised radiated rats, an impossibility in normal animals.

By 1945, scientists and the public alike had become acutely aware of the frightening powers of radiation. John Merrill had been a flight surgeon in the 509th Bomb Group, bombers of which dropped the atomic bombs on Hiroshima and Nagasaki. He and his colleagues well appreciated the sequelae of such extreme injury in humans, in whom the destruction of all rapidly dividing cells in the body led to depression of circulating leukocytes, loss of skin and hair, dissolution of bone marrow and lymphoid tissues, bleeding, and disruption of the lining of the bowel. Fatal sepsis supervened from impaired host defenses.

During the 1950s, several laboratories in Europe and the United States were formed to define more closely the influence of radiation on living tissues and to devise means to control or at least temper its effects. Lead shielding of the white cell–rich spleen or stem cell–rich marrow in the long bones was soon found to salvage heavily radiated animals; the protected cells could divide, multiply, and repopulate the resultant empty areas. Inoculation of the radiated subject with normal allogeneic bone marrow cells often achieved the same end, a technique of obvious potential for future transplantation of that tissue.

The concept that normal lymphoid cells from another subject would proliferate and function in a radiated host whose own white cells had been destroyed was a reasonable one. It was suggested that the administered cells, in combination with occasional host leukocytes that had survived the whole-body radiation, could create a "chimeric" subject bearing both its own and the donor's allogeneic cells. The problem was that many of the reconstituted mice and other experimental animals, although salvaged from the effects of radiation by the living-donor cells, lost hair, became humped and lethargic, and developed copious diarrhea. This often fatal condition, termed graft-versus-host disease (GVHD), in which the active and functioning but foreign cells recognize and destroy the immunologically helpless host, remains a severe clinical problem in bone marrow transplantation.

Despite this unforeseen complication, the idea that total-body radiation could be applied to organ-graft recipients began to appeal to investigators. Allografted tissues were found to be accepted by experimental animals whose immune system had been destroyed—not only those receiving radiation alone, but also those given adjunctive *donor-specific* cells (Figure 3.3). They did not, however, accept the grafts if treated with cells from a genetically disparate "third" party. Such surviving animals were considered to be in a state of "acquired immunological tolerance," specifically unresponsive to the donor tissues but able to destroy tissues from other, genetically different sources.[12]

A young surgeon in London, William Dempster, confirmed in definitive experiments that not only were the cellular and antibody responses reduced in radiated rabbits, but that skin-graft survival could be significantly prolonged. Joseph Murray's research group produced similar results. Perhaps the most compelling data for the clinicians during that period were reported in 1959 by John Mannick and colleagues in Cooperstown, New York. They demonstrated the presence of both donor and host cells in radiated beagles following transfer of

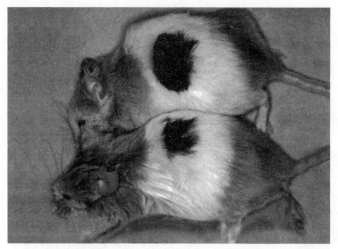

Figure 3.3 Healthy skin allografts on radiated mice recipients

foreign bone marrow.[13] One of these chimeric animals that bore both cell populations, Sam, subsequently received a kidney from the cell donor, Honest John. Sam lived for seventy-three days, sustained by the first "successful" organ allograft in a large animal (Figure 3.4). At the same time, many other experimental subjects died of graft-versus-host disease. Mannick later succeeded Francis Moore as surgeon-in-chief at the Brigham.

Physicians trying to apply these experimental findings to patients soon separated into those transplanting allogeneic bone marrow to correct hematological diseases such as leukemia directly, and those interested in solid-organ transplantation, where infusion of foreign marrow was one part of a strategy to protect the radiated host from the deleterious effects of the radiation injury and to induce graft acceptance.[14] Merrill, who had spent a research year with Hamburger in Paris studying the effects of radiation on the immune system, went further: he hypothesized that a predetermined sublethal dose of x-ray could temporarily impair recipient responsiveness to a kidney allograft (Figure 3.5). The gradual recovery of immunity thereafter could evoke a quasitolerant state through the presence of exogenous bone marrow and/or a few remaining host lymphoid cells regenerating in the presence of graft antigen.

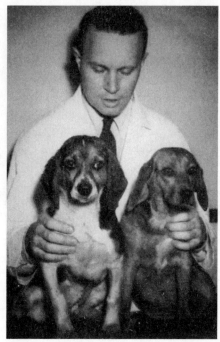

Figure 3.4 John Mannick with Sam,
the chimeric recipient of a successful
kidney transplant

Clinical opportunities to test the theory came quickly. Following the highly publicized success of the Herrick twins and the other identical-twin transplants that followed, patients with renal failure arrived at the Brigham in increasing numbers. As Murray noted, they "had nothing else to look forward to . . . We could only put patients on the artificial kidney three or four times at most because we had to cut down on the artery and vein and insert a cannula each time we did it."[15]

Emboldened by the increased survival of skin grafts they had placed on radiated animals in the laboratory, between April 1958 and March 1962 the physicians treated eleven individuals with total-body radiation prior to transplantation.[16] All received the massive dose as they lay curled on the floor on a mattress within the circumference of the beam. Bone marrow from several sources including his brother's was administered to the first irradiated patient, then a kidney from an unrelated infant. The second received a kidney from his mother fol-

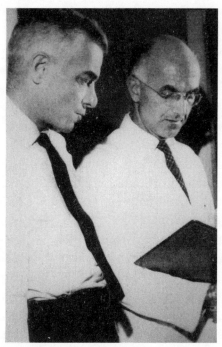

Figure 3.5 John Merrill (left) and
Joseph Murray in 1958

lowing infusion of her bone marrow. The majority of the other recipients were given kidneys from cadaver sources. Each remained isolated in an operating room throughout his or her postoperative course, under the most stringent conditions of sterility. A new pattern of graft behavior emerged: the organs functioned longer than expected and exhibited few microscopic signs of rejection. However, all recipients but one died of sepsis secondary to depression of their immune defenses. It eventually became clear that the source of the infecting "opportunistic" organisms was the individuals themselves and not the external environment. It was a finding that emphasized the power of this type of uncontrolled, nonselective, and overly powerful immunosuppressive modality.

Indeed, with the obvious exception of the identical twins, the suffering and deaths that the allograft recipients experienced were taking an increasing toll on those who cared for them. For nearly a decade, beginning with the nonimmunosuppressed patients in whom Hume and then Murray had placed kidneys, and continuing with those who had received total-body radiation as preparation for their transplant, mortality was virtually complete. Even individuals with renal failure who had not received a kidney could only stay on dialysis for limited periods before running out of access sites. The medical, surgical, and nursing staff became increasingly doubtful about the entire enterprise. The residents and interns treating the patients on a day-to-day basis were particularly despondent. Indeed, one senior medical resident in charge of the ward finally refused to involve himself any longer, telling John Merrill that he had officiated at enough murders. Only Moore, Thorn, Murray, and Merrill continued to push on, having faith that the situation would change.

The dramatic success of the third patient in this series revitalized the thinking of many of the doubters. John Riteris was a 26-year-old male with end-stage glomerulonephritis. His fraternal twin, Andrew, was a willing and understanding donor to an undertaking that he, his sick sibling, and their physicians realized could have only a small chance of success. Although they shared twenty-four of the twenty-five red-cell antigens identified in their blood, they had had separate placentas. They looked different physically. John's prolonged retention of his donor's skin graft was thought to be due to the immunosuppressive effects of uremia. In contrast, his healthy brother promptly rejected two sequential skin grafts from the patient, thereby proving genetic disparity between the two and confirming that the survival of skin grafts, even when placed between closely related individuals, was finite.[17]

The physicians administered the radiation treatment in increments, as the larger single dose had been fatal to the first two patients. They designed the protocol by interpreting data from human radiation accidents, extrapolating the effects of the treatment on experimental animals, and using Merrill's ideas about the production of tolerance in man. Because of the close genetic relationship of the brothers, no bone marrow was given (as it had been in some animal models and to the earlier patients). The transplanted kidney functioned immediately, putting out 32 liters in the first thirty-six hours. A week later, the infected native organs were removed emergently despite a persistently low white-blood-cell count. Intermittent small doses of radiation and adjunctive cortisone, an anti-inflammatory agent, were used to reverse several rejection episodes over the ensuing months that involved both the donor's long-surviving skin graft and the kidney. The patient recovered and lived a normal life over many years without receiving any other immunosuppression, before dying after heart surgery (Figure 3.6).

Like so many altruistic donors since, Andrew had few doubts about giving a kidney to his brother, regardless of the odds. In a letter years later to Joseph Murray, he summarized his thoughts on the subject. "John and I never conversed in a donor-donee context. We were brothers and each other's best friend, and there simply seemed no reason to discuss our personal contributions . . . I always believed, and still do, that the contribution of a donor is not an unusual one. It is nothing more than the rare chance, or fortune, to be a Good Samaritan to one's kin. John might have thought differently, but we never talked about it. The only reference he made to it was in an inscription in a book he gave me one week before his death, 27 years later. The inscription read: 'To Andrew—Thanks for the second drink.' "[18]

The success of this transplant between nonidentical brothers broke the "genetic barriers . . . and became in principle the single most important case, psychologically and otherwise, in the history of the field of clinical transplantation." Within weeks, Hamburger's group in Paris confirmed the Brigham findings by placing kidneys from fraternal twins into their radiated siblings.[19] Like Riteris, immediate function ensued. Although the first French patient died of infection within a few weeks, the second, a postman, lived for twenty-six years before developing bladder cancer.

Over the next two years, kidneys were transplanted into other radiated recipients with and without coincident bone marrow infusion in France, the United States, and the United Kingdom. The results answered whether the genetic closeness of the nonidentical twins contributed to the relative state of host unresponsiveness (as suggested by some animal experiments) or whether success could still occur in more dissimilar donor-recipient combinations. Jean Hamburger, for instance, grafted kidneys from a first cousin and a sibling into their respective radiated hosts. The recipient of his cousin's organ enjoyed satisfactory function before eventual retransplantation; the other

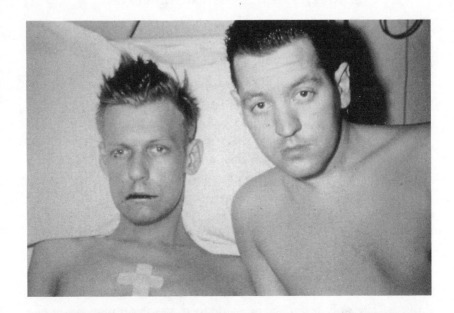

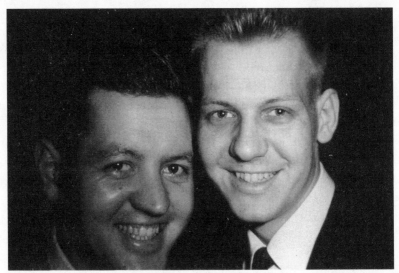

Figure 3.6 A, the Riteris brothers before the transplant in 1959; B, after the transplant. The recipient, John, was immunosuppressed with total-body x-radiation

individual, a member of the French Parliament, remains the world's longest-surviving allograft recipient. In contrast, individuals receiving organs from unrelated sources were less successful. Overall, the French results with radiation were superior to those of the North American units and remained "the principal (and perhaps the only) justification to continue clinical kidney transplantation trials."[20]

The high risks and uncertainties of total-body radiation made obvious the need for a more specific and controllable method of immunosuppression. Despite Merrill's continuing enthusiasm for the treatment, Murray became increasingly convinced that the use of chemical agents would be superior. "It seemed to me, intuitively, that irradiation was not the right way to go. It was too complex and unpredictable."[21] Indeed, there were suggestions that a strategy using drugs was possible. As early as 1916, research workers found that some simple chemical compounds influenced antibody formation in rabbits. After World War I, nitrogen mustard gas and related substances were discovered to inhibit the host defenses of animals. Three decades later, investigators noted that survival of kidney allografts in dogs treated with nitrogen mustard (and cortisone and splenectomy) increased slightly, while at about the same time, use of a related antitumor drug prevented the fatal effects of graft-versus-host disease, generated after administration of bone marrow to radiated mice.

Most significantly, two Boston hematologists, Robert Schwartz and William Dameshek, reported in 1959 that antibody activity of adult rabbits to beef protein could be suppressed by the anticancer drug 6-mercaptopurine (6-MP), which by inhibiting RNA and DNA synthesis diminished proliferation and maturation of all rapidly dividing cells including lymphoid cells. When beef antigen and the drug were administered together, the rabbits remained specifically nonreactive to the foreign protein even after cessation of the agent, but still responded to third-party antigen. The doctors described this state as "drug induced immunological tolerance."[22] Survival of skin allografts trebled in the treated animals, although the accelerated rate of rejection of second-set grafts remained unaffected.

These revelations caused a flurry of activity among surgeons interested in kidney transplantation. Küss had already administered 6-MP to a few radiated patients. Roy Calne, an English surgeon, quickly used the material alone to immunosuppress canine recipients of kidney allografts. As a medical student a decade earlier, Calne had become intrigued with the possibilities of human transplantation, an interest greeted with skepticism by his clinical teachers. Scientists working in the field were no less dissuasive. Calne had attended a lecture by Peter Medawar, who described his work in transplantation biology, specifically the novel phenomenon of tolerance. Although the importance of his findings were evident to many of those considering additional relevant experiments, Medawar's answer to a student's question about potential clinical applications of the observations was a firm "Absolutely none."[23] Undeterred, Calne began to graft kidneys in radiated and then drug-treated dogs. Working outside London at a research laboratory on the grounds of Down House, where Charles Darwin had lived and written his books on natural history and evolution, Calne noted that many allografts functioned relatively normally before the recipients died of drug toxicity. When the dose was reduced, two dogs survived for unprecedented periods of twenty-one and forty-seven days without signs of rejection until developing fatal pneumonia.

Stimulated by the subsequent reports of Schwartz and Dameshek, and by his own marginal results with 6-MP, at Medawar's suggestion Calne arranged to join Murray at Harvard as a research fellow, sailing to New York with his family on the *Queen Elizabeth* in the summer of 1960. On the way to Boston, he visited Doctors George Hitchings and Gertrude Elion at the Burroughs Wellcome Research Laboratory in Tuckahoe, New York. Having previously synthesized 6-MP and similar molecules, the biochemists generously gave him several chemical analogs to test in the Harvard laboratory.[24]

Calne quickly confirmed his earlier findings and those of two other surgical investigators who had treated kidney-grafted dogs with 6-MP. Upon testing the additional materials from Hitchings and Elion, he and Murray found that a chemical derivative of 6-MP, later known as azathioprine or Imuran, seemed the most promising with regard to its immunosuppressive abilities, ease of oral administration, and relatively controllable toxicity. A few of the dogs lived indefinitely in a completely healthy state, supported by their transplanted kidney. One dog, Mona, even had a litter of normal puppies (Figure 3.7). Perhaps

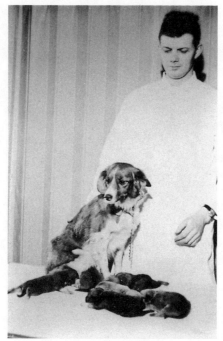

Figure 3.7 An early kidney recipient
treated with azathioprine: Mona and
her puppies

the most convincing demonstration of these unprecedented results
was during Grand Rounds at the Brigham. The surgeons presented the
female recipient of a renal allograft who had survived in excellent
condition for six months. Introduced to the large audience, Lollipop
pranced happily around the room and licked the faces of the professors
in the front row (Figure 3.8). Doing much to persuade the skeptics, she
set the stage for clinical attempts to follow.

Murray put this breakthrough in context: "For a decade in our
laboratory several hundred renal transplants in dogs were performed
using varieties of protocols. Our longest survival had been 18 days.
Within a few weeks after Calne started to work with us one dog was
surviving on a solitary renal allograft for 35 days with 6 mercaptopurine as the only immunosuppressive agent. This was truly a giant
step . . . By 1961, we had reported dogs surviving over 50 days with
normal renal function. It was noteworthy that these animals were not

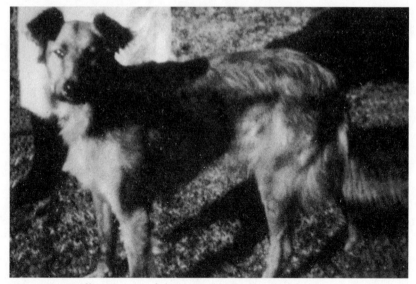

Figure 3.8 Lollipop, one of the original chemically immunosuppressed transplant recipients

sick or debilitated. They ate well, maintained weight, resisted kennel infection, and even procreated normally."[25]

Despite these unprecedented results, half of the 120 canine recipients that Calne and Murray treated with 6-MP or azathioprine died within twenty days of transplantation, and 90 percent of them by three months. Even three years later, the outcomes of more than a thousand dogs treated with twenty-four different drug regimens and combinations had improved only slightly.[26] Although 90 percent of grafts now functioned at fifty days, only 50 percent continued to survive at three months. These early experiments were soon repeated in laboratories in Denver, Minneapolis, and Richmond. The results were similar.

Chemical immunosuppression was quickly instituted in human recipients, however, justified by the occasional but noteworthy successes in dogs. Thomas Starzl, to become a principal figure in the field, later commented on this step: "It was on this dismal record that the clinical kidney transplantation trials of the early 1960s were based. In a display of optimism that would not be tolerated in the clinical research climate of today, the rare exception was given more weight than the customary failure. Thus, the poor results came as no surprise when the drugs were first used for patients in the same way as had been tried in the experimental animals."[27]

But try they did. Spurred on by the "rare exception" among the dogs and the increased efficacy and lower toxicity of drug treatment compared to whole-body radiation, Murray, Merrill, Moore, Thorn, and their colleagues agreed to proceed. Patients were only considered when no other options were open to them. Murray treated the first with 6-MP as the sole immunosuppressant in April 1960. That patient lived four weeks; the second lived thirteen weeks. The first to receive azathioprine was grafted a year later and survived five weeks.[28] After five more failures, success occurred in April 1962. Melvin Doucette, a 24-year-old accountant, received a transplant from a donor who had just died during open-heart surgery. As the body was on cardiopulmonary bypass, the cooled and well-functioning kidneys were removed immediately and transplanted within two hours. Immediate urine flow occurred. Rejection episodes at 39 and 120 days were reversed. Pneumonia, thought to develop secondarily to the effects of the immunosuppression, resolved. A perforated appendix was removed successfully at eighteen months. As the graft began to fail at twenty-one months, Doucette received a second transplant, which also functioned well until he died six months later from hepatitis.

Heartened by the occasional hopeful result, the clinical experience with chemical immunosuppression slowly broadened. Within months the Brigham team had transplanted twenty-seven patients, nine of whom were sustained for at least a year by their functioning graft. Despite the relative success of the French surgeons with radiation, those in the few other existing units also began to use azathioprine. The novelty of the transplant procedure, however, still evoked controversy. Upon his return to London, for instance, Calne began to transplant patients despite opposition by some of the more conservative hospital staff. "Theater Sister would not permit cadavers in her operating rooms so we had to remove kidneys in the open wards. It must of been dreadful for the other patients in the large wards to see the surgeons go behind the curtain and operate on a corpse in bed with blood trickling on the floor."[29]

Late in 1963, all available clinical information was discussed at a conference near Washington, D.C. About twenty-five of the most active participants in clinical and experimental transplantation gathered in a small, hot room in an old building at the National Institutes of Health. Thirteen teams—two from France, five from the United Kingdom, and six from the United States—presented their overall experience with 216 recipients of renal allografts. The results were not propitious: 52 percent of all those receiving grafts from related living donors and 81 percent of those with kidneys from unrelated or cadaver sources had died. Only eight allografts from cadavers, or 4 percent, functioned for more than a year. In contrast, 76 percent of identical-twin or radiated nonidentical-twin recipients were still alive. Murray concluded: "Although the beginnings of clinical success are apparent, strong reservations must be kept in mind regarding the ultimate fate of these patients. Kidney transplantation is still highly experimental and not yet a therapeutic procedure." Hume, now in Virginia, had used a combination of whole-body radiation, azathioprine, and steroids in six patients. He echoed these sentiments: "Renal homotransplantation is showing signs of coming of age but is still a highly experimental procedure."[30]

One clinical report relieved the relative gloom. Thomas Starzl and Thomas Marchioro, two relatively unknown young surgeons from Denver, presented their results with twenty-seven renal transplants performed over the previous ten months—twenty-five from living donors, both related and unrelated.[31] Several in the latter group were prisoners who had volunteered their organs; one such donor, in fact, escaped from the hospital and was never heard of again. Starzl and Marchioro used azathioprine alone as primary immunosuppression, but reversed the virtually inevitable acute rejection episode in over 90 percent of the cases with high doses of prednisone, an anti-inflammatory derivative of cortisone, and actinomycin C, an antibiotic that killed populations of white blood cells. Eighteen of their patients, or 67 percent, remained alive with satisfactory graft function. They repeated this important clinical strategy in dogs: acute rejection was reversed in seven of eight animals by administration of steroids. The genie appeared to be out of the bottle; maintenance immunosuppression with azathioprine and steroids in combination, and the treatment of rejection with high doses of steroids, remained the linchpin of clinical immunosuppressive treatment for the next two decades.

Starzl, to become one of the most visible and consistently productive pioneers in the field and a teacher of transplant surgeons throughout the world, recalled his trepidation during the conference: "At the formal meetings, I found it difficult to speak. It may have been my insecurity in the presence of such important dignitaries which caused me to be uneasy. In addition, I felt like someone who had parachuted unannounced from another planet onto turf that was already occupied. I was the only American transplant surgeon who had no exposure to the Harvard system and experience. However, although I had never been to any other transplant center including the Brigham, I was keenly aware of what had been done by the others who had gathered for the conference."[32]

Both intellectual synergy and competitive forces among investigators and among their institutions drive scientific advances. Transplantation is no exception. Since its inception, professional cooperation and friendly rivalry, in combination in clinical transplantation and transplant research, have not only enhanced knowledge but have attracted financial support. As experience and manpower increased, individual teams began to announce their clinical results, comparing their survival rates for patients and grafts with those of other groups, and touting nuances of treatment. Studies in the biology of transplantation expanded substantially in growing numbers of laboratories.

A spirit of competition became obvious immediately. The two French teams who performed the original cadaver transplants, although from the same hospital in Paris, published their reports in different journals in the same year. Murray stressed, however, that the Boston-Paris rivalry remained communicative and pleasant in contrast to other, often vituperative, medical and scientific claims regarding priority of discoveries or the effects of treatment. Acclaim was comprehensive when Hitchings and Elion were awarded the Nobel Prize in 1988 for their work on immunosuppressive drugs. And elation was widespread when Murray received the prize two years later for opening the field—although some of the French workers, who believed that their seminal contributions had been ignored, were unavoidably distressed. One of Hamburger's colleagues suggested, for instance, that "while we can be proud that Professor Murray was awarded the Nobel

Prize, we deplore the fact that Professor Hamburger was not associated with the nomination." An editorial in *Le Monde* pondered, "We cannot help but be surprised by the decision of the Nobel Jury."[33] Clearly, it is difficult to please everyone by selecting a few individuals from all those involved in a developing field.

Host Defenses and Immunity

4

ONCE THE SURGEONS HAD CREATED AN EFFEC-
tive and reproducible operative technique to transplant a kidney from
human to human, they faced a more formidable barrier. Regardless of
immunosuppression, within a few days most recipients experienced an
intense local inflammatory reaction. The allograft became tender and
swollen. Patients often developed high fevers and general malaise. If
the process could not be reversed, renal function declined inexorably
as cellular destruction progressed. Occasional rupture and hemorrhage of the enlarging organ required urgent surgical removal. If dialysis was unavailable, death was inevitable.

Unique to transplanted foreign tissues, this phenomenon of acute
rejection, as it was termed, became increasingly recognized as a specific
part of the complex spectrum of defense mechanisms protecting an
individual throughout his or her life. Although more detailed biological
definition of the changes occurring in the allografts gathered in parallel
with clinical experience, much of the new information was based on an
older background of experience with infections, their manifestations,
and their control by vaccination and specific antitoxins. What emerged
was the concept that the dramatic events of rejection might also be
modulated or inhibited to allow the foreign tissue to survive. However,
our current appreciation of the relationships between infection, inflammation, immunity, and allograft rejection evolved over centuries.

Infection has always existed as a threat to humans and their place in
the environment. Sometimes raging uncontrollaby, pestilence and epidemics have decimated entire populations and societies. Half the

inhabitants of Europe and over 70 percent of those in cities, for instance, died of the Black Death in the fourteenth century. More indigenous peoples in the New World perished from smallpox, measles, chickenpox, and diptheria brought by those arriving from Europe than from their bullets or whiskey; in recompense, sailors returning in Columbus' ships allegedly carried back a hitherto unknown bane, syphilis. Smallpox, one of the most devastating of man's afflictions, has sprung up periodically throughout the centuries. The British historian Lord Macauley graphically described its devastating effects: "This [was the] most terrible of all ministers of death—filling the church yard with corpses, tormenting with constant fears all whom it had not stricken, leaving on those whose lives it spared the hideous traces of its power, turning the babe into a changeling at which the mother shuddered, and making the eyes and cheeks of the betrothed maiden objects of horror to the lover."[1] The incidence and severity of such scourges in Western countries did not decrease for centuries. A variety of infections still threaten and sometimes decimate those in poorer nations, particularly during periods of war, famine, or natural catastrophe. The swine flu pandemic after World War I and the global AIDS epidemic are modern examples. The current threats of bioterrorism with anthrax and other agents raise new fears. The specter of smallpox decimating unvaccinated populations is particularly unnerving.

Early public health measures finally began to temper the effects of these societal catastrophes. In 1720 Richard Mead, an English graduate of the University of Padua, suggested ways to prevent the spread of infection in his treatise *A Short Discourse Concerning Pestilential Contagion*. But not for well over a century did the implementation of his ideas of quarantine, alleviation of overcrowding, and other improvements in the squalid living conditions of the poor actually affect the course of epidemics. In 1846 William Duncan, a medical officer in Liverpool, used these strategies to contain an outbreak of cholera among Irish exiles fleeing the potato famine, one million of whom were said to live within a single square mile of that teeming city. More conclusively, John Snow, a student of John Hunter, discovered that the great London cholera epidemic of 1854 was spread by means of a contaminated water supply. He identified the source of the epidemic and influenced its outcome substantially by having the handle of the public water pump on Broad Street removed. Discovering the cause of a disease, then influencing the pattern of its spread, although revolutionary concepts at the time, have remained dominant principles in public health as societies grow and populations shift.

Vaccination was an alternative approach to the control of contagion, a means to stimulate the protective responses of one individual by injection of infective material from another who had survived the particular disease, or of a weakened or attenuated version of the responsible organism. The method enhanced appreciation of a cause-and-effect relationship between sepsis and subsequent host immunity, a critical synthesis of the two subjects. One of the great success stories of medical biology, vaccination remains relevant to the concept of immunosuppression of transplant recipients.

Preservation of an individual by external manipulations was an ancient idea. Perhaps the earliest recorded example of purposeful protection against foreign substances was that of King Mithradates, best remembered as thwarting the expansion of the Roman Empire into Asia in about 100 B.C. He defended himself against assassination attempts by eating small doses of lethal poisons and other toxins and building his tolerance to them. The British poet A. E. Housman later described the process:

> There was a king reigned in the East:
> There, when kings will sit to feast,
> They get their fill before they think
> With poisoned meat and poisoned drink.
> He gathered all that springs to birth
> From the many venomed earth;
> First a little, thence to more,
> He sampled all her killing store;
> And easy, smiling, seasoned, sound,
> Sate the king when healths went round.
> They put arsenic in his meat
> And stared aghast to see him eat;
> They poured strychnine in his cup
> And shook to see him drink it up:
> They shook, they stared as white's their shirt.
> Them it was their poison hurt.
> I tell the tale that I heard told.
> Mithradates he died old.[2]

Sadly, a mutiny among his troops led by his own son, Pharnaces II, arose when Mithradates was an old man. Despondent and attempting to end his life, he found that he was totally unaffected by all available poisons. He had to order one of his Gothic mercenaries to kill him with a sword.

The Chinese were reputed to have used vaccination against small-pox as early as the tenth century, the Egyptians from the thirteenth century. Voltaire credits the wife of the British ambassador in Con-stantinople, Lady Mary Wortley Montagu, with appreciating the vac-cination practices of the Turks, who immunized children by inoculat-ing them with material from a "pustule taken from the most regular and at the same time the most favorable, sort of smallpox that could be procured."[3] Her own beauty disfigured by the disease, she had her small son inoculated upon returning to London in 1718. This experi-ence led to the famous Royal Experiment in 1721–1722, in which the Prince and Princess of Wales allowed their children to be vaccinated after extensive testing on orphans and prisoners. By midcentury, En-glish practitioners tempered their use of deep skin incisions, which sometimes resulted in severe smallpox infections and even death. They changed to a technique of superficial skin abrasion and introduction of small drops of lymph from infected persons. This more successful procedure spread throughout Britain and then to the Continent, with English physicians traveling to Saint Petersburg to vaccinate the Em-press Catherine, to Vienna to inoculate the Empress Maria Theresa and her children, and to additional cities and capitals to treat other royalty and disseminate the method.

Across the ocean in Massachusetts, a Puritan minister introduced the novel concept in America's first medical text, *The Angel of Be-thesda*.[4] Cotton Mather had learned about vaccination via a conversa-tion with Lady Montagu in London and descriptions of the practice in Africa from his own slaves. The Boston medical establishment was loath to try such a radical experiment. However, following his tenure as a judge at the Salem witch trials, Mather persuaded Zabdiel Boyl-ston, a local surgeon from the nearby town of Brookline, to inoculate his own son with pus from an active pock. The boy recovered after only a mild case, encouraging Boylston to go ahead with many care-fully documented treatments. Here was a major example of early preventive medicine. As the next epidemic ran its course, it became evident that the majority of those inoculated had become immune. The practice gradually spread to Philadelphia and eventually to Washington's Revolutionary army. In Europe a few years later, Napoleon ordered that his troops be vaccinated.

Edward Jenner, one of John Hunter's pupils, noted that milkmaids infected by their cows never developed smallpox. His conclusion that cowpox, a less virulent disease, would protect against the serious new disease was first reported in England. On July 1, 1796, he vaccinated teenager James Phipps with cowpox. When challenged six weeks later with smallpox, Phipps was immune. As a tribute to this important contribution to humankind, a statue of Jenner sits in a London park. The head of the cow Blossom, from whom the dairy maid Sarah Nelmes contracted cowpox, is carved on each side of the chair. From one of Sarah's skin lesions, Jennifer obtained his vaccination inoculum. Hunter's advice in a letter to his student has encouraged surgical investigation ever since: "I think your solution is just, but why think? Why not try to experiment?"[5]

The understanding that infections could be caused by tiny living organisms did not emerge until the midnineteenth century, despite introduction of the concept by the Roman encyclopedist Varro in about 100 B.C. and its reconsideration during the Renaissance. Anthony van Leeuwenhoek in 1679 in the Netherlands had produced a magnifying glass powerful enough to visualize tiny "animalcules." Still, naturalists were unable to identify minute forms of life until Joseph Lister, father of the surgeon Lord Lister, later invented the compound microscope with achromatic lenses.

Discoveries then came in rapid succession with the appreciation that microorganisms were ubiquitous and played a critical role in the balance of nature as well as in disease. The French chemist Louis Pasteur described their role in the process of putrefaction of animal and vegetable matter in 1857, showing that grapes in the wine industry could neither ferment nor decay in their absence.[6] Shortly thereafter, bacteria identified in the blood of animals dying of anthrax, a fatal disease of sheep and cattle that cost the agricultural economy of the time millions of francs, were found to cause the disease. Robert Koch in Berlin, the other towering figure in the new field of microbiology,

caused the death of experimental animals by infecting them with anthrax organisms cultured in an artificial medium. He subsequently
identified and cultured the tuberculosis bacterium responsible for a
scourge that caused five million deaths a year worldwide. However, his
highly publicized attempts at cure with tuberculin, an extract of the
organism, failed (although the material was later found to be crucial to
the diagnosis). More dramatically, having noted that inoculation of
inactivated virus of chicken cholera protected the chickens from the
disease, Pasteur and his colleagues demonstrated publicly in May 1877
that attenuated anthrax organisms could also prevent the infection in
sheep. Administering live anthrax to a drove of sheep, he inoculated
half the animals with his nonvirulent material. Two days later, at a farm
at Pouilly-le-Fort near Melum, a large crowd of farmers, veterinarians,
reporters, believers, detractors, and doubting colleagues gathered before the two pens of animals. All the unprotected sheep began to
sicken and die. The treated animals continued in perfect health. Within
a few years Pasteur had developed a vaccine for rabies, a treatment
today used the world over. A new era in medicine had begun.

As information on the significance of bacteria and their control
emerged, initially skeptical physicians began to consider further strategies to treat their patients. Substances present in the serum of the
previously infected host were recognized as conferring specific protection against particular organisms. The virtual eradication of diphtheria
and tetanus using antitoxins or antisera from large animals in Koch's
laboratory gained the most publicity. The ability to manipulate host
responses in this manner not only saved people everywhere but also
set the stage for the subsequent flourishing of the related fields of
immunology and transplant biology.

The development of the microbial sciences during this productive
period was driven in no small part by the increasingly sharp and often
vituperative exchanges between the two distinguished microbiologists
Koch and Pasteur.[7] Although their discoveries were often mutually
supportive, the intensity of their rivalry stemmed from differences in
style of the two men and their followers. These were rooted in the
national and cultural characteristics of the Germans and French, and a
smoldering antagonism left over from the Franco-Prussian War of
1870. As he grew older, Koch became an increasingly authoritarian

figure, surgically oriented, and prejudiced in his views by his activities with the war wounded. Supported by his own substantial contributions to the role of specific agents in disease, as well as those of the powerful German school of bacteriology, he stressed that bacteria were pathogens. As such, they should be eradicated. Pasteur's temperament was more composed. Influenced by his experience with French agriculture and the wine industry, he viewed the world of microorganisms as a part of natural ecology. He and the smaller and less well organized French school concerned themselves more with the effects of host immunity on infection; hence his interest in vaccination.

Enormously productive, famous, and acclaimed, these two giants alternately ignored, criticized, and attacked each other's work and conclusions—a situation inflamed by the fact that neither was adequately conversant in the other's language. Although the protagonists emphasized different themes, with Koch making major practical contributions to public health and Pasteur emphasizing protective immunization, their work was fully complementary. The value of their concepts in biology and ultimately in transplantation is immeasurable.

Inflammation has been long recognized as a feature of infection or injury. Descriptions of pus, abscesses, and ulcers are present in Egyptian papyri of 2000 B.C. Hippocrates and his followers defined *erysipelas*, literally "redness of the skin," a term used to this day. Although Galen, the Greek physiologist, and the Roman encyclopedist Celsus noted the cardinal manifestations of inflammation—pain, redness, swelling, and fever—the mechanisms of the process and their role in the body defenses did not broaden until pathological states could be observed through the newly introduced microscope. Several natural philosophers of the Enlightenment discovered that dilation of small blood vessels caused redness in the inflamed area. Hunter offered the radical view that the function of inflammation was to restore the involved tissues to their natural state. The German pathologist Julius Cohnheim enhanced this suggestion in 1882 with his studies of the migration of white cells from blood vessels to a site of injury in the foot webs and tongues of frogs.[8] Others made similar observations (Figure 4.1).

A crucial figure in this emerging biology was Elie Metchnikoff, a Russian zoologist working in Paris (Figure 4.2). Acknowledging the

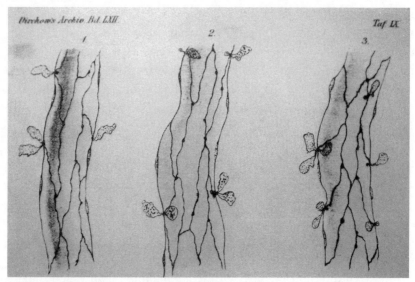

Figure 4.1 White blood cells exiting from the inflamed vessels in a frog's tongue; from the mesentery; from the bladder (J. Arnold, *Virchows Archiv: Pathologische Anatomie*, 1875, 62:487)

seminal contributions of Charles Darwin and Alfred Russel Wallace to the new theory of evolution, he examined the reactions of simple organisms to foreign bodies, then extended his observations up the scale to vertebrates.[9] Noting first that cells in the larvae of starfish "attacked" tiny splinters introduced into their substance, he found that the primitive leukocytes of the crustacean *Daphnia* could destroy fungal spores invading its tissues. Naming these white cells phagocytes, he hypothesized about their protective role in humans. His work on the increasing sophistication of the inflammatory responses up the evolutionary scale and the importance of phagocytosis as a biologic phenomenon formed a critical background for later studies in immunology and transplantation biology.

   Metchnikoff's controversial proposal that host phagocytic cells were instrumental in responding to foreign invaders evoked intense opposition from the "humoral" school of Pasteur and Koch, emboldened by their success with immunization against infectious disease and their conviction that noncellular substances circulating in the blood were paramount in the body defenses. Even the foremost pathologist

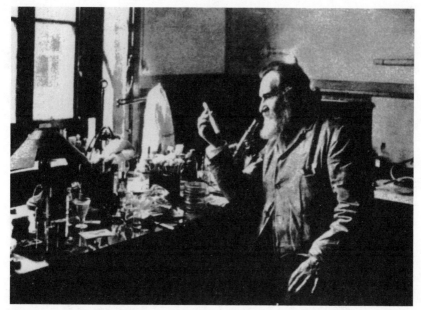

Figure 4.2 Elie Metchnikoff in his laboratory (E. Metchnikoff, *Lectures on the Comparative Biology of Inflammation, 1891*, Mineola, N.Y.: Dover Publications, 1968; with permission)

of the time, Rudolf Virchow of Berlin, warned Metchnikoff to move cautiously in expounding his cellular theories, as "most pathologists do not believe in the protective role of inflammation." It was unfortunate that the announcement of his findings coincided with public enthusiasm for the use of antisera against otherwise fatal infections. As one historian remarked, "the discovery of antibodies pushed phagocytes out of the limelight."[10]

The Silesian-German Paul Ehrlich was a student and close colleague of Koch. Dominant in immunology and immunochemistry, he was another highly visible figure in this debate. Initially staining and identifying circulating leukocyte populations using aniline dyes from the thriving dye industry in Germany, Ehrlich expanded his chemical studies with descriptive cellular pathology. These vital stains bound strongly to proteins in the cell, possibly by inhibiting enzyme activity. Explaining this affinity via the concept of "side chains," Ehrlich postulated the formation of antibodies in the serum that would react specifically against individual foreign antigens. Describing means to neutralize the effects of antitoxins and to transfer immunity from mother to child, he and his colleagues at the I. G. Farben Company in Frankfurt also introduced the concept of chemotherapy, using the drug Salvarsan against syphilis. This agent remained the standard treatment until the advent of penicillin half a century later. Ehrlich believed that four German Gs were necessary for the success of all scientists: *Geduld* (patience), *Geschick* (cleverness), *Glück* (luck), and *Geld* (money).

A series of related discoveries extolled at the turn of the century by chauvinistic German and French scientists included the vital role of antibodies in immunity and the recognition that bacteriocidal proteins are present in normal serum. Peace between the factions was eventually restored when the 1908 Nobel Prize was awarded jointly to Metchnikoff for his cellular work and to Ehrlich for his humoral concepts. Several years later Almroth Wright in London, having already made typhoid vaccine practical during World War I, became a highly vocal advocate for serum factors in combating infections in wounded soldiers.[11] A controversial figure of the humoral school, his polemics against the role of cells in host defenses were so strident that he was held up to public ridicule (as Sir Colenso Rigeon) by George Bernard Shaw in his play *The Doctor's Dilemma*. Wright's subsequent evidence that a coating of serum proteins on phagocytes is necessary to produce full activity against microorganisms silenced the discussion by giving credence to both sides. In retrospect, the intensity of these debates and arguments, which often seemed to reach metaphysical levels, substantially delayed further advances in understanding of immunity.

The complexities of the host responses involved with inflammation and immunity led naturally to consideration of another aspect of the host defenses, the phenomenon of rejection. Appreciation of the reactivity of an animal against foreign tissues arose from studies of tumors. Many investigators recognized that the body would destroy tumor implants before parallel interpretations were made of the behavior of skin or other tissue allografts. Early in the twentieth century, successful tumor engraftment between relatively inbred mice in a closed colony, but not between wild-type animals from the outside, suggested the importance of genetic factors. Antiserum raised in rabbits against mouse tumors killed similar tumors growing in other rabbits.

The leukocyte populations infiltrating the tumors were also associated with their destruction. And as confirmed later with two sequential sets of skin grafts, Paul Ehrlich documented the complete lack of growth of second tumors in animals which had previously rejected the first. "The failure of the second . . . can only be explained by an actively acquired immunity, established on the formation of antibodies resulting from reabsorption of the tumor mass."[12]

Leo Loeb was a high-profile, prolific contributor to the growing subject. A German who emigrated to New York after World War I, he conducted a prolonged series of experiments on the transfer of tumors and the transplantation of a variety of normal tissues between small laboratory animals. These studies included a lengthy analysis of the "individual differentials" between donor and host. In addition, his rudimentary observations of the relationship between infiltrating lymphocytes and graft rejection provided early, barely recognized, and apparently misinterpreted clues to the phenomenon. Despite the overall lack of understanding, the slowly accumulating, superficially often unrelated data were beginning to increase scientific interest in the natural mechanisms protecting the host.

One reason Alexis Carrel removed himself from the field of transplantation may have been that he began to appreciate the complexity of the host responses against allografts and the potential difficulty in altering them. His suggestions that future "research should be directed toward biological methods designed to prevent the body's reactions against foreign tissue" were based at least partly on his knowledge of the work of a tumor biologist in an adjacent laboratory at the Rockefeller Institute in New York. J. B. Murphy had become convinced that the host mechanisms involved in the destruction of tumors were similar to those of transplanted tissues or organs. Increasingly, his studies implicated the lymphocyte—a small, round, rather nondescript white blood cell—as "an important factor in the immunity to cancer." As his peers generally disregarded his well-researched experiments, their significance lay dormant for the next two decades. Even the Johns Hopkins pathologist Arnold Rich, having noted well the presence of lymphocytes in inflammatory sites, decried the lack of understanding about their activities in the body. "The complete ignorance of the function of this cell is one of the most humiliating and disgraceful gaps in all medical knowledge ... Literally nothing of importance is known regarding the potential of these cells." Rich went on to describe them rather dramatically as "phlegmatic spectators watching the turbulent activities of phagocytes."[13]

Appreciation of the role of this population in cellular immunity increased substantially in the 1940s. Experiments showed that transfer of cells isolated from the area of swelling and redness produced in the skin of one set of animals by a tuberculin test or injection of a sensitizing chemical, could create identical skin reactions in other animals as well. The majority of the cells responsible for this so-called delayed hypersensitivity reaction were lymphocytes. Serum from the involved skin injected into other animals, in contrast, had no effect.

The lymphocyte increasingly became the focus of attention of not only clinicians and scientists involved in transplanting organs but also of those studying cancer, viral disease, allergy, and various immune and autoimmune disorders. Several individuals, among them Howard Florey, James Gowans, Peter Medawar, and Paul Terasaki were responsible for promoting understanding of these cells and their functions.

Howard Florey was one of the renowned experimental pathologists of the twentieth century. An Australian Rhodes Scholar, he had become director of the Sir William Dunn School of Pathology at Oxford University in 1935. Recognized primarily because of his 1945 Nobel Prize for the production and therapeutic application of penicillin, his investigations into atherosclerosis, the mechanisms of inflammation, and the physiology of leukocytes also garnered considerable attention. In 1953 a young research fellow began work in Florey's laboratory. Uncertain where to direct his efforts, James Gowans (Figure 4.3) approached the director, who advised him to study lymphocytes, one of his own current areas of interest. Florey said that "lymphocytes had blunted the wits of a number of his colleagues and ... he could see no reason why [Gowans] should be spared a similar fate."[14] Florey suggested that he examine the problem of what was then known as "the mystery of the disappearing lymphocyte," an observation that the numbers of these cells entering the circulation each day from the major lymphatics were ten times those found in the peripheral blood. Existing theories suggested that the discrepancy was

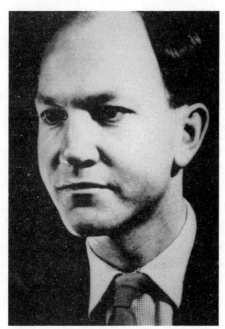

Figure 4.3 James Gowans in about
1960

caused by primitive cells from the bone marrow, which had the ability
to turn rapidly into more specialized populations, or else they were
"end cells," which died in the gut or skin within a few hours of carrying out their unknown functions.

Over the next few years, in experiments involving bulk removal of
lymphocytes from mice and rats via a small plastic tube inserted in the
thoracic duct (the major lymphatic channel in the body), their labeling
with radioactive markers, and their reinfusion into the host animals,
Gowans and his associates showed that many of these cells were long-
lived and recirculated continuously between blood and lymph by migration through the lymph nodes. Other populations remained static
in lymphoid tissues. Contact between the migrating cells and any foreign antigens or bacteria that might invade the animal, it appeared, was
a normal physiological, protective activity. Once a circulating lymphocyte communicated with such a potential threat, additional inherently
reactive populations could receive its message to respond quickly and

effectively against it. Even Peter Medawar, among other skeptics about the recirculation abilities of these cells, became convinced. A lover of opera, he likened the peripatetic lymphocytes to "the chorus of soldiers in a provincial production of *Faust*—they make a brief public appearance and then disappear behind the scenes only to re-enter by the same route."[15]

It took more time to define precisely the role of the lymphocyte in the body's defenses. Although Florey had suggested that their function might become clear if one knew where they went, his point was hardly obvious. Despite increasing information, the Australian immunologist Macfarlane Burnet observed in 1959 that "an objective survey of the facts could well lead to the conclusion that there was no evidence of immunological activity in small lymphocytes." Even in the 1964 edition of Florey's textbook *General Pathology*, this frustrated comment about lymphocytes appears: "A cell which exists in the normal animal in such large numbers and which is mobilized into striking local collections in disease might be expected to possess some obvious and important function. However, the only positive activity in which the small lymphocyte is known to indulge is that of movement."[16]

Evidence gradually arose, however, that the lymphocyte functioned as an "immunologically competent cell," an expression coined by Medawar, who was becoming a leading figure in the emerging field of transplantation biology.[17] Further clues emerged from experiments on graft-versus-host disease. Paul Terasaki, a young Californian working as a research fellow in Medawar's laboratory, first noted that purified immunologically active leukocytes from adult chickens could produce a fatal wasting syndrome after injection into newborn chicks unable to respond to the foreign challenge because of the immaturity of their immune system. Several investigators in Europe and the United States quickly confirmed this observation. Gowans then demonstrated that the recirculating lymphocyte population was responsible, and with other colleagues showed that lymphocytes were involved in the rejection process.

The origin of these cells was also unraveling. In 1961 J. F. A. P. Miller, an Australian working in London, found that the thymus gland, an enigmatic lymphoid organ of unknown function lying beneath the breast bone, was critical in the development of immunity.[18] By surgically removing this organ from newborn mice, he observed that the majority of animals lost weight, wasted, and often died of common laboratory infections. Concluding that the tissue "may be essential to life," he noted that circulating lymphocytes in surviving animals profoundly decreased in number, and that lymphoid organs including spleen and lymph nodes atrophied. Most significant, skin grafts healed and grew hair normally, whereas reconstitution of animals with fetal thymic cells caused acute rejection of the established grafts. Antibody activity was not affected. As removal of the gland from adult mice with already mature lymphoid tissues produced no changes, Miller and the few other investigators examining the thymus concluded that the gland is critical in early life in "training" immature lymphocytes from the bone marrow to become the primary mediators of cellular immunity in the body.

With the increasing excitement about the role of these cells in the immune response, the effect of humoral factors, particularly antibodies, began to fall out of scientific favor. The veterinarian Bernard Glick and his colleagues had observed a few years before that the bursa of Fabricius, a lymphocyte-rich blind pouch connected to the intestine of birds, had immunological functions.[19] After surgical removal of the bursa, young chicks but not adult chickens could no longer produce antibodies against antigens, but they were still able to reject skin grafts. The inference was that specialized lymphoid cells in the bursa, appropriately stimulated, could make antibodies. Although this important fact was not known to most immunologists (the data were published in a rather obscure specialty journal, *Poultry Science*, after being turned down by a more prestigious journal because of "no general interest"), its confirmation several years later in other laboratories provoked considerable enthusiasm. Subsequent search for a "bursa equivalent" in mammals initially implicated the tonsils and appendix but finally settled on lymphoid aggregations in the gut and bone marrow.

These experiments showed dramatically that acquired immunity involved both cellular and humoral host responses. Indeed, they rekindled the controversy between Metchnikoff and Ehrlich, and their rivals, with Medawar becoming a highly visible proponent of cellular immunity and a London geneticist, Peter Gorer, advocating the role of humoral antibodies. Although the dialogue was conducted on a more genteel level than in the previous century, it stimulated promising new lines of investigation. Years before, Gorer had identified the major histocompatibility locus on the mouse chromosome, a site primarily responsible for genetic variability among individuals.[20] His subsequent studies produced the general concept of "histocompatibility genes," which were to open up new areas of research that included tissue matching between donor and recipient. Studies on the genetic and antigenic basis of tumor transplantation followed, embellished by data demonstrating the influence of antibodies against both tumors and transplanted tissues. Gorer became an enthusiastic proponent of humoral immune mechanisms as important not only in destroying foreign tissues but also in inhibiting their destruction under specific experimental circumstances.

As understanding of lymphocytes, lymphocyte classes, and their origins increased, the entire lymphoid system of the body came under close scrutiny. It became apparent that it had developed early in evolution and had attained remarkable functional sophistication in higher animals. Taken in bulk, mammalian lymphoid tissues constitute an organ of considerable size (Figure 4.4). Besides the role of lymphocytes as a defense against many infections, these tissues and their associated populations had another presumed function. They were thought to be involved in the identification and elimination of genetic errors occurring occasionally in rapidly dividing cells that might mutate and become cancerous. Some resident lymphocytes also developed sufficient memory to enable them to respond promptly and forcibly to future challenges of the same sort. This explained the "second-set" rejection of allografts. Further understanding of the role of lymphocytes in the behavior of transplanted tissues evolved at the same time.

Stimulated by these findings, immunology and its related sciences exploded during the 1960s and 1970s. Increasing knowledge about differential lymphocyte function as orchestrated by the thymus and the bursa unleashed a torrent of associated investigations. The concept that different subpopulations of thymus-derived (T) lymphocytes mediated cellular immunity and bursa-derived (B) lymphocytes evoked host humoral activity opened more experimental possibilities.[21] Iden-

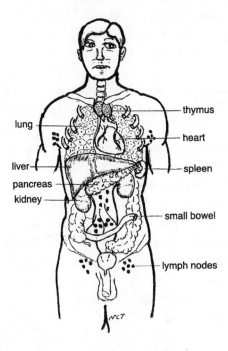

Figure 4.4 Lymphoid tissues and transplantable organs (N. L. Tilney)

tification of histocompatibility antigens directing similarities or differences between humans, and elaboration of their function at both
cellular and molecular levels, unfolded. The increasing availability of
monoclonal antibodies, created in the test tube to react exclusively and
specifically against individual antigens, facilitated characterization of
the intricate cellular cascade mediating allograft rejection; their virtually unlimited variety has enhanced understanding of the actions,
interrelationships, influences, and contributions of cell populations,
subpopulations, and their synthesized products in host defenses. The
more recent outburst of activity in molecular biology, generating the
ability to identify and define a myriad of inflammatory and immunologic mediators, has provoked continuing advances in both experimental and clinical settings.

Peter Medawar summed up the excitement among scientists and
clinicians during those years: "The whole period was a golden age of
immunology, an age abounding in synthetic discoveries all over the

world, a time we all thought it was good to be alive. We, who were working on these problems, all knew each other and met as often as we could to exchange ideas and hot news from the laboratory."[22]

By this time, kidney transplantation was showing promise for patients dying of renal failure—not only the obvious success of identical twins, but also the survival of occasional allografts in immunomodified hosts. Its associated biologies were attracting much interest, even though some pure scientists felt the clinicians were moving too fast. But many of the same individuals were involved in the two parallel areas. Surgeons in particular, having become fascinated with the unremitting challenges posed by transplant recipients, spent time and effort learning and contibuting to the basic information about immune responses— and their ultimate relationship to the phenomenon of graft rejection and other host reactions against foreign tissue. The entire field expanded, meshing perhaps more than any other at the time the life sciences and their potential usefulness in patient care.

The numbers of young scientists and clinicians interested in these biologies increased quickly, commensurate with the emerging knowledge. Surgeons beginning their academic careers discovered they could provide scientists with subjects to investigate that were directly relevant to clinical transplantation, as well as the manual skills necessary to transplant organs not only between dogs but between the increasingly available inbred strains of small laboratory animals. As these technically demanding models became established, data arising from test tube experiments or from skin-graft behavior were translated into the context of vascularized organ allografts.

Despite the continuing postwar austerity in Britain, Medawar attracted to his laboratory a coterie of young investigators from several countries and many backgrounds. All were fascinated by the new biology of transplantation and enthused about the clinical findings emanating from Paris and Boston. During the same period Michael Woodruff and others in the United Kingdom, Jean Hamburger and associates in France, and Joseph Murray, David Hume, and colleagues in the United States began to organize their own groups. Moving around North America and Britain, throughout Europe, and from Australia, these early research fellows worked with and became close to the founders of the field. The lifelong friendships and collaborations that ensued contributed to the spirit and enjoyment of scientific inquiry. These talented individuals later returned to their own countries and universities to found their own units and push forward relevant investigations.

Conditions in many research facilities at that time were, by current standards, relatively primitive. Dogs from the pound were the primary experimental subjects in most surgical laboratories. Anesthesia was usually limited to open-drop ether or other flammable agents. Unwieldy surgical instruments made it difficult to perform delicate maneuvers such as anastomosing small vessels. Sutures of cotton or silk had to be threaded into needles, which in turn were used repeatedly after being sharpened on a stone. Drugs for the animals, particularly antibiotics, were often in short supply. Larger pieces of equipment were castoffs from a hospital. Skin grafts were the primary object of study in small animals; microsurgical techniques and the possibilities of organ grafting did not come into general use until later. Despite such hurdles, the fervor and ingenuity of the young surgeons and their mentors produced definitive original work in transplantation, the findings of which often translated directly to the care of their patients.

One terrifying example of the drawbacks of using worn-out hospital equipment occurred in the surgical laboratory I later joined. It was situated in a Harvard Medical School building across the street from the Brigham. By the early 1960s Murray and his colleagues had grafted kidneys in hundreds of dogs. The standard means of determining whether a renal transplant was functioning was to perform an intravenous pyelogram on the recipient—a test in which a radiopaque dye, injected intravenously, would be excreted by a working kidney. Dye from the functioning organ could be visualized by sequential x-rays. An old x-ray machine, temperamental and only intermittently functional, was available for these studies. While using it one day, a young staff surgeon working in the laboratory suddenly collapsed, pulseless. He had received an electrical shock from the unit that ran through his body to the floor. The highly experienced surgical technician desperately called the hospital for help. He and the research fellows opened the physician's chest with the dog instruments and began to massage his heart. Staff surgeons and anesthesiologists quickly gathered and removed him to the small intensive care unit, where his heart was restarted. For days he lay in a coma so deep that a diagnosis of brain death was considered. Miraculously, however, he gradually revived and went on to a distinguished surgical career. The charred hole in the sole of one of his shoes and a burned patch of linoleum on the laboratory floor attested to the severity of the electrical discharge. The machine still sat in a corner of the room when I arrived a few years later.

The time spent in research was fundamental, both intellectually and socially, to the training of these future academic leaders. A young doctor, already having several years of surgical or medical training behind him, was provided the opportunity to think, read, create, and live in other countries—to interact with unusual personalities, enjoy new cultures, and sample different social mores. At the end of his eighteen-month tenure in Boston, for instance, Roy Calne and his family went on a prolonged camping trip throughout North America, discovering much about the continent and its peoples. Stimulated by this early experience, Calne has remained one of the most recognized international forces in the field. Guy Alexandre, a Belgian who was one of Murray's original research fellows and a major later contributor to clinical transplantation, summed up his own experience: "Looking back at this period of my life, I must confess that it was . . . the most enjoyable and the most exciting." Paul Russell was Medawar's first American fellow and later became a highly regarded leader in transplantation. Soon after Russell arrived in London, Medawar warned him that although conversation and dialogue within his research group were often stimulating, politics were not to be mentioned. "This remark, I later learned, was important as a number of the more distinguished members of the department were active in the British Communist Party and Peter was justifiably worried that a naive, young American surgeon, fresh from a country torn by 'McCarthyism' might make the lively and pleasant conversation at tea time into a free for all. As it happened, I was captivated . . . and generally found my new world completely absorbing."[23] The majority of individuals who transferred themselves and their families across continents, oceans, and hemispheres agreed thoroughly. Over the years this ongoing interchange has broadened with the addition of individuals from Asia who work in increasing numbers in Western laboratories.

On a more personal note, as a resident surgeon I had become increasingly interested in the mechanisms of graft rejection and the other poorly understood phenomena experienced by my transplant patients. I therefore took a prolonged research fellowship with James Gowans at Oxford University during the late 1960s and early 1970s. He and his associates had recently described the recirculation of lymphocytes and their immune capabilities, and they were becoming increasingly interested in the role of these cells in transplantation. I immersed myself in my projects on skin and organ transplants in rats, becoming conversant in the subject but also learning to understand the thinking of basic scientists about interpreting data and designing experiments to answer specific questions. I found out how difficult it is to wrest secrets from Nature! Living in England, savoring its history and its beauties, being associated with an ancient university, and making new friends in a variety of academic disciplines, provided me with exceptional opportunities. Traveling in Europe with my family further embellished my enthusiasms. They have lasted a lifetime.

Many of these laboratory experiences were possible because of the increasing availability of government-sponsored funding after World War II. In Canada, Britain, and various European countries, medical research councils were vital sources of support for scientists. In the United States, government and universities initiated a relationship in the second half of the nineteenth century to develop agricultural research; for many years this remained the only sustained federally sponsored effort. Between the world wars, practitioners carried out most clinically related biologic investigations on a part-time basis, funded by private sources or maintaining their laboratories out of pocket. After 1945, strategies were devised to encourage basic research in universities via a stable source of federal funds, and to concentrate industrial energies on practical applications of the findings. The success of this scheme made the United States preeminent in science. It attracted scientists from both Eastern and Western Europe, as well as taking advantage of the "brain drain" from postwar Britain. The perceived national humiliation engendered by the Russian launching of Sputnik on October 4, 1957, followed by the explosion of America's first rocket on its pad, galvanized scientific development as a U.S. priority. The subsequent advances in nuclear physics and associated technologies are noteworthy examples of the accelerating concentration in the physical sciences.

Medicine and its biologies also thrived under the aegis of the National Institutes of Health (NIH), with emphasis shifting from control of infections to the treatment of cancer, heart disease, and chronic illness. The cold war provided further impetus during the 1950s, with total federal expenditure for medical research soaring from its starting point of $18 million; by 1960 the NIH budget alone had reached $400 million. Private agencies also joined the effort. The philanthropist Mary Lasker, for instance, organized the American Cancer Society, then went on to lobby Congress for ever-increasing funds, believing "that the doctors and research scientists were too accustomed to thinking small."[24] Introduction of the new polio vaccine overwhelmingly relieved public anxiety and encouraged additional spending for studies of human disease. President Richard Nixon increased funding further, promising a cure for cancer within a decade. Similarly, as transplantation captured the public interest, it too gained financial backing. As a result, increasing numbers of young medical scientists entered the new specialty, with their innovative ideas competing with one another for research funding through grants, for clinical activity, and for improved results. Growth of the field accelerated.

No matter how successful an enterprise may be, and regardless of the eager efforts of the participants, an occasional dark side may emerge. It can be fueled by a variety of internal and external pressures to produce, to publish, and to gain fame. One of the most challenging aspects of the advancement of science (more highly developed, perhaps, than in many other areas of human endeavor) is the stringent and ongoing process of review by knowledgeable peers, which can lead to constructive criticism of methods, repetition of experiments, and open debate about results and interpretations. Research findings are presented at conferences and reports are critically examined both before and after publication. The situation in clinical medicine is similar, as preliminary explorations into a new therapy or technique are made by a single investigator or team, repeated in additional units, then analyzed in multicenter or multinational trials if appropriate. The answer that ultimately emerges determines whether the concept, the methods, and the results are acceptable to colleagues and other experts, and whether they will be permitted or denied for public use by professional or governing agencies.

The vast majority of people, regardless of background, avocation, or profession, are honest. But occasional overenthusiasts—stretchers of the truth, those who interpret their results a bit too liberally, or those perpetuating real fabrications—periodically surface. Although his comments could probably be used for many groups, Peter Medawar aptly described the various types of individuals who enter science: "Scientists are people with very dissimilar temperaments doing very different things in very different ways. Among scientists are collectors, classifiers and compulsive tidiers-up; many are detectives by temperament and many are explorers. Some are artists and others are artisans. There are poet-scientists and philosopher-scientists and even a few mystics." He modified this assessment later: "If only I had thought to add . . . 'and just a few odd crooks.' "[25]

Like persons in other highly visible fields, individuals working in laboratories are intelligent, ambitious, often aggressive, sometimes driven, desirous and acquisitive of recognition for their labors and talents, and always interested in funding, promotion, tenure, and other academic perquisites. As a result, preliminary data may be inadvertently (or, rarely, purposely) overemphasized. "As is true in all rapidly moving, competitive and important areas of research, the enormous potential payoff for definitive therapies combined with forces such as competition for scientific eminence and diminished federal support for biomedical research has inadvertently opened the doors a bit to touches of exaggeration, scientific self-delusion and possibly even self-promotion. Some . . . papers, manuscripts and funding applications have in the past sent and at times still send overstated messages of success . . . even in the obvious absence of convincing evidence."[26] Although such transgressions have been few, transplantation has been no exception.

Programs in both clinical and experimental transplantation developed rapidly in the 1970s, with promise of major academic rewards for discovery and innovation. More organs were grafted successfully, intriguing adjunctive treatments were tested, and the possibilities of biological means to increase graft survival were promising. The most obvious of these strategies was suppression of host immunity so that the organ would be accepted, or at least tolerated. An alternative and more theoretical plan was to alter the allografted tissue itself in order to fool the body's defenses into considering the tissue as "self" and not reacting against it. Although a few early investigators had introduced this concept, it had achieved little practical success.

Then a new figure emerged. Working at Stanford, a young physician named William Summerlin was faced with the problem of finding adequate coverage for the denuded body surfaces of burned patients. The use of pig skin as a biological dressing was in vogue. Techniques to culture skin were being explored in nearby laboratories. Reasoning that such an approach might benefit graft survival, Summerlin placed a piece of incubated human skin on a burned patient. The allograft did not appear to reject. Judging that this observation, contrary to all expectations about the behavior of skin grafts, might have been the result of the initial treatment of the graft, he then cultured bits of skin for several weeks and placed them on four normal nonimmunosuppressed volunteers. Again, rejection apparently did not occur.[27] Because of the increasing excitement produced by these findings, the renowned immunologist Robert Good invited the investigator to join his laboratory, first at the University of Minnesota, then at the Sloan-Kettering Institute in New York. By 1973 Summerlin had expanded his culture model to skin grafts transplanted between the same or different species, adrenal-gland grafts in mice, and corneas in rabbits.

News of the supposed success of this novel strategy—the reduction of immunogenicity of tissue to be grafted by incubation in a nutrient medium for days or weeks—spread quickly throughout the transplant community and the press, embellished by the imprimatur of Good and his institution. Others, enthused by the possibilities, initiated similar experiments. However, their consistent failure to reproduce Summerlin's results caused increasing frustration. Several investigators, including one of Medawar's principal collaborators, Leslie Brent, repeatedly requested methodological details. As no answers were forthcoming, in despair Brent finally sent Good all his one-way correspondence to Summerlin.

Later in the year, having reported at a national conference the excellent results of cultured human corneas transplanted into rabbit eyes,

Summerlin was invited to show a rabbit recipient directly to the board of scientific consultants of the Sloan-Kettering, a group that included, among other prominent figures, Peter Medawar himself. Medawar wryly relates the experience: "Through a perfectly transparent eye the rabbit looked at the Board with a candid and unwavering gaze of which only a rabbit with an absolutely clear conscience is capable." Suspicion increased among Summerlin's coworkers, as well as in Good himself. After the NIH, unconvinced by the data, had turned down his grant application, Good asked the investigator to show him the white mice that bore the allegedly successful cultured skin allografts from black donors. Desperate, Summerlin augmented the graft color with a felt-tipped pen, a ploy quickly detected. Suspension and disgrace followed. His mentor and his institution were tainted as well, although Good's reputation recovered as the excellence of his research continued. Summerlin was lost to view. Medawar summarized the episode: "As it is, I am afraid no great truth about scientific behavior is to be learned from the Summerlin affair except that it takes all sorts to make a world." He generously suggested that the initial mouse finding might even have been correct, as many different strains including hybrids look the same and could have been mixed up in the laboratory.[28]

Although usually unimportant in the overall picture, scientific fraud is considered harshly by colleagues who may base their own hypotheses and experiments on erroneous or deceptive data. Reputations, new projects, and career advancement may all depend on the results. Indeed, the entire creative process in science is a continuum. Interesting, ongoing investigations will encourage the individual scientist toward further work, modification, or actual discard. If the results of the background experiments are fallacious, time, effort, and money can all be wasted.

In the Summerlin case, other investigators slowly reexamined the concept of reducing graft allogenicity by culturing endocrine tissues, particularly pancreatic islets and thyroid. They discovered that the survival time of the tissues, after placement on foreign hosts, could actually be increased in mice. At about the same time, prolongation of endocrine grafts from radiated donors revitalized an older theory that donor white cells, retained in and transferred with the transplanted graft, could trigger subsequent host alloresponsiveness to a greater degree than the actual graft tissue itself. It was concluded that culture could, in fact, inactivate or destroy these cells.[29] The strategy of altering the immunogenicity of the organ to be transplanted by this method or by actual donor manipulation, although not yet useful clinically, has stimulated a great deal of subsequent basic research, particularly on T-lymphocyte activation by donor antigens. In the long run, the Summerlin interlude, painful as it was, was not a waste.

5

Peter Medawar and
Transplantation Biology

IT IS DIFFICULT IN RETROSPECT, EVEN FOR THOSE
with a long-standing interest in the subject, to recall how rudimentary
was the understanding of host immune responses against allografted
tissues at midcentury. Only with ever-increasing numbers of wounded
in World War II did it become obvious that theoretical knowledge of
skin-graft behavior needed to be replaced with practical means to cover
denuded body areas. Because of his experience with a badly burned
airman, Peter Medawar (then working in Howard Florey's laboratory)
embarked on a series of studies that were to transform this relatively
obscure subject into a notable new field of scientific endeavor. Too tall
to serve in the Army, Medawar was directed by the recruiting board to
turn toward "service to the military establishment," particularly the
treatment of burns.[1]

His involvement in the subject crystallized one summer afternoon
in 1940 when he, his wife, and their oldest child were sitting outside
their house in Oxford. A British bomber flew low over their heads and
crashed into a nearby garden. One of the airmen sustained third-
degree burns that were ultimately fatal. Taken to a nearby hospital, the
patient endured several weeks of local burn care, removal of areas of
dead skin, and minimal grafting before dying of infection. Anything
more than topical treatment was relatively undeveloped at the time,
and the burned areas were too large for adequate grafting. The frustrated hospital physician caring for the patient asked Medawar for
help, exhorting the young scientist to "lay aside [his] intellectual pursuits and take a serious interest in real life."[2] Establishing to his own

satisfaction that autografts of the individual's own skin—but not the skin of others—would heal permanently, Medawar began to consider the body's remarkable ability to discriminate between its own and foreign tissues.

He was sent by the Medical Research Council to a burn unit in Glasgow to work with a plastic surgeon, Thomas Gibson. They were soon faced with a patient, Mrs. McK, who had been severely burned when she fell against her gas fire during a seizure. After covering the open areas with skin from both the patient and her brother, the investigators took serial biopsies of the grafts. Using techniques learned from Florey, they prepared and stained the tissues for examination under the microscope. Within a few days, they noted that increasing numbers of leukocytes infiltrated the apparently healing fraternal graft beds. In a few more days, the previously healthy-appearing skin had thickened, ulcerated, and become a scab. The autografts, in contrast, continued to appear normal without signs of inflammatory cellular activity. As recognized years before by Emile Holman, J. B. Brown, and others, and as suggested by his colleague Gibson, Medawar confirmed that a second set of allografts from the brother had undergone accelerated rejection. They had evoked an even more intense inflammatory response than the primary grafts, implying that the host could recall the initial stimulus and respond to it more rapidly than previously. In their subsequent report, the investigators postulated that "the mechanism by which foreign skin is eliminated belongs to the general category of actively acquired immune reactions."[3]

Returning to Oxford, Medawar immediately undertook comparable experiments in a large series of rabbits, substantiating and amplifying the clinical findings.[4] His recognition that genetic variations between donor and host evoked differential tissue responses, and Peter Gorer's data on histocompatibility genes and variations in the tempo of tumor rejection in mice of different strains, provided further evidence for the involvement of host immunological mechanisms in the behavior of grafts.

As Medawar's observations on the rejection of skin allografts unfolded, a few surgical investigators were also starting to define the progressive and irreversible events experienced by vascularized kidney grafts, a subject that had remained in virtual eclipse since the work of Alexis Carrel and others decades before. Describing the microscopic changes in transplanted kidney allografts in dogs, William Dempster noted that his 1951 studies were the first to be published since a single report on the subject in 1934. Examining Lawler's clinical experience in detail, Dempster reviewed what was already known, confirming that most allografts experience "complete disintegration at various time intervals."[5] Theorizing on why foreign grafts failed, he enumerated inadequate host nutrients as postulated by Ehrlich, natural immunity based on genetic incompatibility between donor and recipient as described by Gorer, local reaction to destructive cell products in the kidney as suggested by Loeb, and actively acquired immunity as discussed by Medawar.

At about the same time in Denmark, a newly graduated doctor named Morten Simonsen was examining the role of systemic host responses in acute rejection of organ grafts. During his internship in a country hospital in Jutland, Simonsen initiated experiments designed ultimately to provide a new kidney for patients dying with renal failure. Conditions were primitive. He used his own salary to buy the experimental animals. "The noisy dogs had to be installed in the yard of a nearby municipal workhouse, and the inmates were not supposed to mind." Unaware of Medawar's work, he independently arrived at the theory of acquired immunity in a convincing series of studies that included the accelerated rejection of a second kidney from the original donor. He admitted that such concepts were not universally accepted, particularly in the United States, apparently because of the prolific work of Loeb, whose "system of ideas is impenetrably metaphysical to most investigators."[6]

The increasing perception that skin grafts behaved in a manner different from vascularized organ grafts posed additional questions. An unexpected discrepancy in host responsiveness to the various tissues caused Medawar himself to note later that "kidney grafting rescued us from the tyranny of the skin graft." Immunosuppression, when it became available, was not only relatively ineffectual in prolonging the survival of skin allografts, but even autografts healed slowly after placement because of the delay in reestablishment of their blood supply. Organ grafts, in contrast, were without blood flow only as long as it took the surgeon to remove them from the donor and join their vessels to those of the recipient. "Skin ... grafts invariably are subject to severe traumatic inflammation associated with primary healing and the establishment of a circulation."[7] In fact, the important differences in behavior between skin and organs turned out to be more complex than originally thought and are still not completely understood.

Many in the field believed increasingly that rejection represented a specific lymphocyte-mediated immunological event evoked by the recipient to destroy selectively the transplanted foreign tissue. Yet some researchers still felt that the immunological basis of graft destruction was hardly proven, much less controllable. One eminent New York plastic surgeon, for instance, found "no evidence [that Medawar's] immunization theory should apply to man," concluding that the changes described in skin grafts were specific to rabbits, which are particularly disposed to develop "anaphylactic inflammation." At the same time he expressed a fear pervasive during the cold war era of the 1950s by poignantly emphasizing the increasing "urgency of developing skin banks . . . In the case of atomic attacks upon our cities, these banks could serve in emergency use."[8]

Despite such doubts, investigators were considering strategies to temper the immune responses and prolong graft survival either by inhibiting host immunity directly or by reducing the antigenic character of the organ so that host cells would not respond to it. Some devised means to diminish the activity of the large mass of immunologically active leukocytes present throughout the body of the recipient animal by using vital dyes, metabolic poisons, total-body x-radiation, or the new corticosteroid drugs. Others designed experiments to exploit the protective effects of some antibodies on foreign grafts, as suggested by Gorer and some of his colleagues. Still others, until the Summerlin affair decreased their enthusiasm, attempted to reduce the immunogenicity of tissue grafts by culture alone or with host plasma. A few groups tried to make the kidneys less reactive to host attack by freezing, heating, or immersing them in chemicals. Alternative approaches included cold storage, perfusion with oxygenated substances, and administration of anti-inflammatory agents "to protect the kidney from immune reactions."[9] Success was infrequent.

In contrast to this plethora of nonspecific treatments, Peter Medwar, his first research fellow and close colleague Rupert Billingham, and their new graduate student Leslie Brent stirred the imaginations of

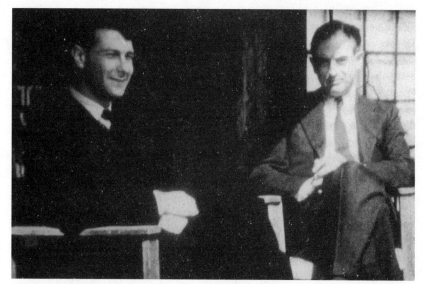

Figure 5.1 Leslie Brent and Sir Peter Medawar in the early 1950s (P. I. Terasaki, with permission)

many in the early 1950s with their innovative experiments on host tolerance (Figure 5.1). Tolerance is a state in which an animal or even a patient can be made selectively unresponsive to the antigens of a given graft, while the remainder of the immunological defense mechanisms remain intact. Few discoveries in science arise de novo, however, as potentially relevant findings of previous investigators take time to be uncovered. Tolerance was no exception. At the beginning of the twentieth century, for instance, biologists inoculated embryo toads and newts with frog cells, then later showed that the adults bore normally growing frog xenografts in their bodies. Rat tumor cells flourished in chick embryos, but could be destroyed by injection of spleen fragments from adult chickens.

More relevant clues arose to explain the concept. The ancient Greeks and Romans had recognized that the male offspring of cattle twins were normal but that the females were sterile. John Hunter called these "free-martin" cattle an "experiment of nature" when describing the observation to the Royal Society in 1779. In more modern times, the phenomenon was finally explained in answer to the concerns of cattle breeders. In Chicago before World War I, F. R. Lillie conjectured that when the twins were of different genders, the cow was invariably sterile because sex hormones had crossed from the male to the female twin via their fused placentas in the maternal uterus. R. D. Owen in Wisconsin reported that each member of a pair of free-martin cattle twins carried not only his or her own red blood cells in the circulation but also those of the nonidentical sibling.[10] The chimeras were mutually tolerant to each other's comfortably coexisting cells.

About the same time, Macfarlane Burnet and an Australian colleague, Frank Fenner, speculated in their book, *The Production of Antibodies*, on how animals could recognize their own tissues ("self") and not react against them while responding briskly to foreign ("nonself") stimuli.[11] They surmised that during fetal development higher organisms were endowed with an entire panoply of cells able to respond to every stimulus that might be encountered throughout life. After birth, however, all cells which could react against self proteins were eliminated by "clonal selection"; only those cells with the potential to respond against nonself proteins were retained. Tolerant subjects like the cattle twins, which had been exposed to each other's antigens during fetal life, could not tell the difference.

Evidence that such animals could accept the tissues of others was also mounting. In 1929 investigators at Stanford University had transplanted skin between newly hatched Rhode Island Red and Plymouth Rock chickens. In some cases, patches of different-colored feathers grew normally on their new hosts. However, the findings were wrongly interpreted as reflecting a constitutional similarity between the two breeds. Grafting the immunologically innocent chick at the time of hatching produced occasional successes. No transplants survived on older birds with a more mature immune system.[12]

After World War II several important papers in Russian (with German summaries) came from an eminent Czechoslovakian immunologist, Milan Hašek. These revealed that surgically joined parabiotic chick and chick, or chick and duck, embryos whose circulations had united at the point of juncture, not only became red cell chimeras but also accepted each other's skin grafts. In the repressive atmosphere of Eastern Europe at the time, the imaginative scientist was forced to explain his observations in a manner acceptable to the highly political and powerful Lysenko school of biology. This scientific propagandist and his party-approved followers had radicalized and incorporated into prevailing Communist dogma the belief of the eminent early-nineteenth-century biologist Jean-Baptiste de Lamarck that environmental influences are responsible for genetic changes in new generations of an organism. Because of Lysenko's revisionist theories, Medawar later condemned him as "an evil genius . . . who single-handedly arrested the teaching and practice in Russia of . . . genetics and brought about the disgrace of its principal practitioners."[13] These included Hašek, whose career was destroyed after the Russian invasion of Prague, a political catastrophe that led to his eventual suicide. Two groups in Britain soon confirmed Hašek's concept, however, by demonstrating that "natural tolerance" could exist in humans. One cited an example occurring in a pair of nonidentical twins with both group A and group O red cells in their circulation, the other described brother and sister twins who were red cell chimeras and accepted each other's skin grafts.

Medawar synthesized these rather diffuse data into controlled and pertinent experiments after an initially unexpected finding. In 1947, relaxing over drinks during a microbiological congress in Stockholm, he and a Scottish geneticist, H. P. Donald, discussed the difficulties in distinguishing between identical and fraternal cattle twins. "In the rather spacious and expansive way that one is tempted to adopt at international congresses," Medawar stated dogmatically, "my dear fellow—in principle the solution is extremely easy: just exchange skin grafts between the twins and see how long they last. If they last indefinitely, you can be sure these are identical twins, but if they are thrown off after a week or two you can classify them with equal certainty as fraternal twins."[14] In answer to Donald's later acceptance of Medawar's rather airy statement "that I should be happy to demonstrate the technique of grafting to his veterinary staff," Medawar and Billingham drove to a farm forty miles away to perform the appropriate experiments. To their surprise, all the cattle twins, identical or not, accepted each other's grafts—a striking exception to the acknowledged doctrine regarding skin graft behavior. When the same results were obtained after repeating the study, the researchers reasoned that the tolerance of the cattle to each other's skin must lie in the comingling of the circulation of the twins before birth via their fused placentas.

Supported by their reading of Burnet and Fenner's book, which referenced the work of Lillie and Owen, the two investigators, now joined by Leslie Brent, tried to duplicate this unexpected and puzzling observation in laboratory animals. After they failed to inject adult cells intravenously into chick embryos, a colleague drew their attention to Hašek's parabiosis experiments. The technique worked, and soon the scientists had produced chimeric chickens bearing each other's skin and feathers.

A critical part of their success was that the scientists could obtain fine hypodermic needles to inject newborn mice, now their experimental model. The growing availability of various genetically pure strains of inbred mice created by many generations of brother-sister matings also provided the opportunity to undertake comparable well-controlled experiments. Finally, by 1953, Billingham, Brent, and Medawar were able to describe adult mice, injected with foreign spleen cells as newborns or even as fetuses, with healthy donor-specific skin allografts.[15] Skin from third-party animals was rejected quickly. Studies on "acquired immunological tolerance" were repeated by other investigators and soon induced in other species. The three investigators were soon designated the Holy Trinity by their biblically literate colleagues; the Holy Grail of tolerance was an expression of Medawar's oft-stated enthusiasm for Wagnerian opera. His receipt with Burnet of the 1960 Nobel Prize for Medicine and Physiology added to the enduring luster of acquired immunological tolerance.

Interest in tolerance—"a central failure" of host immunity and a manifestation of Burnet's clonal selection theory—has increased substantially over the years. Laboratory experiments potentially more clinically applicable were undertaken in the late 1960s with the introduction of microsurgical techniques to transplant whole organs such as heart, kidney, and liver between inbred strains of rats and even mice. Indeed, over time, every new immunosuppressive modality and concept has been compared to the state of tolerance. The few successful clinical examples have been examined and reexamined, and ever-broadening experimental variations on the theme considered. The majority of current clinician-investigators feel that the model of neonatal tolerance in mice described almost a half century ago remains the standard against which all other immunological manipulation must be measured. Indeed, the phenomenon continues to serve as a beacon of achievement, as yet unobtained, for the entire field.

Medawar's accurate definitions of acute rejection, the second-set response, and immunological tolerance; his clarity of observation and ability to organize data into a comprehensive whole; and his speaking and teaching talents made him a central figure in the new science of transplantation biology. His experiments were so incisive that they immediately challenged other investigators to repeat and amplify them, and they did much to break down the barriers between basic scientists and clinicians involved in the transplantation of patients. Medawar suggested that "the scientific method," the highly publicized tool of the researcher, does not exist. In reality, investigators must experience false hypotheses and dead ends before a phenomenon such as the burned airman can galvanize a line of research. In conjecturing why Medawar was so influential, one analyst noted that experiments in tissue transplantation had flagged: "Much work was forgotten and . . . Medawar's studies . . . were received as 'new' discoveries." The field needed "new data, new technologies and, above all a new point of view to rekindle . . . interest."[16] During the years that followed, the subject provoked an outpouring of productive effort from laboratories in Britain, Europe, North America, and Australia to examine, define, and elaborate the role of host immunity against transplanted tissues.

In considering Medawar's contributions, Rupert Billingham queried eloquently whether science is a highly programmed and logical process open to a relatively few imaginative and creative individuals, or whether it develops by chance, in unpredictable fits and starts (Figure 5.2). Transplantation, he suggested, is an excellent example of parallel and not mutually exclusive forces, to which investigators in basic biology and scientifically oriented physicians and surgeons contribute equally while seeking answers relevant to their patients. Emphasizing that progress and dissemination of new ideas stem from the ability to think clearly and communicate well, Billingham praised his colleague's remarkable ability to express and translate his findings in his lectures. While the experiments Medawar described in one presentation, for example, had often arisen by serendipity, the sequence of events he portrayed bore no relation to their actual chronology; false starts were

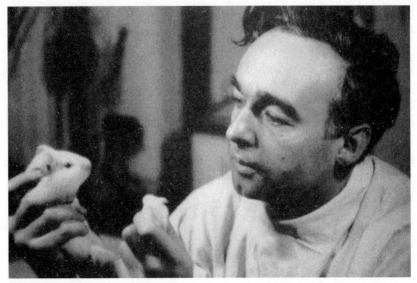

Figure 5.2 Rupert Billingham in the early 1950s (P. I. Terasaki, with permission)

ignored, some of the studies had been carried out for different reasons, and "luck" was not a factor. His arguments were persuasive and logical, his hypotheses unassailable, his reasoning impeccable. Members of the audience, despite their diverse backgrounds, sat hypnotized. It never occurred to anyone that the smoothly flowing story represented a beautifully crafted reinterpretation of the true history of the project, "despite the meticulous honesty with which the observations were treated."[17] For Medawar, science was a creative and deductive art form from which came ideas for experiments to prove or disprove theories and concepts. Because of his enduring stature and critical contributions, he has remained the seminal figure in the development of transplantation biology.

The use of experimental animals has allowed the definition of normal physiological states and the understanding of abnormal ones, the testing of pharmacological agents, and the creation of surgical procedures to correct a variety of developmental or pathological abnormalities. New medications can rarely be administered to humans before preclinical trials are completed, analyzed, and accepted. Gastrointestinal,

urological, and vascular operations, cardiac and pulmonary procedures, joint replacements, and neurosurgical innovations have all been
developed in animal models—especially dogs, pigs, and monkeys.
Clinical transplantation of abdominal or thoracic organs and the gen-
esis of immunosuppression have become realities because of animal
availability. For highly controlled basic studies, inbred strains of rats
and mice are necessary; these are the species responsible for many
advances in immunology and transplant biology. More recent developments in molecular biology and genetics would have been impossible without animal cells. For these reasons a discussion of the use of
animals, and the continuing opposition to it, needs to be included in
this account of the evolution of transplantation.

Animal experimentation has roots in the ancient world, as described by early scholars including Herodotus, the medical historian,
and Erasistratus, the great Alexandrian anatomist. Galen made many
of his anatomical observations in animals. By the sixteenth and seventeenth centuries, leading European scientific figures were performing
occasional studies on living animals.[18] The new field of experimental
biology arose in France and Germany early in the nineteenth century
and yielded significant discoveries about the behavior of organs and
organ systems. These advances began to open opportunities for students hoping for scientific careers in university settings, where active
professors were becoming increasingly available.

One of these in particular, the influential French physiologist
François Magendie, used animal subjects to produce substantial new
knowledge, particularly about the function of the spinal cord. At the
same time, his practices evoked substantial criticism from his peers because of his public demonstrations of cruel operative techniques. Physiological studies became more common after the introduction of anesthesia, as pain could be controlled and related variables diminished. For
most Continental investigators of the time, vivisection became a means
to understand both normal bodily functions and dysfunctions based
on pathological conditions, as well as to define and answer questions
regarding mechanisms of disease. Claude Bernard, for instance, the
greatest physiologist of late-nineteenth-century France, produced an
abundance of knowledge about the workings of the gastrointestinal
tract (Figure 5.3).

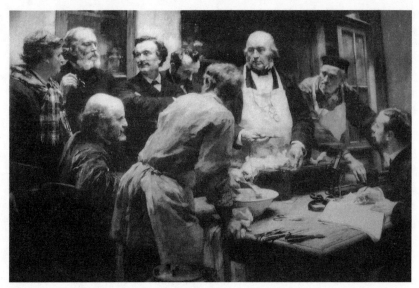

Figure 5.3 The French physiologist Claude Bernard performing an experiment (Novartis, with permission)

In contrast, experimental physiology remained a relatively minor subject in Britain. Much of the medical establishment was loath to accept the importance of laboratory research over the traditionally strong clinical areas of physical diagnosis and human anatomy. In 1870, however, the field suddenly changed. Investigators making basic contributions to the new subject started major research schools. The Royal Colleges of Surgeons demanded more specialized knowledge about the normal behavior and function of the body from those taking their qualifying examinations. Medical schools opened their own laboratories and recruited physiologists to run them. As a result, experiments on living animals rose sharply, along with appropriate controls and restrictions. Much of the interest accrued from the publication in 1873 of *The Handbook for the Physiological Laboratory*, which described in detail standard experiments on animals. Highly regarded by the scientific establishment, this widely available book triggered a storm among both antivivisectionists and individual physicians threatened by the new influences in medical education.

The abuse of animals, including their use in investigations in the life sciences, has been a sensitive and emotional topic for centuries. Particularly in Britain, voices were raised consistently against accepted cruelties. In the eighteenth and early nineteenth centuries, for instance—an age of bull baiting, dog and cock fighting, inadequate care of animals in husbandry and as beasts of burden, and rare instances of animal experimentation—distinguished artists and writers decried the practices, sometimes on humanitarian grounds, sometimes from an antiscience stance. William Hogarth graphically portrayed common examples of maltreatment in London in his painting *Four Stages of Cruelty*, hoping to correct "the barbarous treatment of animals, the very sight of which renders the streets of our metropolis so distressing to every feeling mind." Mary Shelley noted disparagingly that Victor Frankenstein had "tortured the living animal to animate the lifeless clay" as a step toward creating his monster.[19]

The poet Alexander Pope and the essayist Joseph Addison added their voices to the chorus. Samuel Johnson emoted against the use of animals in science, writing in remarkably current tones and presaging the increasingly powerful antivivisectionist movement a century later.

> Among the inferior professors of medical knowledge is a race of wretches, whose lives are only varied by varieties of cruelty . . . What is alleged in defense of these hateful practices everyone knows, but the truth is . . . knowledge . . . is very seldom attained. Experiments that have been tried are tried again . . . I know not that by living dissections any discovery has been made by which a single malady is more easily cured. And if knowledge of physiology has been somewhat increased, he surely buys knowledge dear . . . It is time that universal resentment should arise against these horrid operations, which tend to harden the heart, extinguish those sensations which give man confidence in man, and make physicians more dreadful than gout or stone.[20]

Reforming zeal and moral crusades on behalf of causes ranging from the political to the social and religious filled the second half of Queen Victoria's reign. This was the era of the original antislavery movement and the rise in humanism, evangelicalism, romantic poetry, and fiction. The uproar against Darwin's theories continued unabated. In addition to religious and moral disagreement with the perceived direction that science was taking, antagonism broadened toward the experimental use of animals. So even as public interest in the results of experimental physiology was growing, the antivivisectionist movement was evolving into a national and international force, gradually spreading from Britain to other European countries and to North America.[21] Hospitals that supported experimental medicine in nearby animal laboratories inflamed public antipathy and suspicions about human experimentation. Even the vaccinators and microbiologists did not escape notice. Koch's inoculation of animals evoked adverse comment. And Pasteur's work on rabies vaccine was derided, though many of the complainers were presumably dog lovers.

The British antivivisectionists gathered allies among writers and artists. Tracts, pamphlets, short stories, and magazine articles on the subject were common. In his novel *Heart and Science* (1883), Wilkie Collins described the suicide of an experimentalist after his scientific objectives had been thwarted by two antivivisectionist physicians. In *A Physiologist's Wife* (1890), Sir Arthur Conan Doyle portrayed a cold and overdirected animal experimenter who considered the workings of the lachrymal glands as his wife wept on his shoulder.

Two books especially whetted public suspicion of science, scientists, and vivisectors: Robert Louis Stevenson's *Dr. Jekyll and Mr. Hyde* (1883) and H. G. Wells's *Island of Dr. Moreau* (1896). The protagonists were not portrayed handsomely in either of these popular stories, written during a time of intense debate between those celebrating the advances of medical science and those highly suspicious of its aims and methods. Stevenson described the associations of the nefarious Jekyll with dissection and experimentation. Although Wells was a vocal proponent of science and author of a popular textbook of biology, he characterized Moreau as a dark and driven torturer aiming to humanize his animal victims by the transplantation and reconstruction of body parts. "You forget all that a skilled vivisector can do with living things ... It is a possible thing to transplant tissue from one part of an animal to another, or for one animal to another, to alter the chemical reactions and methods of growth, to modify the articulations of its limbs, and indeed to change it in its most intimate structure."[22] The book was not only a parody of Darwinian selection but also an uncomfortably close description of the methods of renowned physiologists. An entire genre of Victorian painters led by Sir Edwin Landseer fueled the fires further by depicting animals with sentimental human qualities.

Many in the United States also expressed their feelings on the subject. In 1866 the American Society for the Prevention of Cruelty to Animals was established in New York by individuals distressed at the maltreatment of horses. The movement spread, encouraged by its success abroad and stimulated by the increasing use of animals in research in the new life sciences and in medical education. In Massachusetts, public hearings on the subject captured so much attention that several distinguished scientists and physicians attended to support the aims of the experimentalists. President Charles William Eliot of Harvard argued forcefully about academic freedom and education and debated against his antivivisectionist opponent who "said he was here to represent the dumb animals. I should like to be permitted to represent here some millions of dumb human beings . . . It is for them that the scientific biologists are at work. It is to save them and their children from disease and death that the gentlemen who have testified before you are at work."[23]

Such arguments continued unabated in the new century, with much of the public and most scientists and academically oriented physicians taking one side, and a vocal minority of reformers and private practitioners taking the other. The antipathy toward animal experimentation began to interfere with advances in medical treatment. The innovative technique of lumbar puncture to diagnose meningitis in children, trials with antisera in rabbits to develop diagnostic tests for syphilis, and the tuberculin test to assess prior exposure to tuberculosis, all produced intense discussions. Even Alexis Carrel became a primary target of the antivivisectionists. The press only inflamed passions. An article in the *Washington Post* in December 1913 opened with the startling headline "Doctors of Death," followed by equally emotive section headings: "Humans Murdered by Vivisection, speakers claim / Called victims of poison / English physician bitterly assails injections of serums / Girls and little children inoculated with germs of loathsome diseases in the name of science / Practices like Spanish Inquisition."[24] In this atmosphere, rational debate was difficult.

The majority of biological scientists were and are seriously concerned with animal welfare and make sure that those in their laboratories act responsibly toward their charges. Yet irregularities have undoubtedly arisen. While organized medicine at the turn of the century stressed advances in medical science and prepared guidelines for animal use, not until 1966 were minimal standards formulated in the United States, with subsequent regulations from the NIH and other federal bodies becoming progressively more stringent. In Britain, Germany, and other European countries, the restrictions are even more severe; laboratory licenses are difficult to obtain. But painful instances arise in which activists liberate animals from laboratories, destroy results of investigations, break equipment, and burn buildings. Lives of research workers have been threatened, letter bombs and car bombs have caused injury, homes have been vandalized.

In spite of these ongoing differences, the basic and applied sciences have improved the lot of not only ill patients but of animals as well, with significant advances in veterinary medicine and attention to comfort and quality of life. While thoughtful individuals continue to hope that biological knowledge can be gained without the use of animals, the prospect seems unlikely in the foreseeable future.

Some advances have been made. The cosmetics industry, for instance, no longer uses rabbits to test its products. Because of public pressure, the dog has been largely replaced by the pig or sheep for large-animal experiments. The higher primates are used less frequently as subjects of investigation. Ethical questions, particularly surrounding the risks to nonhuman primates in xenotransplantation, and in AIDS and other viral research, continue to be discussed and refined, not only by those directly involved but in public forums as well.[25] Still, few fields in medical biology could progress without animal experimentation. The development of organ transplantation is an obvious example.

6

Innovation and the
Struggle for Legitimacy

THE 1960S AND EARLY 1970S WERE YEARS OF TU-
mult. In Britain disquiet and anger emanated from the oil crisis, high
levels of unemployment, and police intolerance. After years of national disputes involving Algeria and other social ills, ten million
French workers struck in March 1968 for better working conditions
and higher wages. The United States endured a series of political assassinations, fears of nuclear war, sporadic riots among the inner-city
poor, and the national agony of the Vietnam War. The disgrace of
Watergate forced the President from office. Events influencing daily
life seemed out of control.

Hospitals and laboratories were hardly immune to the pressures,
although the sick continued to be cared for and science continued to be
pursued. Teaching hospitals were particularly affected. With the draft
mandating that all physicians up to 35 years of age must enter the
military, the incessant coming and going of residents and speciality
fellows challenged the continuity of training programs and altered
individual career plans. Some young doctors served in military hospitals in the United States; many went to Vietnam. Others were assigned
as research workers to various military facilities or to the National
Institutes of Health, to investigate topics relevant to the war effort.
Interested individuals who had finished their service commitment pursued transplant-related research in laboratories in Europe, Australia,
and North America before returning to clinical responsibilities. I was
one of those.

The turmoil of the period that encouraged unorthodox or

iconoclastic ways of thinking about society and its aims also produced a series of innovations in transplantation, despite the persistent skepticism of many outside the field. Thomas Starzl summarized a philosophy that seems particularly relevant to this dynamic and uncertain era. "Progress consists of a series of great and small revolutions against authority. A great advance necessitates the overthrow of an established dogma, and when that occurs the advance itself becomes the new dogma to which advocates flock. It is natural for these disciples to become protectors instead of improvers of the status quo, guardians of the past instead of seekers of the future."[1] In this fast-moving discipline, however, the "improvers" continued to drive the "protectors." Stimulated perhaps by the overall restlessness in society, the more imaginative investigators in clinical transplantation, transplantation biology, and related sciences spurred each other on through individual efforts and by mutually productive collaborations. With discoveries in the laboratory accelerating in parallel with patient-based activity, and in spite of differences in terminology and techniques, researchers were increasingly confident that scientific understanding could be related directly to the problems posed by graft recipients.

Scientists, physicians, patients, and institutions became increasingly receptive to developments in this novel venture. The burgeoning information on the subject was pooled, and details of methods and treatments were shared more fully than in many other specialties. Communication was open. The first international transplantation conference in 1954 in New York was attended by a group of about twenty-five participants who represented much of the existing expertise in the field.[2] By 1966, the seventh conference had been held. As the number of participants grew to several hundred, a new society was created. The Transplantation Society, with Peter Medawar as its first president, convened the following year. Meeting every two years thereafter, its present membership has soared to more than three thousand physicians and scientists from sixty-seven countries around the world. This society, together with national and regional organizations formed over the next decade with their related journals and proceedings, continue to stimulate innovations and disseminate emerging data.

In the 1972 meeting, information on hundreds of transplants from cadavers and living donors was presented, beginning with the first clinical experiences in the 1950s. Unaccountably, French patients were excluded. Advances were obvious, particularly with kidneys from living related sources; the rate of function had improved to 75 percent at one year. Results with cadaver organs increased from 25 percent to 45 percent, a relatively mediocre figure that was to remain static over the next decade. A few long-surviving patients had returned to normal lives.[3] Of equal interest, perhaps, was that the data now came from 220 transplant centers around the world instead of the original handful.

With slowly accumulating clinical successes and intriguing scientific findings, a series of new strategies were initiated in hope of improving the results further. Care of individuals with end-stage renal disease became better understood. Tissue matching, with its potential of offering the best organ to the best recipient, appeared full of promise, particularly as hope increased that the dosages and toxicities of the existing immunosuppressive modalities could be reduced. New methods of preservation and storage allowed more time to transfer a kidney to a well-matched recipient, even in a distant city. More effective dialysis techniques sustained more patients as they awaited a transplant. The possibilities that organs other than the kidney could be grafted successfully piqued the surgical imagination. Increasing numbers of young doctors entered both the clinical and the experimental arenas in search of intellectual and academic fulfillment. More institutions initiated transplant programs. Progressive understanding of the biology of the host immune responses, and the realization that a variety of chemical and biological agents could modulate their activity and increase the survival of foreign organs, focused investigative efforts.

The handful of immunosuppressive drugs available by the mid-1960s included antimetabolites such as azathioprine that interfered with cell division, cytotoxic agents that killed cells directly, and inhibitors of protein synthesis that slowed cell proliferation. The common action of these agents, albeit via different mechanisms, was to attenuate or destroy rapidly dividing cells throughout the body—particularly lymphocytes, which were by this time recognized as critical in mediating the process of acute rejection. Among the primary immunosuppressants tried clinically, azathioprine became widely established as the most satisfactory. Its efficacy was notably increased by the addition of corticosteroids. (Although steroids had been discovered three decades earlier, full appreciation of their ability to inhibit inflammation and downregulate host immunity took years.) The earliest compound recognized, adrenocorticotropin (ACTH), in the 1940s was shown to prolong skin-allograft survival in a burned patient.[4]

Further clues subsequently emerged that these agents might have a role in transplantation: the inflammation from chemically induced delayed hypersensitivity responses in the skin of small laboratory animals could be diminished by treatment, antibody production reduced, wound healing inhibited, and skin-graft survival increased. The dramatic histological changes in rejection of renal allografts in dogs were modulated by administration of one of the new anti-inflammatory steroids, cortisone.[5] As a result of these and similar findings, maintenance azathioprine and steroids in combination were to remain standard immunosuppressive therapy for transplant recipients over the next twenty years.

But this type of treatment of transplant recipients had a downside. Azathioprine and the other powerful primary drugs had potentially fatal side effects that included bone marrow depression, denudation of the gastrointestinal tract, and general reduction of the host defenses. The sequelae of steroids became increasingly evident as clinical experience accumulated. One of the penalties of trying to improve graft survival was overuse of these agents, a problem that recurred again and again in the ensuing years. This danger became particularly obvious when the steroid "pulse" came into popular use—a regimen in which extremely high doses of the compounds were administered over several days to treat episodes of acute rejection. The ultimately misguided philosophy was that rejection, no matter how severe, could be reversed by increasing the amounts of these anti-inflammatory agents. In considering this explosive early period, one clinician presciently noted, "One of the most interesting things that could come out of all this will be observations of what may turn out to be new diseases in some of these long range survivors."[6]

Complications of steroids were the first manifestations of the "new diseases." All of us caring for the generally oversuppressed patients during this period, although encouraged by occasional graft successes, were increasingly concerned, frightened, and horrified by the effects of the treatment. Patients developed moon faces, buffalo humps, and protuberant abdomens. Thinned skin bruised and tore easily. I vividly remember firmly shaking the hand of a transplant recipient and inadvertently stripping off a patch of skin with my thumb. Wounds did not heal. Healed incisions broke down. After weeks of unexplained fever, the bland-appearing incisions of some individuals would suddenly open and discharge copious amounts of pus. Occasionally the vascular anastomoses connecting the graft and recipient vessels became infected, leading to acute rupture and life-threatening hemorrhage. Even repaired vessels occasionally opened, as in the case of Joe Palazola. Infections, often with unusual and relatively unknown bacteria, fungi, and viruses, were prevalent. Mysterious pneumonias developed, impervious to the most powerful antibiotics. Systemic fungal infestations were common and virtually impossible to treat. As a result, the early mortality rate of recipients of cadaver-donor kidneys was over 25 percent in many centers, including our own.

The effects of maintenance steroids administered over the long term to retain a functioning graft were no better. Chronic use of the drugs contributed to the development of hypertension, diabetes, and increasing levels of serum cholesterol and other blood lipids. Normal growth of children was inhibited. Bones broke. Cataracts developed. Some patients, distressed by what was happening to them, either stopped their medications and returned to dialysis or committed suicide. Despite the benefits to graft survival provided by the addition of steroids and other adjuncts to azathioprine, the results remained unsatisfactory and the treatment sometimes appeared worse than the original disease.

Many of us in the field investigated various adjunctive biologic means to reduce host immunity. Like the chemical agents, most of these measures were designed to inactivate or destroy immunologically competent lymphocytes. As some experimental data had suggested that surgical removal of lymphoid tissue could prolong graft survival, excision of the spleen was carried out in many early recipients before or during kidney transplantation. The thymus gland was removed in others, to prevent development of mature peripheral lymphocytes. The ineffectiveness of these invasive procedures curtailed their transient popularity. The magnitude of the operations was also too threatening: the first surgery involved a major abdominal operation to remove the spleen, and the second often entailed splitting the breastbone of the fragile transplant recipients to isolate and take the thymus. Bulk removal of recirculating lymphocytes by prolonged drainage of the thoracic duct (the large lymphatic vessel in the neck) was carried out by several groups based primarily on James Gowans' experimental data with rats and mice. Indeed, for a period during my training, much of my time was spent attempting to locate and isolate this delicate and filmy structure, then place a plastic tube into it for drainage (Figure 6.1). We removed up to one hundred liters of lymph from some patients over days or weeks. While initial results were encouraging, the technique was never really effective.

Nonoperative strategies also were tried. One imaginative idea was "antigen competition," the theory that a powerful antigenic stimulus separate from that produced by the transplanted organ might compete with the host immunological responses so effectively that the foreign graft would be spared. To evoke this stimulus, we administered typhoid antigen. The unfortunate patients not only sickened dramatically from the bacterial product, but continued to reject their grafts. Local x-radiation of the allograft to destroy infiltrating cells became popular. A system of extracorporeal radiation was devised in which the peripheral blood was pumped around a radioactive cobalt source to inhibit the immunologic competency of the circulating leukocytes. Although these measures often appeared effective in animal models, they were not helpful in human patients. Their use reflected both overoptimism of clinicians regarding their efficacy and naive underappreciation of the breadth and power of the immune responses of the host.

A more lasting strategy involved the administration of antibodies destructive to white blood cells. Antilymphocyte serum (ALS) and its various permutations, antilymphocyte globulin, antithymocyte and antisplenocyte serum and globulin, and other antisera from several animal species, engendered much interest as potentially potent immunosuppressive adjuncts. The concept stemmed from the observations of Elie Metchnikoff, a half century before, that transfer of rat lymphoid cells into guinea pigs would stimulate production by the host

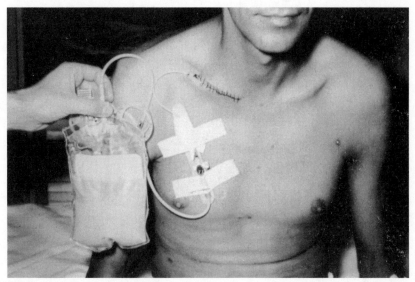

Figure 6.1 Removal of lymphocyte-rich lymph via a thoracic duct fistula

animal of an antirat lymphocyte antiserum, which in turn could kill circulating lymphocytes when injected back into the donor.[7]

During the next decades, others confirmed the cytotoxic potential of such antisera. "Antireticular cytotoxic sera" were extensively studied in Russian laboratories, although their effectiveness was never clear. By the 1950s, researchers noted that ALS could inhibit cutaneous delayed hypersensitivity reactions. The later demonstration by Michael Woodruff that skin-graft survival could be increased in rats receiving the material emphasized the potential relevance of these immunosuppressive proteins in transplantation. Investigators then prolonged kidney grafts in treated dogs. Coincident administration of donor bone marrow could also, under some circumstances, evoke specific unresponsiveness (some called it tolerance) in grafted mice. Produced for clinical use by inoculating a horse, goat, or rabbit with human lymphoid cells, the resultant antihuman cytotoxic antibodies caused a sharp drop in numbers of circulating lymphocytes when injected intravenously into human subjects.

These and other findings triggered a stampede to test the materials further in small- and large-animal models, and soon in patients. Early clinical trials were optimistic. Within a few years, however, most of those involved agreed that although potent ALS or related preparations reduced the number and severity of early acute rejection crises, ultimate graft survival was not materially affected. Indeed, like the other immunosuppressants, these preparations yielded unexpected disappointments and complications. The production of antibodies by the graft recipient, directed specifically against the administered foreign antibody, often diminished its efficacy. Important batch-to-batch variations in potency occurred regardless of the source of inoculating cells, the protein type, or steps in the manufacture. Patients hated the severe side effects: redness, pain, and swelling at the injection sites; fever; malaise; and skin rashes. Systemic and sometimes fatal infections occurred. Occasionally those receiving the proteins reacted violently against them with anaphylaxis, shock, or death.

With the slow but progressive improvement in the clinical results of transplantation, primarily related to better patient care before and after graft placement, it became increasingly problematic to rationalize the general use of these difficult agents. (Some groups still administered them in relatively short courses as induction therapy.) In retrospect, perhaps their main contribution was to act as a forerunner of various monoclonal antibodies directed against specific lymphocytes or lymphocyte products—a newer generation of more refined and safer agents that have gained some clinical acceptance.

Immunosuppressed recipients of kidney grafts were quickly determined to be at high risk not only from unusual infections, but also from a more sinister type of life-threatening condition that was barely understood. As transplanted patients began to live longer, hints arose that the incidence of cancer was surprisingly high, and that its presence might be linked to diminished host immunity. Paris yielded the first suspicion in 1960. René Küss was working with a 36-year-old patient with carcinoma of the kidney, a M. Coq. Although his other cancerous kidney had been excised three years before, the tumor now involved the remaining organ. At the family's insistence, Küss removed the diseased kidney, radiated the patient, and transplanted an organ from his sister in January 1960 (Figure 6.2). The graft functioned well, but Coq died four and a half months later of multiple metastases, a hint that depression of the immune responses (in this case by radiation)

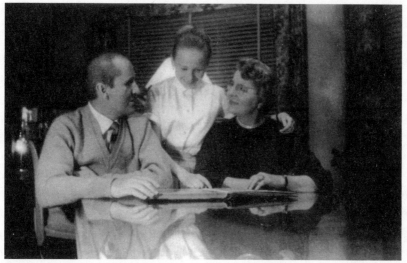

Figure 6.2 M. Coq, his daughter and his sister, the kidney donor, in 1960
(P. I. Terasaki, with permission)

might accelerate the cancer spread. A comparable situation occurred
four years later with Joe Palazola. Shortly thereafter, David Hume in
Virginia described a patient who developed a liver tumor with lung
metastases three years after transplantation with a kidney from a cadaver donor who had died of the same condition. Once again, cessation of the chemical immunosuppression and sacrifice of the organ led
to complete remission. After several months, a second kidney was
placed and immunosuppression restarted. There was no recurrence.[8]

Within a few years, four more such patients were reported. One
received a kidney from a donor who had died of breast cancer. Although the transplant was quickly removed at day 5 because of infection, large deposits of malignant breast cells were found unexpectedly
upon examination of the organ under the microscope. In another patient, nests of thyroid cancer cells extended throughout a kidney, excised from the new host after seven days because final examination of
the remaining donor organs had shown multiple metastases from an
unrecognized primary thyroid tumor. An especially vivid connection
between the use of antilymphocyte globulin and neoplasia was suggested by a renal recipient who developed a sarcoma in his leg at the
site of injection of the antibody.[9]

The growing disquiet about the subject was accelerated by the 1975 report of Starzl's first 483 transplant recipients: 27 had developed cancer, an occurrence one hundred times higher (6 percent) than that of the general population in the same age range.[10] Almost in passing, it was recognized that the frequency of cancer among relatively immunodepressed dialysis patients was twice the normal. This increased incidence of malignancy in those with abnormal immune responses has continued to the present day and includes more than ten thousand afflicted persons.

The tumors have been divided into three types. The first were inadvertently transmitted with the organs of donors with cancer. The only donors in this group who have become acceptable in current practice are the rare individuals with primary brain tumors. These do not metastasize. The second type occur in recipients from whom cancers were removed months or years before and considered cured. These may recur after grafting and the initiation of immunosuppression. M. Coq is a striking example. The third type includes transplanted patients with tumors arising de novo, the most common being of the skin and the lymphoid system.

Several causative factors have been implicated. Depression of the host responses combined with overexposure to sun are critical risk factors for the development of skin cancer, an important epidemiological problem (particularly among light-skinned transplant recipients living in warm climates). Some viruses may be responsible for lymphomas and other lymphoproliferative tumors, an association recognized when an unexpectedly high proportion of the first patients to receive Cyclosporin A developed B-cell lymphomas. The preferential inhibition of T cells by the immunosuppressive drugs presumably allows an unbalanced proliferation of B cells responding to viruses. This unregulated and activated lymphocyte population may ultimately transform into lymphomas. Conversely, the preexistence of antiviral antibodies may confer immunity against development of this tumor after grafting.

The unexpectedly high incidence of cancer in transplant recipients prompted researchers to review past clinical and experimental work for clues. The incidence of scrotal cancer among chimney sweeps in England had, for instance, been known for nearly a century to be unexpectedly high. The soot collecting in the bodily folds and crevices of these unfortunate boys sent up narrow chimneys was later found to be carcinogenic because of its content of coal tar. Experimentally, the material produced similar tumors when painted repeatedly on the backs of mice. Ehrlich and his followers then investigated the behavior of host animals against foreign tumors. Accumulating evidence that tumor growth could be increased by various topically applied chemicals or other external stimuli, or in animals whose immune responses had been altered by cortisone, ALS, or total body x-radiation, was later broadened into the context of transplantation. One investigator noted, "The phenomenon of homograft rejection will turn out to represent a primary mechanism for natural defense against neoplasia."[11]

Most relevant to immunosuppression was Macfarlane Burnet's theory of "immunological surveillance" by the lymphoid tissues of the body, which represent "a system . . . to cope with the occurrence of somatic mutation and potential neoplasia in large, long-lived animals with many cell systems involved in life-long proliferation." Rapidly dividing cells may occasionally produce a mutant or its clone which, if left unchecked, may become cancerous. The immune defenses of the host are critical in identifying and destroying potentially carcinogenic cells. Much of this activity, he felt, centered around the thymus-derived T lymphocyte, "an important agent of defense against tumor growth." When such a surveillance system is impaired, the incidence of cancer increases. The relatively high number of lymphomas and Kaposi's sarcomas in immunodeficient AIDS patients is a striking current example. Burnet went on to suggest that cancer is relatively common at the two extremes of life because the immune system is immature and relatively ineffectual in newborns and is atrophied and worn out in older people. Transplant patients whose immune system is suppressed with drugs are at similar risk.[12]

Genetic differences between individuals are the greatest barrier to successful transplantation. We have noted that blood cannot be transfused between persons of differing ABO blood types because of the presence of red cell antigens. Tissue antigens produce the same effect. After its definition in the mouse, the major histocompatibility locus (MHC) in humans was characterized. This discrete area resides on a single chromosome in each species and encodes for a large number of antigens, including "transplantation antigens" expressed by an allograft. In the 1950s a French hematologist and future Nobel Prize winner, Jean Dausset, defined a system of human leukocyte antigens (designated HLA), entirely separate from red blood cell antigens and critical in determining differences between donor and recipient. Collaborative work on the differential rate of rejection of skin grafts in a large series of human volunteers supported his conclusions.

Interest in this new subject, immunogenetics, increased over the next decade, which saw standardization of the names of the different antigens, improvements in matching techniques, and the availability of sera of known anti-HLA specificities for use in the growing numbers of tissue-typing laboratories involved in organ matching and distribution. Other advances in this new science included computer analysis of serological reactions to white cell donors and the initiation of a standard method of tissue typing using a plastic microcytotoxicity tray. The introduction of monoclonal antibodies and newer molecular methods have allowed further dissection of this remarkably complex genetic system, intrinsic to the discrimination by the host between self and nonself, and differentiation between individual members of the same species.

What were the practical ramifications of these advances for organ transplantation? One of the few surgical investigators examining the differences in behavior between kidney allografts and autografts in the 1920s had conceptualized the then-unknown subject of tissue typing: "It is unfortunate that the lower animals, such as the dog, do not possess a blood grouping like that of man. In the future, it may be possible to work out a satisfactory way of determining the reaction of the recipient's blood serum or tissues to those of the donor and the reverse; perhaps in this way we can obtain more light on this as yet relatively dark side of biology." In 1954 Billingham, Brent, and Medawar amplified the impressions of earlier investigators by demonstrating precisely that the broader the reactivity of the host against donor lymphocytes in a test tube, the more rapid was the tempo of skin-graft rejection between mouse strains. This relationship was confirmed subsequently in humans by inoculation of the skin with normal lymphocytes. With further experience, many in the field began to appreciate the potential significance of tissue matching between kidney donor and graft recipient.[13]

Understanding of the critical importance of circulating antibodies in the recipient before placement of a donor allograft was a related advance. In 1964 a brother-to-sister transplant was performed on closed-circuit television for those attending a small conference in Los Angeles. After a technically perfect revascularization, the kidney became pink for a few minutes, then rapidly turned blue, then black, then died. This was the first case of hyperacute rejection in a recipient with, as it turned out, preexisting circulating antibodies directed specifically against the donor.[14] Seven more cases were subsequently reported, six of which occurred in women with prior pregnancies who had formed antibodies against their husbands' cells and, by inference, against similar donor antigens. As it soon became apparent that graft recipients whose sera killed donor lymphocytes in the test tube inevitably developed hyperacute rejection of their transplant, Paul Terasaki and his colleagues at UCLA developed the standard cross-match as a tool to prevent such a catastrophe. This test and its refinements, since that time performed routinely before operation, has been so effective that the disaster of hyperacute rejection has become extremely rare.

Because of increasing enthusiasm about the cross-match and HLA matching as ways of improving the results of organ transplantation, the 1970s were halcyon years for tissue-typing laboratories. Many studies were carried out to show the efficacy of the concept, funding became available, and facilities and personnel expanded. Dialogue increased about the sharing of highly matched organs across countries and even continents. "A cottage industry of clinical tissue typing based on the assumption that matching would have a profound influence on transplantation had sprung up world wide, mostly funded by contracts or grants by the NIH or other governmental agencies."[15] Some countries even began to write laws requiring specific matching parameters for transplantation between a given donor and a given recipient.

Unfortunately, the practicalities were not that simple. Terasaki created a sensation in the last of his several presentations at the 1970 Transplantation Congress in The Hague. He started off slowly. In the first of his talks, he described serological techniques and their reproducibility. In another, he noted the benefits of matching in living-related donor-host combinations and stressed the sharing of histocompatibility data throughout all transplant centers to assess outcome. However, in a third report, he failed to show any correlation between tissue typing and the results of cadaver transplantation in pooled data throughout the United States. Terasaki also mentioned the "center effect," whereby better results were achieved by the most experienced units. As many new units were opening at the time, those involved received this concept unenthusiastically. There was little applause and much argument; his paper was the only one from the entire conference denied publication. Finally published elsewhere, it was accompanied by a warning editorial.[16]

Two special conferences were quickly called to analyze all available international tissue-typing data. The conclusions were equivocal. Within weeks, a group from the NIH agency responsible for the contract supporting Terasaki's laboratory gathered for a visit on site. On Christmas Eve they withdrew his federally sponsored funding. Shortly thereafter, Starzl, who had publicly defended the data, also received a site visit from the NIH and transiently lost his research funding.[17] Fortunately, Terasaki's laboratory was able to survive primarily by selling to all typing laboratories throughout the country his plastic tissue-typing tray, in which the reactions of large numbers of lymphocytes from potential recipients with donor sera could be compared simultaneously. The NIH offered its version of the trays gratis. Yet colleagues throughout North America generously supported Terasaki, ultimately turning the venture into a lucrative business that sustained his laboratory for years. The tissue-typing enterprise continued relatively unscathed by these findings, although many were outraged by the negative data. Few surgeons were bothered, as they felt compelled to use every appropriate organ for their waiting patients. They resented the extra laboratory time required to obtain matching results, as it lengthened the storage interval before transplantation and potentially increased graft injury. They also feared that the number of kidneys going to their units could be reduced because organs might be transferred to better-matched recipients out of their region. For them, a negative cross-match was sufficient.

In retrospect, there were several reasons for Terasaki's unexpected findings. The data supporting the efficacy of tissue typing had been based primarily on results from living-related transplants; few cadaver donors were in the original series. Methodology was limited, and understanding of genetic complexities rudimentary. In 1970 only eleven

HLA antigens and their associated specificities had been identified; more than seventy are presently recognized in a continuously expanding system.[18] In addition to the established role of tissue typing in bone marrow transplantation, its major value in organ grafting has been to target the best matches between living-related donors and their recipients. The overall influence of the tissue match on the survival results of cadaver-donor recipients has not been striking, at least over the short term—with the exception of HLA identical combinations that are matched at all recognized antigenic sites. While constituting only about 20 percent of cadaver transplants, the results are consistently superior to those employing mismatched organs. Despite vast efforts worldwide, the full potential of tissue typing has yet to be realized, although long-term results may depend on the number of antigenic matches or mismatches.

The prospect that a satisfactory tissue match would improve results of transplantation also implied that an optimal organ could be offered to a chosen patient, even if it had to be shipped over a long distance. Before any type of preservation strategy had been devised, the interval between removal of the kidney and placement into the host had to be minimal or the cells of the isolated organ would die from lack of blood. As the use of brain-dead, heart-beating donors had not yet been considered, kidneys were taken from cadavers and transplanted as soon as possible. Surgeons even sat with the dying donor to be ready to move swiftly after cessation of the heartbeat.

Although there had been a few sporadic attempts to cool or even freeze kidneys before transplantation, only when a young Dutch surgeon, Folkert Belzer, joined the staff of the University of California in San Francisco in 1964 were detailed investigations into kidney storage initiated. Although living-related donation was ongoing in this unit, Belzer's task was to instigate a cadaver-donor program, often using kidneys removed at hospitals some distance away. Considering how he could optimally protect the stored organs, he reasoned that introducing fluid via a pulsatile pump would best simulate the normal arterial circulation to the organ, that blood would be the most physiological perfusate, and that the isolated kidneys should be cooled to slow their metabolism. He and his group soon noted, however, that the unexpectedly increasing perfusion pressure of dog kidneys could be reduced by switching from blood to cell-free plasma. Yet no transplanted kidney survived after twenty-four hours of storage, even with the use of a membrane oxygenator and perfusion pump. In experiments designed to uncover the reason for these poor results, the researchers ultimately found that removal of one component of the plasma, the lipoproteins, made the resultant perfusate less injurious to the tissue and allowed 100 percent survival of autografted kidneys transplanted as much as seventy-two hours after their removal. It turned out that aggregates of unstable lipoprotein molecules in normal plasma clogged the tiny vessels of the perfused organs, driving up perfusion pressure and destroying their function.[19]

Belzer was soon faced with a patient urgently needing a kidney. The only one available had been perfused for seventeen hours. Transplanted, it functioned immediately. To exploit this positive experience, he created a large perfusion machine that fitted into the back of a rented truck used to collect organs from around the city. Within a few years, he had devised several portable preservation units. Their efficacy was demonstrated clearly on Christmas Eve 1974, when Belzer carried a perfused kidney from San Francisco to Leiden in the Netherlands for transplantation. The small machine performed nicely while sitting in a first-class seat in the aircraft. After thirty-seven hours of perfusion, the kidney was grafted into a 42-year-old Dutch truck driver, sustaining him for seventeen years (Figure 6.3).[20] Such units soon became commercially available, particularly as it was apparent the kidneys from nonheart-beating cadavers did better when preserved by machine perfusion than when stored in the cold. Parallel attempts to store livers, however, proved ineffectual.

Geoffrey Collins, a surgeon working with Paul Terasaki, introduced an alternative approach to organ preservation by reasoning that machine perfusion would be unnecessary if the metabolism of the organ could be slowed by an effective cold-storage solution. Such a practical, inexpensive method would facilitate transplantation of matched kidneys from cadaver sources to a large national and international recipient pool. Antagonism toward such a simplistic approach was high, however, as a virtual industry using machine perfusion had sprung up in the United States. Yet the point was proven when a series

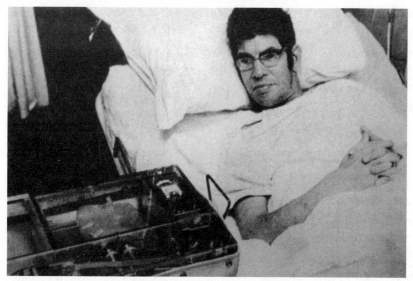

Figure 6.3 1974 recipient in the Netherlands of a machine-preserved kidney from California (P. I. Terasaki, with permission)

of dog kidneys from California were flushed with an effective cold perfusate, shipped in ice in small cardboard boxes around the world, and grafted successfully in laboratories as far apart as Israel, England, and Australia.[21]

With additional reports of successful transplantation by the French of large numbers of nonperfused, cooled human kidneys, the technique became accepted throughout Europe. Because of its complexity and expense, use of machine perfusion began gradually to decline in the United States. By 1980, as improved perfusates became available, about three quarters of all kidneys were cold stored. It should be noted that interest in the pumping technique has recently resurfaced because of its benefit in organs of less-than-ideal donors and in the prediction of viability of potentially suboptimal kidneys.

The years between the first use of chemical immunosuppression in 1960 and the advent of Cyclosporin A two decades later comprised a time of growth, innovation, and trial and error in organ transplantation. The emotions of those of us dealing with the allograft recipients and their families during this period ranged between depression and elation. Although the rates of mortality, morbidity, and unexpected complications remained high, they were declining with refinements in patient care despite the relative lack of substantative improvement in the results of the grafts themselves. The occasional successes drove us all to further efforts, as both increasing clinical experience and new and potentially relevant findings in transplant biology were considered to hold great future promise. At the same time, innovations in thinking increased with investigations of new departures in treatment. Developing during a time of social restlessness, this era of modern transplantations seemed to reflect the ongoing disquiet outside the walls of hospitals and laboratories.

The early experience also highlighted a potentially problematic divergence in interests and loyalties, one that is still faced constantly by many productive clinical investigators and their teams. At best, conundrums arising at the bedside and answered by applied research in the laboratory directly benefit patients. The resultant changes in clinical care, or unexpected experimental findings, often provoke even more questions, which may amplify existing research projects or offer new avenues for study. In reality, the two objectives may at times produce conflict in the minds of those caring for the graft recipients, particularly when the desire for direct benefit to the patient blurs with the ability to obtain new scientific knowledge or increase research funding, or when side effects of a given agent mask its purported efficacy. As those involved in transplantation investigations recognize all too well, it may be difficult to resolve these equally compelling demands. The pressures have only magnified as success of the treatment has increased.

Prolongation of Life and of Death

7

THE HISTORY OF SCIENCE IS REPLETE WITH IN-
stances in which a discovery or advance in one subject suggests an
alternative approach in an associated area, or provokes the development of an unrelated specialty which in turn may stimulate advances in
the two fields. Both the specialized support of patients with organ
failure and the transplantation of organs exemplify this relationship by
introducing a spectrum of ideas ranging from novel technologies and
treatments to reappraisal of long-held medical, cultural, and ethical
beliefs. Some of these changing perceptions have included concepts as
unusual as extension of life by the dialysis machine, or as startling as
prolongation of death by the respirator. The first involves a practical
mechanical means to sustain the lives of individuals with irreversible
renal disease. The second challenges the long-accepted tenet that death
is synonymous with the cessation of heartbeat and changes it to one
less intuitively obvious, that the condition occurs when the brain dies
and the patient is no longer a sentient being. In the context of transplantation, the viable organs can at this time be removed from the dead
to replace those that have failed in the living. These two subjects are
considered in this chapter, as they are curiously related.

The support by chronic dialysis of the lives of individuals whose sole
infirmity is that their kidneys have failed has become common and
accepted practice. It involves being connected to a large filtering device
for several hours, three times each week, for as long as life lasts. Existence sustained in this way may be a burden for some because of

143

persistent malaise, fatigue, dietary limitations, and the substantial time commitment. Many rescued from a premature death by the machine, in contrast, live relatively stable and productive lives. The experience of one of my colleagues who developed renal failure as a premedical student in the early days of the treatment illustrates the difficulties confronting those afflicted. Becoming a professor of medicine, my friend remained on dialysis for twenty-five years before receiving a kidney transplant. When this failed after five years, he returned to dialysis.

> It came as a surprise . . . the fact that I had terminal kidney failure. I had no idea what hemodialysis was or what it would require, but at 22 years of age, with little idea of my pending demise, I looked forward to life. I wanted to be a doctor. After 2 years of premed studies resisting worsening uremic symptoms . . . what I was being told on that late afternoon in February of 1966 was that my kidneys were almost finished. I had a choice: dialysis or death. Only a short time before, I didn't have an option. For me there was no suitable related kidney donor, and chronic dialysis was not available at Stanford at the time. If I agreed, I would go to Seattle, Washington . . . If this is what I have to do to live, so be it . . . I remember my first dialysis. My [new] shunt was clamped, disconnected, and hooked up. I don't recall what I felt as the bright red blood coursed out of my leg under the pumping pressure of my heart into the dialyzer and back again. I had little understanding of what was happening and no idea whatsoever of what lay ahead. In my mind, I suppose it was simply a matter of "putting one foot in front of the other," taking what came, and making the best of it. My goals were still in sight, but I had no idea of what others might be thinking of my future . . . I was fortunate to have had the opportunity because many others of my age, younger and older were dying simply because of the lack of money to pay for dialysis.

He goes on to describe difficulties and complications over the years, noting that he was dialyzed 4,100 times and spent 2,400 hours on treatment through his years of residency and professional life. He concludes: "There exists a remarkable human adaptability to trying circumstances."[1]

Hemodialysis became an integral and indispensable corollary to renal transplantation after its development during World War II by the Dutch physician, bioengineer, and inventor Willem Kolff. There was some background on which the concept was built. A Scottish professor of chemistry had coined the term *dialysis* in 1861 by demonstrating that a semipermeable membrane of parchment coated with a soluble protein, albumin, would allow diffusion of crystalloids—low-molecular-weight salts in solution—from high to low concentrations, but not colloids—large nondissolved protein particles in suspension. He had also showed that urea, one of the body's waste products which is normally filtered from the serum into the urine by the kidney, could traverse the membrane into a surrounding water bath. Although he predicted that such an approach might have medical applicability, fifty years elapsed before investigators in the pharmacology laboratory at the Johns Hopkins Medical School described a technique by which "the blood of a living animal may be submitted to dialysis outside the body, and again returned to the normal circulation" via a series of glass cylinders glued together.[2] Terming this apparatus the artificial kidney, they suggested its use in humans.

Unfortunately, the advent of World War I curtailed their experiments by prohibiting the importation of hirudin, an anticoagulant derived from the saliva of leeches, which prevented the blood from clotting. "When the Great War came it was no longer possible for us to get leeches as these anilids ('Hirudo Medicinalis') were imported by us in quantities of 1500 or more from Hungary. Shortly after the outbreak of the War indeed I had a consignment of 1500 leeches lying at Copenhagen. The English Foreign Office ruled that this consignment was of 'enemy origin' and the leeches were left to die." During the 1920s Georg Haas, a German physician unaware of the work in Baltimore, dialyzed the first two humans following preliminary trials with dogs.[3]

Years later Kolff became interested in using the technique to treat patients with uremia. He appreciated not only that small molecules like urea could cross a semipermeable membrane such as cellophane depending on their respective concentrations, but that excess water could be removed from the circulation if the solution in the dialysis bath was more concentrated. The blood therefore had to move continuously across a membrane surface.

In a letter to Francis Moore, Kolff recalled his early experience building the apparatus.

One of my first patients was a young man suffering from chronic nephritis and slowly dying of renal failure. He was hypertensive, had headaches, became blind, and was vomiting every day. His old mother was the wife of a poor farmer, her back bent by hard work, dressed in her traditional Sunday black dress, but with a very pretty white lace cap. I had to tell her that her only son was going to die, and I felt very helpless. Gradually the idea grew in me that if we could only remove 20 grams of urea and other retention products per day, we might relieve this man's nausea, and that if we did this from day to day life might still be possible. This was in 1938 ... There were only a few papers published about hemodialysis ... In order to determine how much cellophane I would need to make an artificial kidney, I took a piece of cellophane tubing, commercially available as sausage casing ... I fixed this on a small board and rocked it in a saline bath. I added 400 mg percent of urea to the blood and found that after one-half hour of dialysis all the urea had passed out of the blood ... I had built several apparatuses, and I had to pay for these machines myself; none was well enough constructed to be applicable clinically ... On the 10th of May, 1940, the German Armies invaded the Netherlands ... Four days later from the upper floor of the hospital we saw a large mushroom cloud rise over the City of Rotterdam, which had been set alight by the incendiary bombs of the German Luftwaffe.[4]

Upset and disrupted by the Nazi invasion, the suicides of his Jewish professor of medicine and his wife, and their replacement by a Dutch Nazi as head of his department, Kolff left his large university hospital for a small hospital in Kampen, a city to the north. Once there, he and an engineering colleague developed a usable rotating dialysis machine (Figure 7.1). They dialyzed their first patient early in 1943, a 29-year-old woman whose vision was failing from the effects of hypertension and uremia. On admission she was anemic and short of breath. Her heart was enlarged. The improvement with dialysis, particularly after removal of large amounts of fluid, was obvious: "she was strikingly well and her mind was perfectly clear." Her vision improved so that "she could read the paper without any difficulty."[5] After twelve consecutive treatments, she died because she ran out of peripheral vessels to connect to the machine. At autopsy, both kidneys were shrunken and scarred.

Emboldened by this success, Kolff went on to dialyze seventeen individuals, two of whom survived. During those grim years under the Nazi occupation, he and his colleagues contended with technical prob-

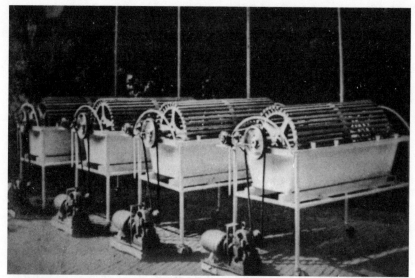

Figure 7.1 Willem Kolff's original dialysis machines (Novartis, with permission)

lems and equipment shortages. Rubber tubing was used and reused as plastic tubing was not available, heparin (a recently introduced anti-coagulent more effective than hirudin in preventing blood clotting) and penicillin were difficult to obtain, needles became rusty and dull.

Others built their own devices, including Gordon Murray and colleagues in Toronto, who dialyzed a patient with a coil-type kidney in late 1946. But not until the physicians and engineers in Boston had substantially modified Kolff's rotating machine did dialysis become accepted in the United States (Figure 7.2). The prototype was refined and used in various hospitals throughout Europe despite local reservations about this novel departure in treatment. Britons were actively hostile toward it. Frank Parsons of Leeds was the first in England to dialyze patients with acute renal failure. Having spent time at the Brigham, he requested permission from British medical authorities to bring a Kolff-Brigham kidney to Leeds upon his return. Their response was succinct. "Our advisors say there is no place for an artificial kidney in British medicine." The head of the committee went even further: "Parsons, try it, but remember that the country is against you."[6]

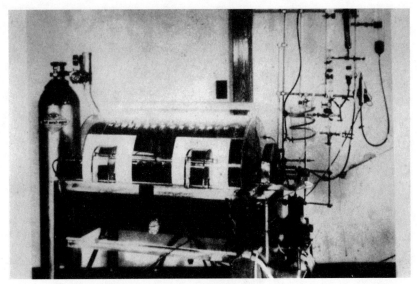

Figure 7.2 The Kolff-Brigham artificial kidney

Despite such doubts and antipathies, more effective dialyzers were developed in the ensuing years. The increasing availability of antibiotics, safer blood transfusions, and better means to access the circulation enhanced the success of the new method. Public recognition of the technique grew. The machines came into use in the Korean War to treat badly wounded American soldiers; the innovation was initially resisted by those in military command but was successfully pushed by physicians. Indeed, the 95 percent mortality rate of wounded soldiers who had developed renal failure before the institution of dialysis fell to 35 percent thereafter.

A critical advance was the creation in 1960 by Belding Scribner at the University of Washington of the external arteriovenous shunt, a device to connect the circulation of the patient to the tubing of the machine as needed.[7] Up to that time, glass or plastic tubes had to be placed in appropriate arteries and veins in the arms and legs before each dialysis. A few clinicians had tried to retain these accesses throughout several treatments, but infection and clotting inevitably precluded their sustained use. When patients ran out of appropriate vessels, dialysis was no longer possible and death ensued. The new shunt was composed of tapered hollow Teflon tips inserted into the vessels and connected to nonwettable tubing through which blood flowed. Heparin was administered to prevent clotting in the device. The tubing was clamped when not in use, but could be opened after connection to the dialysis machine. Their first patient with a successful shunt, a machinist named Clyde Shields, survived on dialysis for eleven years.

Over the following decade, surgeons began to join an artery and vein at the wrist to create an internal arteriovenous fistula, a significant advance in technique. Enlarged and engorged by arterial flow, the dilated vein in the forearm could be easily punctured through the skin. The most effective method to date, fistulas often function for years and are relatively resistant to infection. Synthetic tubular grafts, running beneath the skin between an artery and vein, are also used frequently. While convenient for needle placement, they are difficult to keep open as they tend to clot. Indeed, the most common cause of hospitalization for dialysis patients in the United States at the present time is failure of access caused by venous narrowing, clotting, or infection. Maintenance of the devices remains an expensive unsolved problem.

With improvements in dialysis and its increasing availability, the growing numbers of patients began to outstrip the existing facilities. How to offer adequate care and meet the substantial costs of this technology were difficulties that became paramount. The only two centers willing to provide dialysis in 1960 approached the problem differently. Both were in the United States, one at the University of Washington and the other at the Brigham. The dialysis program in Seattle soon became overwhelmed with patients seeking help—not only those living locally, but also individuals from areas that did not offer such treatment (as exemplified by my colleague at Stanford). The financing of this effort was helped initially by a small grant from a private foundation, and the NIH offered modest support. Public fund drives became necessary. As sustaining even one patient cost thousands of dollars each year even at that time, the numbers of acceptances had to be limited. By the mid-1960s physicians were arguing desperately against legislators, who denied any problem: "At the present time in the United States, there are not more than 50–100 patients on transplants plus chronic dialysis—yet in the last four years, since these techniques have become available, 10,000 or more ideal candidates have died in this country for lack of the treatment, so obviously rigid selection of one sort or another must take place." The cries from patients and those trying to care for them became increasingly desperate.[8]

An Admissions and Policy Committee (the "death committee") was quickly formed; its brief was to triage or screen candidates for placement into available openings. Composed of physicians and laymen meeting anonymously to consider who was to be chosen and who was to be refused, the position of the group became increasingly untenable. While in other areas of medicine the choice to refer or not refer an individual to a specialist, or to continue or discontinue treatment, was a private matter between physician, patient, and family, the dilemma facing the Seattle committee received national attention through a *Life* magazine article entitled "They Decide Who Lives, Who Dies: Medical Miracle Puts a Moral Burden on a Small Committee." The article noted that factors for acceptance or exclusion included "sex of patient; marital status and number of dependents; income; net worth; emotional stability . . . ; nature of occupation, past performance and future potential." Divorce or diabetes subtracted further points. It was a task for Solomon to decide whether the life of a minister was worth more than that of a mechanic, a school principal more than a policeman, or a businessman more than a housewife and mother.[9]

The dialysis program at the Brigham also started with a few patients, selected on a case-by-case basis. However, rapid demand soon outpaced the available places. The only other facilities available were in a small state hospital on the outskirts of Boston. No other institution in the region would take on such a commitment. Pushed by desperate patients, three Brigham nephrologists including John Merrill, with the blessing of the hospital administration and the medical school dean, opened a small unit. This freestanding facility and others like it began to grow steadily; indeed, it quickly became clear that dialysis treatments there could be carried out more efficiently and more cheaply than in the hospital.

Although this particular endeavor arose out of expediency, the fact that it eventually became a company with stockholders including the relevant physicians stirred considerable controversy. One of the targets of those raging against established norms and institutions in the troubled 1960s was the perceived exploitation of the helpless by commercial interests. As publicity about the dialysis arrangements widened, vocal reaction against several aspects of business entering medical care became strident. Community activists cried that the professionals were not saving the patients but torturing them for monetary gain. They complained about a mercantile advantage to the parent hospital and the medical school, preached that doctors who referred their own patients to their own companies had a major conflict of interest, and considered that such an arrangement was a monopoly—even though no other choices were available.

More broadly, many students and their supporters were upset that occasional university-based faculty-scientists were taking paid consultant posts with companies associated with medicine and medical care. The Brigham administrators increased the pressure by complaining that the hospital was not receiving some of the grant money allotted to care for its patients, despite their treatment in free-standing units outside the Brigham's purview. Although the Brigham and Harvard Medical School eventually disengaged their interests and John Merrill resigned from the facility to retain his hospital position, the remaining physicians lost their faculty rank. They rose to direct the company, National Medical Care, which was to grow into a huge international concern.

The fundamental differences in values arising during this early period are still not resolved. The lines continue to blur, and for-profit business-run hospitals and hospital chains have become increasingly common.

As other dialysis units emerged, the obstacle of cost for the increasing numbers of individuals with renal failure who presented themselves for care became ever more pressing. Although some of the original patients had to pay for their treatments out of pocket, Rhode Island and Massachusetts were prompt to provide funds via existing disability and rehabilitation laws, an innovative approach that set a precedent. Eventually, some support for the dialysis population came from the states themselves, and some from federal monies funneled through the states.

Problems with payment began to affect the transplant recipients. The early Brigham patients had to produce a substantial stipend even to be considered for transplantation, although with the advent of chemical immunosuppression in the early 1960s, the NIH helped bear the cost of care as well as of testing the efficacy of the available modalities. But by the end of the decade, "stories were common of desperate acts to finance the dialysis or transplant care of loved ones in private centers. Failing these efforts, crimes sometimes were committed to raise money. A national scandal was in the making."[10]

The equitable distribution of restricted resources in medicine poses an accelerating problem as technology and applied knowledge outstrip both available facilities and money to pay for treatment. Questions posed by this unresolved dilemma and faced by patients with organ failure have only become more unanswerable as time has progressed. "Shall machines or organs go to the sickest, or to the ones with the most promise of recovery; on a first come, first served basis; to the most valuable patient (based on wealth, education, position, what?); to the one with the most dependents; to women and children first; to those who could pay; to whom? or should lots be cast, impersonally and uncritically?"[11]

To ease the situation among their patients in Boston and Seattle, the physicians who were involved developed less expensive home dialysis programs. At the Brigham, groups of patients and their families formed the Kidney Transplant Dialysis Association. Raising money through bake sales, raffles, and other efforts, the group bought equipment for the dialysis unit, created a patients' lounge, and organized social contacts and exchange of information. By the early 1970s, this venture had grown sufficiently that financial aid to needy individuals could be considered. Grants were allotted for transportation, dialysis, rent, food, medicine, clothing, and other necessities. Similar programs grew quickly in various areas of the United States. Other countries reacted differently, with solutions ranging from those that provided the services without cost to the individual, to those that offered hemodialysis only to the few who could pay privately. And physicians treating patients with chronic renal failure were forced to face the relatively new concept that they could prolong life through much effort and large cost, but they could not affect the disease process itself.

In 1972 the U.S. Congress passed HR1, an act that provided financial recompense under Medicare to patients with kidney disease; such insurance coverage had previously been reserved only for persons older than 65 years who received Social Security. The singling out of this relatively small patient population was due in no small part to extensive lobbying by individuals afflicted with kidney failure, national patient organizations, interested physicians, and dialysis and transplant units throughout the country trying frantically to finance their operations.

The law was created just in time. In 1967 about 5,000 patients in the United States were known to have died of chronic uremia. By 1973, 24,000 people diagnosed with renal failure who otherwise could have received treatment died for lack of facilities. But as a result of the support afforded by Medicare, the number of persons identified as requiring treatment accelerated far beyond the expectations of the original planners. Currently over 300,000 patients are on chronic dialysis—about half of whom are waiting, realistically or not, for kidneys.[12] The average annual cost to sustain each individual is more than $50,000. As the number of kidney transplants remains relatively stable at about 13,000 per year, most patients will remain on dialysis. The expense of treatment for all with end-stage renal disease, including those on dialysis and following transplantation, today is roughly $18 billion, with the federal government paying 75 percent. By 2010, about 600,000 individuals are expected to require renal support, with the necessity for a proportionate increase in funds. Worldwide, the numbers and the costs become staggering.

Difficulties in caring for this ever-enlarging patient population continue to broaden, particularly as the transplants performed annually constitute only a relatively small portion of the whole. As might be expected perhaps, with the availability of federal money for maintenance support of renal failure over the long term has come increasing commercialization of dialysis and entrepreneurial interest in the monetary possibilities of a life-sustaining, device-driven business enterprise. As technology has improved and manufacture of machines and disposables burgeoned, there has been a coincident rush to open new units, not infrequently owned by doctors encouraged to enter the field for its professional and financial opportunities.[13] Indeed, the evolution of dialysis was the first example of a now-common phenomenon, the increasingly close relationship between hospitals, medical schools, and industry. At the same time rapid movement took place toward both private and public providership—almost ownership—of the patient population and the income it generated.

An unbecoming aspect of this increasingly bleak picture has been the specter of "turf wars over the control of the uremic patient."[14] In the best units, surgeons and physicians have worked together for the benefit of the sick. In others, surgeons have competed with physicians controlling dialysis who refer only the sickest patients for transplantation as an often irreversible answer to an insoluble problem. Although countries with centralized health systems have experienced fewer of these entrepreneurial machinations, some have developed their own solutions to controlling the considerable cost of the new technologies by not offering treatment alternatives if a patient is too old or has a serious concurrent disease.

Many published reports throughout the 1970s compared the two modalities, emphasizing that the results of transplantation were considerably less satisfactory than those of dialysis. It took years for a more cooperative relationship to evolve between specialists toward comprehensive therapy of those with end-stage renal disease and their increasingly recognized physiological complexities. The modern multidisciplinary team has been the result, with its global approach to these difficult patients. But even now, controversy persists regarding cost cutting, reuse of dialyzers, safety issues, decreasing numbers of physicians and nurses to care for patients, and lack of oversight of the entire effort. Although dialysis sustains many individuals with an otherwise fatal chronic disease, the existence it provides is often difficult. The population is growing progressively older; the mean age of dialysis patients in the United States is presently over 60 years, compared to a preponderance of individuals in their 20s and 30s in the earlier experience. As older patients often have comorbid conditions such as arteriosclerosis, hypertension, or diabetes, not only is the quality of their lives problematic, but their overall rate of death is more than 15 percent annually.

One poignant reminder of a present and future supported by a machine was written by a patient in 1971.

The Travenol salesman wears glasses and a dark suit:
"Do you
Take this Machine
In sickness and in health
Till death do you part?"
I do.
Reclining
On the nausea-green hospital chair:
Below me children, playing in the street;
Above me old men, dying of coronaries.
I am
The final essence of the technological age,
Flesh conjoined with plastic, vessels with steel,
Coils, alarms, twisted tubing turning scarlet
Deep within the machine dark blood
Mixing with fluid, cellophane-separated, plugged in and turned on.
"Dear God
Purify me."[15]

Although dialysis machines keep people alive, other machines defer the moment of death to allow retrieval of functioning organs for transplantation. Whereas the first sustain life and hope, the second are called upon when hope is lost. While those who die are buried, mourned, and missed, few tragedies can be as overwhelming to family and friends as the sudden and unexpected death of a loved one. Regardless of whether it is a parent, spouse, or child, life can never be the same for those who remain. In relatively few cases and if circumstances allow, however, the family can have a feeling of continuity when the spirit of the donor lives on in others.

Acceptance of the state of brain death has been a departure from established concepts about the end of life. The patient usually looks normal. Only the action of a respirator gives a clue to the gravity of the situation. In contrast to cadaver donors, whose hearts have stopped and whose organs no longer have a blood supply, those with brain death provide healthy and well-perfused tissue for transplantation. The following remembrances of the wife of a donor summarize the emotions faced by family members caught in the tragic but potentially redeeming circumstances of organ donation.

"Suzanne, I just saw a program on organ donation the other night and it moved me so that I want you to promise me if I die you will donate my organs!" At that time all I could think of was that my handsome, healthy, and young husband was out of his mind. Why was he torturing me with thoughts of his death and the unthinkable task of donating his organs? What about my feelings in the matter? Oh well, I thought, it's important to him so I'll agree in order to end this disconcerting discussion.

"Mrs. Aiken, you are needed at the hospital. Your husband is in full respiratory arrest and you must come immediately . . . We are sorry, Mrs. Aiken, but your husband is dead. We did all that we could for him . . . It is very difficult to explain to you since he was only 38 years of age. We are all in shock." There I stood looking at the man I loved so dearly, wondering what in the world was happening. He can't be dead, we are about to have our third child in thirteen days! Open your eyes, David, look at me! How will I tell my girls their father is dead? What in God's name do I do first? . . . After my farewell, preparing to leave the hospital, I remembered my promise. I frantically called for a nurse to ask how to fulfill what my husband had so strongly urged me to do . . . I was reassured that it was not too late to grant what would be David's last and most important request, and that I would be contacted later that day. "Mrs Aiken, this is Mike from the New England Organ Bank. We are so sorry for your loss and do not wish to disturb you at this difficult time, but we must if we are to help you. We will be as brief and respectful as possible. We are grateful for the gift that you are giving to others in great need of donations." I was struck by his sincerity. He was efficient with the tedious information that had to be dealt with. He was kind and I know he was grateful. David would have liked him. David was sincere.[16]

For millennia, the idea of death and the mystique surrounding it varied little, not only among individuals but across populations, cultures, and religions. Primitive man considered the condition to be a kind of deep sleep, an inexplicable transition from one state to another. The fear and superstition it engendered were controlled, dissipated, and tempered by ritual. The individual was assisted on his journey to the next world. The Greeks and then the Romans described the barrier that the dead must cross from the land of the living by personifying Charon the boatman ferrying the departed across the river Styx; the journey was paid for by coins placed on the eyes as the body was prepared. Later Christian writers took up the theme: Dante portrayed it graphically in the *Inferno*, Milton in *Paradise Lost*. In the nineteenth century, Tennyson recapitulated these events in *Crossing the Bar*. More recently, C. S. Lewis characterized the journey by bus from a Hell-like place to Heaven in *The Great Divorce*. Such traditions continue in contemporary Western culture. Most common is the simple service in church, synagogue, or funeral home during which the dead person is mourned and remembered. The other extreme occurs in state funerals, with plumed black horses pulling the caisson on which the body lies. One remembers the funerals of John F. Kennedy in 1963 and Winston Churchill in 1965, and the panoply surrounding the 1998 farewell to Princess Diana.

Burial, a Paleolithic rite centering around the placement of the corpse into the ground and its removal from the sight of man, was initially conceived as a means to achieve closeness to the Earth Mother. In some cultures, bodies were buried upright in the fetal position; in others, the arms of the dead were bound to prevent their return to earth to do harm. Interment in more formal tombs depended on how important or powerful the individual had been in life. Huge monuments were created in older civilizations, most obviously those of the Egyptians and Incas. The elaborately mummified body was placed in these structures, surrounded by possessions and treasures to ease the journey into the next world. The artifacts found in the elaborate memorials of those from such cultures are sought increasingly by archaeologists and, regrettably, looters. Terra-cotta armies of horses, chariots, and foot soldiers guard long-dead emperors in Xian and other ancient cities in China. The early Christians included crucifixes in the coffin. In medieval times the Eucharist was added. Rulers, statesmen, ecclesiastics, and other personages of note are portrayed in elaborate marble effigies in churches and cathedrals, or lie in stately sarcophagi. Cemeteries, gravestones, and mausoleums are common in modern societies. The tradition continues even in "godless" states: Lenin remains entombed grandly in Red Square in Moscow; Mao lies in splendor in Tienanmen Square in Beijing.

The ability to diagnose death reliably was debated for centuries. For a time, putrefaction was considered the ultimate determinant until the presence of local gangrene made even this interpretation insufficient. The "death watch" became important as physicians and others attending appreciated increasingly that life did not always end abruptly but sometimes ebbed inexorably over time.[17] The eighteenth century, an age of quackery and medical incompetence, saw tales of corpses awakening during their funerals or after burial. These, in turn, were fueled by rumors of exhumed bodies found to have clawed the lids of their coffins. In the mid-nineteenth century Edgar Allan Poe enumerated several such instances in his story *The Premature Burial*, while later Mark Twain noted that morgue attendants had attached a bell by a string tied to the finger of the deceased, in case he awoke.

The inability to differentiate actual death from deep coma following stroke, head injury, or epilepsy continued to cloud the issue. The invention of the stethoscope in 1819 finally allowed physicians to detect cardiac or pulmonary activity. With this diagnostic tool, most people accepted that when respiration and heartbeat ended, all parts of the body including the brain ceased to function. The heart was the central organ: when its motion stopped, life was finished.

As technology that could support the end of life advanced in the twentieth century, however, the very concept of death became increasingly complex, both physically and philosophically. Two trends changed accepted beliefs: first, mechanical innovations could sustain cardiopulmonary function in severely afflicted individuals; second, the need for viable organs for transplantation forced reconsideration of the issue of death. Support of the respiratory abilities of those in coma or near death had a long history, perhaps beginning in the Renaissance with Vesalius. "But that life may . . . be restored to the animal (a sow), an opening must be attempted . . . in the trachea into which a tube of reed or cane should be put; you will then blow into this, so that the lung may rise again and the animal take in air." In the eighteenth century, mouth-to-mouth resuscitation was described, then various external breathing machines produced. Apparatuses introduced in the United States and Denmark in the early 1930s allowed paralyzed polio victims to breathe. Applying the principle of external negative pressure ventilation, the "iron lung" saved large numbers of patients.[18]

These devices became obsolete during the 1951–1953 polio epidemics, when positive pressure ventilation could be transmitted to the lungs directly via a cuffed tube placed in the trachea through the mouth or by a tracheostomy. This newer arrangement provided effective extended support of those in respiratory failure. Two kinds of ventilators became available: pressure-limited devices tripped or assisted by the patient, and volume-regulated respirators that controlled the breathing rate of heavily sedated, anesthetized, or paralyzed individuals. The latter machines could also mediate the respiration of patients with irreparable brain injury who were unable to breathe.

At about the same time, pacemakers to regulate the heart rate were becoming available. Means of defibrillation were devised. The introduction of ways to analyze oxygen and carbon dioxide levels in the blood, and increasing knowledge of blood chemistry, improved the metabolic care of complex patients. Although its diagnostic capability was much debated, the electroencephalogram (EEG) enhanced the ability of clinicians to diagnose the extent of brain activity or injury— or even, it was suggested, to define the limits of life. Cessation of all electrical activity by EEG, "cerebral silence," was taken by many as death both of brain and of patient, with increasing numbers of scientists beginning to agree "that the personal and social meaning of the word 'death' applied to irreversible brain death regardless of the state of other tissues or organs." The development of cerebral angiography allowed physicians to confirm readily the absence of blood flow to the brain.[19]

While these technical advances opened new avenues for maintenance of severely ill patients in intensive care settings, they also provoked difficult philosophical questions relating ultimately to the transplantation of organs. Asked in 1958 by a group of anesthesiologists for guidance on the ethics of prolonging life by medical means, Pope Pius XII concluded that although vital functions of a deeply unconscious patient may be maintained over time by artificial life support, the declaration of death must be left to the physician. It was not, he noted, "within the competence of the Church" to define death. What he made clear was that the interests of the individual and the family were paramount, and that opportunities for research or benefits to other patients should not be considered.[20] Contradictory versions of the statement were published widely. The true definition of death continued to be debated by professionals and public alike.

The brain-dead cadaver donor has become virtually the linchpin of modern transplantation, without which the field would hardly exist. Indeed, brain death probably would not have become an issue if a need for organs had not arisen. Brain death was not, however, a new idea. In 1800 the French anatomist M. F. X. Bichat had emphasized the dynamics of death by describing "vegetative functions of life which stopped at the very moment of brain death and organic functions of life which persisted for a longer period of time." Not until 1959 was the subject again raised by several French neurophysiologists who depicted "coma dépassé," a state of irreversible coma.[21] Although the French studies were not generally familiar to English-speaking physicians, discussion of the subject expanded, particularly among those in the United States who required organs for transplantation.

The concept of death as a continuum rather than a discrete event became increasingly considered. While a dialogue between neurologists, neurophysiologists, legal scholars, and surgeons held relatively early in the transplant experience did much to solidify the various points of view of brain death, as well as to open debate about legal access to the body, many in the field continued to question the wisdom of considering brain-dead patients as organ donors. In discussing such a case in 1963, Roy Calne noted: "Although . . . criteria [of brain death] are medically persuasive, according to traditional definitions of death, he [Calne was referring to Guy Alexandre, the Belgian surgeon who first transplanted a kidney from a heart-beating, brain-dead donor] is, in fact, removing kidneys from live donors. I feel that if a patient has a heartbeat he cannot be regarded as a cadaver. Any modification of the means of diagnosing death to facilitate transplantation will cause the whole procedure to fall into disrepute."[22]

As usual, practical considerations outpaced philosophy. Surgeons in Belgium and France demonstrated unequivocally that the quality of kidneys from "heart-beating" cadavers compared favorably with those from living donors. A 1965 U.S. law stated that removal of organs from these donors was allowed as long as the closest relatives had given permission. A later act mandated that all brain function had to cease before death could be declared. Donations of this type were officially authorized in France. In Britain, opposition to kidney removal until after the heart had stopped remained strong until 1976, when the concept of brain death became accepted.

In December 1967 Christiaan Barnard, a surgeon in Cape Town, transplanted the heart of a young woman with a massive and irreversible head injury to a patient with terminal cardiac failure. The worldwide publicity surrounding this event pushed the donor issue to the forefront and caused many to rethink their beliefs about death and to consider the state of brain death for the first time. "Almost overnight, the organs of the irreversibly comatose had become targets for procurement." Indeed, beneath all the enthusiasm and media frenzy concerning Barnard's operation lay public skepticism about the ethics of the procedure, mistrust of the autonomy of the medical profession, doubt about the use of patients in irreversible coma as donors, and even more primitive fears of premature burial. The widely quoted comment "You're dead when your doctor says you are" summarized the public ambivalence.[23]

As a response to these pressures, the dean of Harvard Medical School quickly formed an ad hoc committee to define "irreversible coma." The members included an anesthesiologist/ethicist, a neurologist, a physiologist, a lawyer, a psychiatrist, a theologian, and a transplant surgeon and physician. A crucial reason for such careful definition of the condition was that "obsolete criteria for the definition of death can lead to controversy in obtaining organs for transplantation." The chairman elaborated further: "One can distill two major conclusions. The first is that it is clear beyond question that a time comes when it is no longer appropriate to continue extraordinary means of support for the hopelessly unconscious patient. Pope Pius XII spelled this out. Secondly, a strong case can be made that society can ill afford to discard the tissues and organs of hopelessly unconscious patients so greatly needed for study and experimental trial to help those who can be salvaged. This can come about only with the prior concurrence of those involved, the agreement of society and finally approval in law."[24]

Although the use of organs from brain-dead patients has become routine in most Western countries, the subject continues to make many people uncomfortable. Nonacceptance of the concept in several societies has forced many afflicted with end-state renal disease to buy organs from living donors in other countries. In 1980 an adverse report on brain death, aired on the British television program *Panorama*, reported four anecdotal and totally inaccurate cases of "brain death" in North America, from which each patient reputedly recovered. In retrospect, none of the accepted criteria for the condition were fulfilled. However, the audience did not know this, and no retraction was ever aired. The rate of cadaver organ donation in the United Kingdom therefore fell by 50 percent during the next six to nine months. The transplant surgeons interviewed on the program received hate mail, often from nephrologists in dialysis centers.

The marked decline in the numbers of donors following this and subsequent "exposés" in other countries attests to the fragility of the donation effort. True definition of the time of death has resulted in occasional court cases and has even led to the prosecution of a few surgeons for murder; in fact, between 1984 and 1991 eight medical teams remained under investigation for kidney and pancreas transplants they had performed. Although legal in Japan since 1996, cadaver donors are rarely used. And it continues. In 1997 a popular news program, *Sixty Minutes*, presented a piece entitled "Not Quite Dead," which charged that patients in a major medical center in the United States were being killed for their organs. As allegations are inevitably more sensational than rebuttals, the program was hardly advantageous to the transplant effort. Occasional popular books such as Robin Cook's *Coma* (and the film based on it) have provoked nervous laughter among those involved in organ transplantation and the public. Even those who routinely remove organs from brain-dead patients must overcome an inherent sense of disquiet that does not abate over time.

The necessity to use organs from the dead to save the living must supersede any emotional feelings a surgeon and his or her team may have about the circumstances surrounding individual donors. All of us who deal with such matters sometimes recall our sad professional experiences more vividly than our successes. The often tragic memories of individual organ donors remain particularly vivid. Some whose organs I transplanted especially stay in my mind, tempered by acknowledgment of the remarkable sacrifice they made unknowingly and their families made unselfishly and deliberately. I remember grafting a kidney from a young woman who died unexpectedly from a brain hemorrhage, leaving behind her husband and young children. I used an organ from the talented son of a distinguished politician who had been killed by a drunk driver, and that of an elderly male dying after a massive stroke; his kidney, by serendipity, went to his own son waiting on dialysis. Very young donors in particular endure in my consciousness. One boy, playing Tarzan with a rope in a tree, accidentally hanged himself. Another was strangled in his own garden by his two dogs playing tug-of-war with his scarf. Despite these heartbreaking tragedies, and the professional ambivalence that sometimes accompanies them, these donors provide the means that allow others to live. But the ghosts remain.

8

New Departures

THE TRIUMPHS OF RENAL TRANSPLANTATION OF identical twins and the occasionally successful forays into immuno-suppression encouraged a few surgical enthusiasts to consider replacing other abdominal viscera such as the liver, the pancreas, and even the small bowel. However, transplantation of organs in the chest—particularly that most symbolic of structures, the heart—generated the greatest excitement. The perception of the heart as the site of the more tender emotions, as the center of spirituality, as a vital force and a mystical place where noble sentiments are retained, has been invoked throughout the ages in poetry, literature, and the arts. The ancients conceptualized it as the seat of the soul. Entire lexicons built around it were tinged with the most intense human feelings and included *heart-ache, heartbroken, heartfelt, bleeding heart, tenderhearted, heartless, heartsick, heart of a lion*. Hippocrates and Aristotle believed it to be the center of intelligence, although Galen disagreed because gladiators often maintained their mental faculties during the hours they endured an ultimately fatal cardiac wound. The hearts of heroes and of saints were sometimes buried separately or enshrined more visibly than other remains. Sushruta long ago stated that the hearts of individuals killed by poison did not burn, a concept that passed into later Roman thinking. Indeed, in a more modern context, as the body of the drowned poet Shelley was cremated on a beach in Italy, his undamaged heart was plucked from the ashes and presented to his wife.[1] More than any other organ in the body, the heart has symbolized the traits and character of personhood.

With this emotive overlay, surgical innovators were loath to exploit their creativity and boldness in operating on the heart, particularly as any tampering was considered to result inevitably in death. The excessive mortality from cardiac wounds had convinced many throughout the ages that injury to the organ would quickly be fatal. This belief was so enduring that those in the learned societies of the late sixteenth century were shaken and perturbed when Ambrose Paré described a man wounded in the heart in a duel who managed to chase his adversary 230 yards before collapsing.[2] Doubts were also raised by later descriptions of myocardial scars in anatomized subjects who had been hanged, proving that the injured muscle could heal.

The challenges of human conflict and violence give impetus to surgical innovation, regardless of the age in which they are raised. Baron Larrey, a principal surgeon of the Napoleonic wars, successfully drained blood under pressure from the pericardium (the sac surrounding the heart) of a French soldier. By the end of the nineteenth century, a cardiac stab wound had been repaired in a patient, a feat possibly based on prior reports of the closure of lacerations in rabbit hearts. Constrictive pericarditis was also relieved surgically, while a French surgeon, with the help of Professor Wilhelm Roentgen's new x-ray technique, removed a bullet adherent to the heart muscle of a young officer. Despite such anecdotes, Theodor Billroth, one of the foremost surgical figures of the time, stated dogmatically in 1882 that no practitioner might "preserve the respect of his colleagues if he would even attempt to suture a heart wound."[3]

As the new century began, few surgeons could summon enthusiasm for operative repair or reconstruction of the human heart, regardless of the occasional excitement engendered by experiments on dogs. But rare clinical reports of operations on the cardiac walls were beginning to garner interest: by 1904 fifty-six cases had been compiled, 40 percent of which recovered.[4] In spite of the general lack of acceptance by most practitioners, awareness was growing that the beating heart could be manipulated surgically and that the heart muscle, the myocardium, could successfully hold sutures. The times were auspicious to take the obvious step from repair of accidental wounds to correction of existing abnormalities.

Advances in surgery of the great vessels of the heart increased before World War II. A variety of congenital anomalies in infants and children were successfully reconstructed, procedures that followed inevitably on progressive improvements in pulmonary operations for tuberculosis, safer anesthesia, the use of blood transfusions, and other adjuncts. Related developments and refinements in patient care broadened the scope of treatment. The new technique of cardiac catheterization provided a comprehensive means to correlate physiological and anatomical abnormalities, to appreciate the significance of pressure across valves, and to document precisely the need for operative intervention. Combat experience increased surgical expertise, particularly the ability to remove pieces of shrapnel from within or near the heart and great vessels of wounded soldiers. Means of exposure of various portions of the organ and approaches to entering its chambers evolved from this experience. By the 1950s, intracardiac defects in children were being closed, and more invasive techniques in adult heart surgery developed with attempts to repair tight or insufficient heart valves. Direct replacement of affected valves was increasingly considered over the following decade. Bypass of blocked coronary arteries evolved, and surgical reconstruction of diseased or deformed hearts became routine.

Few complex cardiac operations can be performed, however, while the heart continues to beat; a still heart in a bloodless field is usually necessary for precise and delicate manipulation. Investigators became convinced that support with an external cardiopulmonary bypass machine, connected to the patient via a major vein and artery, would be necessary to maintain normal circulation of oxygenated blood to the brain and other vital organs after cessation of ventricular function. With the background of direct blood transfusion attempted in the seventeenth century and appreciation of the necessity for the oxygenation of tissues by gas exchange in the lungs in the eighteenth century, the concept of extracorporeal circulation was suggested early in the nineteenth century in France. "If one could substitute for the heart the kind of injection of arterial blood, either naturally, or artificially made, one would succeed in maintaining alive indefinitely any part of the body whatsoever."[5] Charles-Edouard Brown-Séquard, putting aside his investigations into the efficacy of glandular extracts, reversed rigor mortis in the limbs of guillotined criminals by running his own blood through their vessels. German workers later built equipment to nourish isolated organs with venous blood oxygenated outside the body by bubbling the gas into it. Before World War II, Carrel became interested in the cultivation and perfusion of isolated organs via small circulation pumps. The introduction of heparin made such techniques feasible.

In 1953, after two decades of research on extracorporeal circulation, John Gibbon in Philadelphia used his apparatus to close successfully an intra-atrial septal defect in the stopped heart of an 18-year-old girl, a feat he was never able to repeat. In collaboration with his wife, he had worked single-mindedly on his pump oxygenator despite prevailing pessimism about its future among his surgical colleagues. Francis Moore recalls visiting Gibbon to see how the

> Great Machine was coming along . . . We trooped in, 10 or 15 of us, and were asked to take off our shoes and put on rubber boots . . . We were then ushered into the operating room of the Gibbons' laboratory. At that time the pump oxygenator was approximately the size of a grand piano. A small cat, asleep to one side, was the object of all this attention. The cat was connected to the machine by two transparent blood filled plastic tubes . . . The contrast in size between the small cat and the huge machine aroused considerable amusement among the audience. The bulk of the machine was not required for pumping but rather for adding oxygen to the cat's blood and removing the carbon dioxide . . . Watching this complicated procedure, concentrating mostly on the cat, whose heart was about to be completely isolated from its circulation, opened, and then closed, we began to sense that we were not walking on a dry floor. We looked down. We were standing in an inch of blood. "Oh . . . I'm sorry" said Gibbon, "the confounded thing has sprung a leak again," but his machine opened an entirely new era in surgery.[6]

Improvements soon allowed prolonged (up to forty-six minutes) extracorporeal support of dogs, with satisfactory survival. As Thomas Watson happened to be the father-in-law of one of Gibbon's colleagues, the vast resources of his company, IBM, played a significant role in refining the oxygenator. Investigators primarily in the United States, France, and Britain subsequently improved the apparatus to a state in which open-heart surgery became reality.

Although Christiaan Barnard's dramatic surgical feat in South Africa burst on the world in December 1967, experimental efforts toward the possibility of heart transplantation had been under way for several years, based on even earlier work. Alexis Carrel and Charles Guthrie transplanted hearts to the neck vessels of canine recipients in 1905. Comparable studies in the 1930s showed that the organs transferred between dogs could quickly regain ventricular function once their blood supply had been reestablished. Such grafts functioned for only about four days, however, before they became swollen and filled with host white blood cells. They were thought to have failed because of "some biologic factor which is probably identical to that which prevents survival of other homotransplanted tissues and organs." While research groups during the 1950s examined physiological, metabolic, and pathological changes developing in hearts transplanted to the neck of other animals, a few investigators began to move the isolated organ into the chest of the recipient to study its function in its normal location. In an extensive series of experiments, the Russian surgeon V. P. Demikhov developed methods to graft a donor heart in parallel with the native heart, eventually showing that the auxiliary organ could supply the entire canine circulation.[7] Within a few years, workers in the United States, Europe, and India, among others, achieved similar results.

Interest in the subject remained sporadic, however, until Norman Shumway began to examine methods to protect the myocardium following his arrival at Stanford in the late 1950s. While training in surgery at the University of Minnesota, he had become interested in ongoing studies to improve heart-lung bypass techniques and on the effect of cold on cardiac muscle. In his Stanford laboratory he refined methods of myocardial preservation and simplified the pump-lung apparatus for both clinical and laboratory use. Shumway and Richard Lower, a surgical resident, began to examine "topical hypothermia," in which the stopped hearts of animals sustained on bypass were cooled by local application of cold saline or ice, preserved as long as seven hours, and allowed to recover.[8] Although perhaps not verbalized at the time, such studies also suggested strongly that cessation of heartbeat was not synonymous with the end of life.

The investigators considered what coincidental projects they might undertake. Lower began to remove the cooled heart and replace it in its normal location as an orthotopic autotransplant, arriving at a relatively simple technique by which a cuff of both left and right atria was retained in the recipient animal. Thus, instead of the ends of the donor and recipient vena cavae and pulmonary veins being joined separately with six different suture lines, it was only necessary to sew the muscular walls of the two atria, then the pulmonary artery and aorta in sequence. Within a year, the two men had successfully used this method to transplant a heart allograft into a dog, the first of several such experiments.

These procedures generated little interest among their colleagues, as noted by Shumway when commenting on Lower's presentation at a surgical meeting in October 1961. "When Lower and I presented our first heart transplant results in the dog to a very important Congress, there was nobody in the room . . . except me listening to Lower speaking from the rostrum and the projectionist behind his slide projector. Even the Chairman had left his chair." The researchers persisted, and in a series of subsequent reports they described the two-year survival of animals whose hearts had been autotransplanted. They noted that the cardiac rhythm was normal, the organs had become reinnervated, and that physiological functions, at least those of the right side, were unremarkable.[9]

By 1965 Shumway and Lower were able to suppress acute rejection of cardiac allografts with a combination of 6-mercaptopurine (6-MP), azathioprine, and prednisone, showing also that decreasing voltage on electrocardiogram was a reliable means to identify rejection.[10] They subsequently reported that twenty-nine of thirty-two dogs recovered from the operation, and that one immunosuppressed recipient remained healthy after eight months. Other long-term animals, however, developed fatal blockage of their coronary vessels, a manifestation of the unanticipated phenomenon of chronic rejection. This process of gradual arterial closure, now termed graft arteriosclerosis, remains the critical unsolved problem in cardiac transplantation.

Overall, evidence that the heart could be effectively transplanted was compelling. The investigators hoped that this relatively simple muscular pump would be less immunogenic and less prone to rejection than other physiologically more complicated organs, thereby reducing the need for a suitable match between donor and recipient. Shumway discussed such expectations in broad terms: "[The heart is] a far less complex tissue than either skin or kidney and perhaps therefore less antigenic. Also, the heart is a large dose of antigen and conceivably could force an antigen-antibody stalemate. Finally, teleologically, perhaps the animal would be reluctant to shed such a vital foreign tissue!"[11] None of these conjectures turned out to be true.

With the expansion of information about heart transplantation in experimental animals, a few cardiac surgeons were quietly preparing to try in humans. James Hardy and his colleagues at the University of Mississippi had been perfecting the technique in large animals and in human cadavers for several years. In January 1964 they accepted a 68-year-old patient with generalized arteriosclerosis and terminal and irreversible heart failure as an appropriate recipient. At the same time, the family of a young man dying of incurable brain disease agreed to donate his heart after death. As the donor lingered, the failing patient was placed on cardiopulmonary bypass to keep him alive. In desperation, Hardy and his team substituted the heart of a chimpanzee from the laboratory, perhaps encouraged by the surprisingly successful results of two kidney transplants carried out between this primate species and humans in New Orleans the month before. Unfortunately, because of the relatively small size of the animal's heart, it was only able to sustain the larger host for twenty-four hours.

Others too—including Shumway at Stanford, Lower (now with Hume in Richmond), and Adrian Kantrowitz in Brooklyn—felt ready to move to human patients. All were completely surprised by the news from South Africa. Christiaan Barnard had quietly prepared himself by spending two years at the University of Minnesota examining the possibilities of open-heart surgery using cardiopulmonary bypass and developing a prosthetic aortic valve. In 1967 he was an observer in Hume's kidney transplant unit for three months, and also watched Lower perform a cardiac transplant in a dog. He then went to Denver to learn about antilymphocyte serum as an immunosuppressant. Returning to Cape Town, he started the first open-heart program on the African continent and later opened a renal transplant unit as preparation for his cardiac patients, grafting a single kidney.[12]

In the planning for a heart transplant, requirements for declaration of death had to be considered and criteria for the suitability of both donor and recipient established to the satisfaction of the hospital administration. Barnard had accrued extensive clinical experience with open-heart procedures and experimental expertise with cardiac transplantation in baboons, the most common laboratory animal in South Africa. He and his team were ready on December 2, 1967, when a potential donor was admitted: a 25-year-old woman struck by an automobile and sustaining irreversible head injury. Although her heart continued to beat, she was declared dead by the neurosurgeon. The donor team waited for cardiac arrest to occur before she was placed on bypass to cool her heart before removal. The recipient, Louis Washkansky, a 53-year-old diabetic with progressive and irreversible cardiac insufficiency from previous heart attacks, was prepared for transplantation in an adjacent operating room. Within two hours, Barnard and his team completed the procedure. The new heart functioned quickly and supported its host.

And support him it did. Within twenty-four hours the previously moribund patient was talking. By two days his heart failure had disappeared (Figure 8.1). By eleven days he was out of bed. He was treated with local radiation to the new organ and with azathioprine and maintenance corticosteroids, standard immunosuppression at the time. For a rejection episode on day 9, his steroid dose was increased and an additional cytotoxic agent administered. Unhappily, fatal pneumonia supervened on day 18 as his white blood cell count plummeted. Despite his death, his course did much to stimulate future events in this intriguing field. The surgery took place only thirteen years after the first identical-twin kidney transplant and seven years after the initial use of chemical immunosuppression.

Within days, four more heart transplants were performed.[13] Indeed, Adrian Kantrowitz had almost scooped the South Africans. By the summer of 1966, he had gained hospital agreement to use an anencephalic baby as a donor; these infants, born lacking much of their brain, do not survive. The opportunity for transplantation soon presented itself. Parental permission for both donor and recipient were in place. Everything was ready. But because of last-minute objections on the part of the anesthesiologist toward removing a beating heart from the donor, the team had to wait until cardiac arrest occurred. The organ became unusable, and the transplant was canceled. The child who was to receive the heart died within weeks.

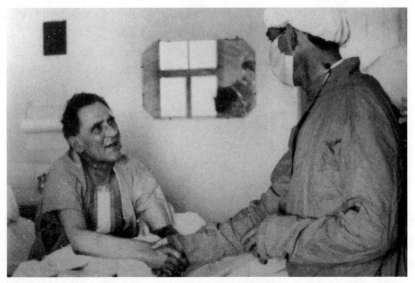

Figure 8.1 Louis Washkansky, Christiaan Barnard's first heart-transplant recipient in 1967 (P. I. Terasaki, with permission)

By late 1967, preparations for another transplant were under way. Five days after Barnard's operation on Washkansky, Kantrowitz performed the world's second transplant, grafting the heart of an anencephalic donor to a 17-day-old baby with severe congenital heart defects. The infant died a few hours later.

Barnard then carried out his second, the world's third, heart transplant on January 3, 1968, placing the heart of a 24-year-old "mixed blood" male into a 58-year-old white dentist, Philip Blaiberg—a racial combination that was to provoke political and ethical discussions, not only in apartheid South Africa but throughout the world.

Within a few days, Norman Shumway, who had laid so much of the groundwork for the procedure, performed his first heart transplant on patient Mike Kasperak. Perhaps as a premonition of discussions to come, the complex care of this individual included four operations and 210 units of blood at a cost of nearly $30,000. He survived only two weeks. During the same month, Kantrowitz transplanted a heart into a 57-year-old male, Louis Bloch, who died a few hours later.

Although Barnard was not one to shun attention, no one anywhere was prepared for the explosion of public interest generated by his first procedure and those that followed. Carrel, Lawler, Murray, and others had experienced blazing headlines and editorials, the comments of ecstatic radio personalities, and the hyperbole of television news-casters. Yet the outpouring of enthusiasm engendered by the first hu-man heart transplant was unprecedented. Barnard, an attractive and articulate figure, became highly visible. He was interviewed every-where and traveled from continent to continent for speeches and hon-ors, as interest in his case catapulted the subject to unrealistic heights. His success evoked serious animosity toward him from those Ameri-can surgeons who had lost the race; they felt that they had done much of the preparation and should have received more credit for their efforts. As Shumway allegedly answered a colleague who asked him for his reaction to Barnard's transplant, "Does anyone know who was the second person to fly across the ocean?"

Obviously, excessive media dissection does medicine and science little service. Distortion of the facts, false hopes, and overinterpreta-tion of difficult and incomplete data can be the only result. The "hype" has continued to accelerate in recent years, as constant reporting of new "cures" and "breakthroughs" emblazon the pages of our news-papers and the screens of our television sets.

A brief but frenetic period of clinical activity now began, apparently driven by a combination of intense publicity, surgical machismo, and national chauvinism. It brought little credit to those in the field. Fol-lowing the next heart transplant in France in April 1968, the first in Europe, the floodgates opened. The public was besieged by reports of patients from centers as geographically disparate as Sidney, Sapporo, Houston, Cleveland, Pittsburgh, Montreal, São Paulo, and Leningrad. Even Britain succumbed to the atmosphere. One of my surgical col-leagues, in London at the time the heart donor was conveyed to the hospital where the first British recipient waited, recalls the scene viv-idly: "I remember the whole ghastly triumphalist charade. The press had been tipped off by one of the physicians involved. The donor was to be brought to the National Heart Hospital by ambulance. The paparazzi set up their tripods. Someone shouted 'Roll' and the am-bulance appeared preceded by a Daimler owned by one of the team. The procession moved rather slowly and with decorum appropriate to this new national milestone, watched by mystified but enthusiastic crowds. Thirty-four years later, I think I can see good humored police holding back the exuberant spectators." Francis Moore, present at the time, described the mood following this heart transplant: "The surgeons, in full operating regalia, appeared on the steps of one of the London teaching hospitals to the shouts of cheering crowds, bands playing 'Britannia Rules the Waves' and 'God Save the Queen' with the waving of flags, guardsmen in bearskin busbies hovering around on horseback. British reserve was cast into those waves that Britannia rules."[14]

Two important consequences emerged from this extravaganza. First, organ donation, such as it was at that time, virtually stopped because the public took offense at the hullabaloo. Second, a group of transplant surgeons and physicians advised the British government that intact donors should never again be transported to the recipient hospital.

Only a few surgical investigators in experienced centers appreciated the biologic intricacies of transplantation. The majority of the cardiac surgeons climbing on the bandwagon were unschooled on immunosuppression and ignorant of the responses of the host immune system that become activated against a vascularized foreign graft. They thought their technical abilities and expertise could transcend such theoretical matters. Lacking laboratory experience or background, many joined the race to demonstrate that they, their institutions, and even their countries had scientific and clinical resources comparable to those of the leaders. Before satisfactory preservation techniques were available, potential recipients were relocated to the donor hospital to ensure optimal freshness of the organ to be transplanted. One potential kidney donor arrived at the Brigham in this manner. As doubt was voiced about his neurological status, he remained in the intensive care unit overnight. The next morning, to the embarrassment of some and the undisguised delight of others, he was found sitting up in bed reading the *New York Times*. No comparable donor was ever again considered, sight unseen. Alternatively, private or chartered airplanes ferried the isolated donor heart to the waiting recipient.

By the end of 1968, this "year of the transplant," 102 such procedures had been performed, 26 in November alone and over half in the United States. Within two years, 64 additional teams in 22 countries had joined the bandwagon—54 of which carried out three or fewer such operations, 38 performing only one.[15]

Several new adventures were also forthcoming, enlivened by continuing media excitement and possibly leavened, at least in the United States, by the optimism engendered by the first person to orbit the moon. In contrast to the continuing national crises, disruptions, and self-doubts of that period, apparently positive medical "miracles" caught the public interest and improved its mood. The highly experienced Houston cardiac surgeon Denton Cooley placed a sheep heart into a patient, also grafting a second heart into an individual who had rejected her first. The kidneys, the heart, and part of a lung from the first multiorgan donor were transplanted into three recipients, again in Houston. Cooley performed his first heart-lung transplant. Thomas Starzl in Denver grafted a heart and a kidney into the same recipient.

Still, there were legal troubles. In Cape Town, a heart was removed from a black donor, apparently without permission. In Richmond, Richard Lower was exonerated of a charge of murder after using the heart of a young man dying from severe head injury; it was the first time a jury had been asked to consider brain death as a legal definition of the end of life. In Sapporo, a similar accusation was lodged against an eminent Japanese professor; because of the sustained public outcry, his heart transplant in August 1968 until recently remained the only such operation ever carried out in that country.

By the close of the year, hard lessons had been learned. Only a handful of the recipients transplanted worldwide survived more than six months. Although more patients were doing well over the short term, it was becoming evident that many were dying from coronary artery disease of their grafts, which progressed far more rapidly than the arteriosclerosis in their native vessels. As a result, the Montreal Heart Institute in early 1969 announced a moratorium on further transplants until the mortality rate could be improved. The lead surgeon, Pierre Grondin, had compiled an enviable record. At six months, seven of nine patients were ambulatory; all but one had survived more than thirty days after operation. Initially opposed to stopping his program, he became increasingly persuaded as he watched the recipients die one by one of coronary insufficiency.

As news of the moratorium spread, those associated with heart transplantation became polarized. At a conference in the United States a week later, a prominent cardiac surgeon declared a halt to his small transplant program, decrying "the time, the effort and the money used for a handful of patients and the unrelenting and harmful publicity the subject was receiving."[16] Many agreed. But vehement dissenters cited the remarkable success of the living patients and noted, not unreasonably, that knowledge could only accrue with further experience. Indeed, almost lost in the gloom was the fact that several individuals continued to thrive, including Philip Blaiberg in South Africa (he was to live nineteen months before dying of coronary artery insufficiency), Father Boulogne in Paris (who would live fifteen months), Louis Russell in Richmond (more than six years), Betty Annick in Milwaukee (nine years), and Emanuel Vitria in Marseille (over eighteen years). Some recipients achieved at least some relative normalcy. Pictures of Blaiberg swimming, for instance, were published widely (Figure 8.2). However, the quality of his life extension was questionable, as described by the physician who had cared for the donor: "He [Blaiberg] was left with considerable disability . . . A syndicated photograph of him lying in the sea happily splashing in the waves appeared in the world's press as testimony to his remarkable recovery . . . [A] distinguished politician . . . had, by chance, taken a stroll along the same beach that day and stumbled on Blaiberg's venture into the sea. He was carried into the water, the entourage stepped back, cameras flashed, and he was hauled out before he disappeared helplessly under the waves."[17]

Although these early results were comparable to those in the original kidney transplant experience, the patients and their surgeons were more visible; the stakes were higher with no fallback to dialysis; and the heart, an enduring object of mysticism, spirituality, and emotionalism, was a more prominent, newsworthy, and dramatic organ.

Representatives from various medical and legal fields and from government and philanthropic organizations soon met at the NIH to discuss the existing state of transplantation. They considered the experience with all organs transplanted up to that point and made several recommendations, including some for the heart. "Cardiac transplantation, still in an early stage of development, shows promise for the

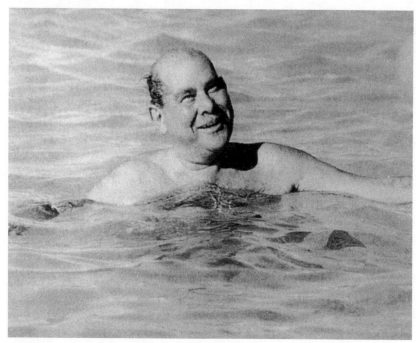

Figure 8.2 Dr. Philip Blaiberg "swimming" after his heart transplant in 1968 (Novartis, with permission)

future treatment of many people with severe heart disease; it should be conducted by surgeons with proven capability in cardiac surgery, physicians experienced in all phases of cardiology, and with the collaboration of persons experienced in immunosuppression and transplantation biology . . . The need for new knowledge from *basic and applied research* for the continued improvement of all transplantation is emphasized." An important member of the committee, less sanguine about what had happened, wrote in an editorial about the "disadvantages in emotional publicity and rush to reckless adventures in heart transplantation efforts by incomplete teams where ambition exceeds multi-disciplinary balance. The recurring theme of heart transplantation 'in the early stage of development . . . and promise' must be limited to a few sophisticated centers with a broad spectrum of capabilities embracing donor selection, heart surgery, and rejection suppression. It should constitute firm restriction to future experimental adventures."[18]

Only Shumway continued to broaden his experience by performing a limited number of heart transplants (Figure 8.3). Through carefully considered laboratory and clinical refinements, his results contrasted strikingly with those of most others who continued. Within a year he had performed twenty-seven transplants; nine of the recipients survived. The next largest unit, in Houston, had no survivors among twenty-three patients. The message that the committee had delivered seemed warranted.

The numbers of heart transplants decreased markedly as realism overcame enthusiasm. The formidable mortality rate permeated public consciousness, and opinions from the same press that had depicted the surgeons as heroes began to disparage their procedures. Following the death of Britain's first recipient at forty-five days, the *Times* noted: "There can be no justification for an operation that carries such a devastatingly high mortality rate and the performance of which is more or less equivalent to a death sentence . . . If the medical profession is not prepared to act itself then Parliament must step in." Many teams were influenced not only by their own dismal results and by increasingly adverse media coverage, but also by the lack of support of prominent physicians and surgeons. An eminent New York cardiologist, for example, decried "the circus trappings and glitter created by the first human transplant," commenting that heart transplanters were treated as heroes "in an international race to be a member of the me-too brigade."[19]

The death of Blaiberg, at that time the world's longest survivor, added to the gloom. The shortage of heart donors accelerated as public opinion shifted. Even the number of potential recipients declined. *Newsweek* summarized the general feeling, describing Cooley's unit in Houston: "Just a few months ago, as many as a dozen desperately sick patients lay in the wards anxiously waiting for heart transplants . . . Last week, not one patient was waiting for a new heart. . . . 'People are choosing to stay at home' says . . . Cooley . . . 'Either they have lost their interest or their courage. And whether it's negativism or loss of confidence, doctors don't refer patients to us.' Everywhere it seems, heart transplant surgeons are beset by distrust and doubt."[20] In fact, Cooley soon stopped his program. By November 1970 cardiac transplantation had ceased throughout the world.

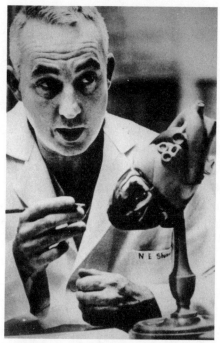

Figure 8.3 Norman Shumway
(Novartis, with permission)

The clinical moratorium provided a pause, the chance to catch a collective breath. The few patients surviving on their new hearts continued to provide hope for the future, but at a huge cost in effort, manpower, and money. Indeed, the entire field seemed receptive to the step it had taken. Roy Calne, setting up a liver transplant program in Britain, requested "more cooperation [within] the profession and a return of the good will and charity of the public toward organ transplantation, which suffered so severely following the unfortunate and often inaccurate publicity surrounding so many of the cardiac transplantation operations."[21]

Beyond the commitment of surgeons to the welfare of their individual patients, and their personal high standards and intense drive, common sense began to prevail. A respite was called until clinical results could catch up with scientific and technical improvements.

At the same time, the public mood was shifting against other societal adventures. More and more voices demanded cessation of the

Vietnam War, the arms race, and the use of nuclear power. Undeniably, the burst of activity with heart transplantation had opened an entirely new avenue of progress. But a delay in the proceedings permitted a more secure foundation for the considerable advances which followed.

The lung, a less conspicuous organ than the heart but equally vital, had long been part of the surgical purview. Allegedly, the oldest operative procedure, referred to repeatedly in the writings of Hippocrates, was thoracentesis, the drainage of fluid, pus, or blood from the chest cavity to the outside. Later Roman physicians used metal cannulae or trocars for the purpose. They also identified the coincident danger of pneumothorax, collapse of a lung by air entering the thoracic cavity, although treatment of this condition was not perfected until World War I. The novel art of percussion and the invention of the stethoscope in the late eighteenth century allowed accurate physical diagnosis of chest disease. While pulmonary function was first measured in the mid-nineteenth century using a spirometer, chest abnormalities could not be precisely diagnosed until x-rays became available. Investigators in London defined bronchopulmonary anatomy in 1889. The inventors of the bronchoscope confirmed their findings a half century later in New York.

Definitive understanding of the anatomy and physiology of the bronchial tree and the lungs themselves emerged during the 1940s. In 1948 in England, new knowledge about the segmental anatomy of the lung allowed limited resections for a variety of pathologic conditions and the eventual transplantation of individual lung segments. The unique double circulation to the organ—the pulmonary artery carrying unoxygenated venous blood from the body via the right side of the heart and the smaller bronchial artery supporting the lung tissue with oxygenated blood—became evident; the importance of the blood supply to the bronchus itself was to be emphasized during the development of lung transplantation.

Always innovative, James Hardy performed the first lung transplant in a human seven months before he grafted the heart of a chimpanzee. In addition to his investigative cardiac work, he and his associates had carried out an extensive series of reimplants and single lung grafts in dogs. Some of their experiments followed those of Carrel;

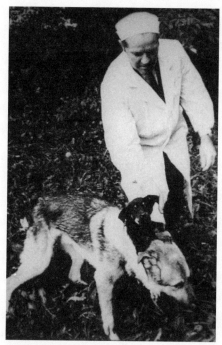

Figure 8.4 The Russian transplant surgeon V. P. Demikhov and his two-headed dog

others continued the work of the indefatigable Demikhov, who had performed numerous lung transplantation experiments in the late 1940s, and transplanted a dog's head to the neck of the recipient (Figure 8.4).[22] Several investigators from Italy, France, and the United States described operative techniques for lung reimplantation and the placement of pulmonary autografts and allografts in primates, dogs, and sheep.

With this background, Hardy and his group refined their surgical approach, devising a reproducible animal model with which they were able to investigate several compelling issues.

1. The effect of division of individual vital structures at the base of the lung on pulmonary function, including the pulmonary artery, pulmonary vein, and bronchus.
2. The importance of lymphatic disruption and regeneration.
3. The ability of the reimplanted or grafted lung to support an animal

whose opposite pulmonary artery had been ligated or the entire opposite organ removed.

4. The effect of storage on function and survival.

5. The influence of immunosuppression on lung allografts.

Although the reimplantation response of all grafted lungs produced dramatic initial physiological changes and functional deterioration, these normalized or at least stabilized within a few days. Autografts continued to improve. In contrast, allograft function deteriorated, as acute rejection intervened despite use of all immunosuppressive strategies available at the time. As confirmed in experimental reports, the allografted lung supported only an occasional dog for prolonged periods; the majority of recipients died within four to five weeks. Transplantation of both lungs in the dog gave even worse results, particularly inasmuch as the bilateral procedure was found to interrupt a nerve reflex essential for respiration. In single lungs such reflexes could be preserved by leaving the nerve supply of the retained native organ intact.

Frank Veith, a surgical investigator in New York, substantially expanded and broadened these observations. He formulated the physiological demands on a new lung, realizing that, like the heart, it must assume full respiratory responsibility from the moment of its placement and continue these functions indefinitely. He and others in the small field improved or corrected persistent technical problems, which included clotting at the atrial suture line, pulmonary artery narrowing, and necrosis of bronchial cells with resultant leakage at the bronchial suture line. He was particularly optimistic about the ultimate clinical potential for lung transplantation, enthusing in a review of the subject: "If kidneys and hearts, why not lungs."[23]

Despite the striking lack of success with experimental animals, the desire to move to patients was stirring. Hardy had carefully established "stringent preset technical and moral criteria for the procedure." These included consideration of patients with irreversible end-stage disease whose life expectancy would not be shortened by lung replacement, and the insistence that no existing functioning pulmonary tissue could be sacrificed.[24] A careful thinker, he had already turned down many potential candidates. Thus, he was ready when John Russell presented himself.

This patient was terminally ill with cancer of his left lung, a respiratory cripple barely able to function. He had been transferred to the hospital from prison, having been sentenced to death for murder some years before. Rejecting the possibilities of radiation, Russell agreed to a lung transplant. Indeed, the possibility that his death sentence could be commuted was raised; the "authorities in the state government . . . indicated that a favorable attitude might be adopted if the patient were to contribute to human progress in this way."[25] In June 1963 he received the left lung of a donor dying of a massive heart attack. The new organ functioned well for seventeen days until Russell developed fatal kidney failure. Under the microscope the grafted lung appeared normal.

This potentially encouraging experience was supported by data from Russian surgeons, who described seven patients with asthma from whom they had removed and reimplanted a lung.[26] Five, including one in whom both lungs were reimplanted, survived. Although not acceptable treatment in the West, the experience proved that lung transplantation was possible and that one or even two lung replacements could support a patient indefinitely.

Surgeons in the United States, Canada, and Europe performed about forty single-lung transplants between Hardy's operation in 1963 and the end of 1980. Not unexpectedly, all recipients died from a series of technical complications, respiratory insufficiency, or infection. However, a single striking success gave hope to those struggling in this difficult field. Fritz Derom, a professor of surgery in Ghent, Belgium, transplanted a single lung into a 23-year-old sandblaster with advanced pulmonary silicosis in late 1968, treating him with azathioprine, prednisolone, and antilymphocyte globulin. Despite two reversible acute rejection episodes, the patient, Alois Vereeken, improved progressively; by three months his new lung had reached 80 percent of normal function. It continued to perform for ten months before he died of pneumonia. At autopsy, the organ showed minimal signs of rejection.[27]

So progress did occur despite the setbacks. The operation was technically feasible. A transplanted lung could function well in a human over both the short term and the relatively long term. Acute rejection episodes could be reversed. Other lessons, however, were less encouraging. The site where the donor and recipient bronchi were joined remained a potential hazard, with cell death, leakage or disruption, narrowing, bleeding, or infection occurring all too commonly. These devastating complications were blamed on several factors, including ischemia of the bronchial stump and the nonhealing effects of the steroids necessary to prevent rejection. As experience slowly broadened, the threat of opportunistic infections—not only bacterial but also from an increasingly recognized virus, cytomegalovirus (CMV)—became ever more prevalent, possibly because a lung, like a bowel allograft, is always open to the outside environment and more at risk from external hazards than truly internal organs. Even with potential resolution of these acute problems, an unexpected and deadly entity occurred over the long term. Bronchiolitis obliterans, characterized by progressive airway obstruction and probably representing a type of chronic rejection, became a major unsolved problem in lung transplantation.

Interest in replacing a single lung revived in the early 1980s, encouraged by introduction of the new immunosuppressive drug Cyclosporin A, and initial successes in heart-lung transplantation. Indications for the procedure became more sharply defined, particularly in patients with fibrosis, emphysema, and chronic obstructive disease, although the advantages for other pulmonary conditions were less obvious. The use of adjunctive cardiopulmonary bypass to facilitate the operation became more widespread. By 1990, 290 cases were listed; patient survival reached 65 percent at one year, 54 percent at two years.[28] At the same time, techniques for double-lung transplants were improving. The 130 cases described were carried out mostly in patients with emphysema or cystic fibrosis. Although transplantation of the lung has progressed at a slower rate than that of other organs and long-term success remains limited, the procedure gives hope to certain individuals with terminal respiratory disease.

The enthusiasm surrounding Barnard's first human heart transplant quickly encouraged three clinical attempts to graft heart and lungs in combination. That this extravagant surgery was even undertaken is interesting in light of the singular lack of success initially with lung allografts. In 1968 Denton Cooley in Houston, ever daring, performed a heart-lung transplant in a 2-month-old baby with severe congenital anomalies. She died after fourteen hours.[29] One year later, surgeons at the University of Minnesota unsuccessfully transplanted heart and lungs into a 43-year-old patient with emphysema, and in 1971 Barnard undertook the third such procedure, grafting the heart and lungs of a black donor into a man of "mixed race," Adrian Herbert. Several complications including necrosis of the bronchus caused Herbert's death within three weeks. The case was clouded by the donor's widow, who claimed that she had not been informed about the removal of her husband's thoracic organs—despite a law in South Africa at the time that allegedly precluded the necessity for such permission.

Experimental precedent for these attempts had been minimal. Carrel's 1907 report of the placement of the heart and lungs of a kitten into the neck of a cat was often quoted. In the 1940s and early 1950s, Demikhov placed donor heart and lungs in parallel with the native organs of unsupported anesthetized dogs, later excluding the host organs. Two of sixty-seven animals lived over five days, with most deaths occurring from pneumonia.[30] A decade later, recipient dogs survived six hours after circulatory arrest and central cooling, an interval improved to twenty-two hours and to six days by 1961 by using a simplified tracheal anastomosis. The subsequent discovery by several groups that the primate, unlike the dog, could maintain normal patterns of respiration despite denervation of both lungs energized research on the subject.

In 1980 Bruce Reitz and his associates at Stanford described thirty-seven Cyclosporin A–treated monkeys with heart-lung transplants who lived for several months, one for several years.[31] These critical experiments established not only the efficacy of the operative technique and the importance of the new agent, but also the fact that recipients of this huge organ complex could survive for indefinite periods. Based on these unprecedented results, Reitz and Shumway quickly performed heart-lung transplants in four patients: one survived for four years, one for three years, and two for two years. These investigators introduced the novel technique of needle biopsy to diagnose cardiac rejection and to detect early rejection of the lung. An intriguing fact which emerged was that the heart and the lungs (like the liver in combination with other abdominal organs) do not always experience rejection at the same rate.

By 1990, 785 heart-lung transplants had been performed world-wide with a one-year survival of 60 percent and a two-year survival of 45 percent, results that have continued to improve in the relatively few transplants carried out annually.[32] Indications for the procedure now are better defined for both adults and children. On the negative side, the unsolved problem of bronchiolitis obliterans continues to lurk.

Related procedures have included a coincident heart-lung and liver transplant by Calne, thoracic plus abdominal multivisceral replacements by Starzl, and the introduction of a "domino" transplant by surgeons at Johns Hopkins, whereby the healthy heart of a heart-lung recipient was transplanted into another needy patient. Although still replete with uncertainties and complications, a combined heart-lung transplant has become a dramatic, often reasonable treatment for selected individuals with end-stage pulmonary disease.

The Dracula of Modern Technology

9

ON GOOD FRIDAY OF 1969 IN HOUSTON, DENTON
Cooley implanted an artificial heart into Haskell Karp, a patient dying
of cardiac failure. After being sustained by the device for sixty-four
hours, he received a heart transplant. The donor was flown by chartered air ambulance from Lawrence, Massachusetts, in response to
a nationwide appeal by Karp's wife on television and radio and in
the newspapers. Her eloquence was striking: "Someone, somewhere,
please hear my plea. A plea for a heart for my husband. I see him lying
there, breathing and knowing that within his chest is a man-made
implement where there should be a God-given heart. How long he can
survive one can only guess. I cry without tears. I wait hopefully. Our
children wait hopefully, and we pray . . . Maybe somewhere there is a
gift of a heart . . . Please."[1] One day after the transplant her husband
died of kidney failure and pneumonia.

The development of the artificial heart involved a complex interplay of
ideas, technologies, and self-aggrandizement on the part of the participants, their colleagues, and their institutions—all tempered with professional and personal competition, feuds, and the eventual destruction of several careers. It must be emphasized, however, that a central
theme running through these often less than appealing events, as
throughout the entire story of transplantation, is that of talented and
imaginative surgeons trying desperately to salvage their dying patients.
At such a climactic moment, rarely encountered by those outside of
medicine, external considerations of philosophy, religion, or societal

187

approval become irrelevant. The surgeon in particular must occasionally make rapid, definitive decisions from which there can be no turning back. Debate about correctness or appropriateness must be left to the future.

In the case of the heart, normal function is so central to the viability of the entire organism that its failure demands urgent and often dramatic attempts at correction. In response to such needs, a few surgical innovators contemplated creating an artificial heart for use in patients. The shift from a theoretical concept to a distinct possibility occurred during the late 1960s in the United States, a period during which arguments about national priorities were frequent and vituperative, and societal aims were questioned and derided. A confused and disenchanted public sought solutions. Expectations were high that technology, one of the country's strengths, would provide answers.

The artificial heart has a relatively long history. German workers had discussed the idea in the nineteenth century. In 1928 English physiologists designed and built a pump to function like an entire heart. Carrel and Lindbergh described a "mechanical heart" in the 1930s, an apparatus that perfused organs via a rotary valve reproducing a pulse. Compressed air drove the pump (Figure 9.1). Having refined it from Carrel's original prototype to preserve organs outside the body, they also considered its ultimate use as an aid for heart surgery. In Russia, Demikhov repeatedly suggested the benefits of an artificial heart.[2] By the end of the 1950s several groups, particularly in France, had mechanically supported the failing hearts of dogs. A balloon, designed to be placed inside the aorta and to inflate and empty with each heartbeat, increased perfusion pressure and blood flow to the coronary arteries and brains of patients with failing hearts. Cardiopulmonary bypass, improving throughout the 1960s, became a routine (albeit temporary) means of circulatory support for open-heart surgical procedures. Because medical and pharmacological solutions to heart failure remained inadequate, left ventricular assist techniques and biventricular bypass devices were introduced and investigated in a variety of large animals, primarily calves and goats, in laboratories in the United States, France, Italy, Argentina, Germany, South Africa, and Japan.

It should be remembered, in discussing these mechanical adjuncts, that the normal functioning heart essentially comprises two separate

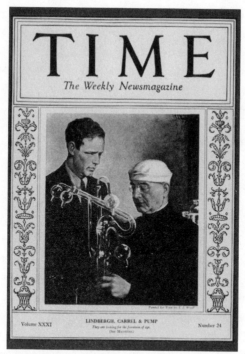

Figure 9.1 Alexis Carrel and Charles Lindbergh with their so-called mechanical heart, *Time*, July 1, 1935 (TimePix, with permission)

pumps. One, the left ventricle, distributes bright red oxygen-rich arterial blood via the aorta to all organs of the body. Cells extract the oxygen to provide them with energy to carry out their various roles. The oxygen-poor blue venous blood leaves the tissues and enters the great veins, which in turn empty into the right side of the heart. The right ventricle then pumps the venous effluent via the pulmonary artery through the lungs where reoxygenation takes place. This "fresh" blood enters the left side of the heart and is again distributed to the rest of the body. Both cycles occur simultaneously with each heartbeat. The mechanical devices considered here are designed to replace one or both of these functions.

In 1962 Michael DeBakey founded a new artificial heart program at the Baylor and Rice Universities Laboratory in Houston. The National Heart Institute (NHI) had awarded a grant of $4.5 million to

DeBakey, one of the pioneers of cardiovascular surgery, chairman of the department of surgery, and president of the Baylor College of Medicine. Among others his team included Domingo Liotta, an experimental surgeon from Argentina experienced in such research. Having produced a left ventricular bypass pump to assist canine circulation transiently until a poorly functioning left ventricle could recover, the investigators used it in 1963 to support their first patient for four days. Within four years, an improved version functioned successfully for ten days in a 37-year-old woman with severe cardiovascular disease, allowing her to recover from her short-term ventricular failure and live normally for several years thereafter.

The team had also attempted to create a biventricular artificial heart as a bridge to further therapy for totally failing hearts. The development of such a device became more urgent with the emergence of heart transplantation late in 1967, and the group soon designed a double-ventricle pump "for study of the control mechanism required for maintaining proper balance of both pulmonary and systemic circulation and adequate cardiac output and perfusion during total mechanical replacement of the heart." Liotta implanted the first such apparatus into a calf in January 1969. Curiously, he had the day before submitted an abstract to be considered for a major scientific conference of the American Society for Artificial Internal Organs, claiming that the artificial heart had successfully sustained ten calves between twenty-four and forty-eight hours. DeBakey, unknowingly listed as one of the five coauthors, did not learn of the abstract until a few days before the meeting was held, three months later. When the devices were eventually placed in seven (not ten) animals, all but one died within a few hours; the remaining calf, surviving for forty-four hours, was "virtually cadaver from time of implantation."[3]

Cooley, one of DeBakey's principal surgical associates, worked in an adjacent hospital. He approached Liotta during this period to collaborate in developing an artificial heart for clinical use.[4] Liotta was enthusiastic but did not tell DeBakey of the proposal. He persuaded the Rice University engineer who had designed the power source for the heart, and whose salary was paid by DeBakey's NHI grant, to build a duplicate machine on the side. Unaware that such a unit was for a human instead of for calves, the engineer agreed to collaborate because of the opportunity to work with Cooley and the chance to refine his instrument relatively inexpensively. Indeed, when he delivered the console to the hospital in early April, he included a note stating that it was untested and should be used only for experimental animals.

Meanwhile Liotta, now acting director of the university laboratory, was assembling several more artificial hearts. Although uneasy at the unfolding events, the technicians assumed that these had been authorized. The next day, the devices were taken to Saint Luke's Episcopal Hospital, where Cooley and Liotta prepared to implant one into a human for the first time. They informed no one, including the cardiopulmonary pump team, of the scheme. As the designated patient, Haskell Karp, opposed a heart transplant, they planned a "myocardial excision with ventriculoplasty," removal of the nonfunctioning cardiac muscle, and repair of the cardiac wall. However, little normal ventricle was seen when his heart was exposed at operation: "an extensive area of fibrous transformation [scarring] of the left ventricle and septum was excised and ventriculoplasty [closure of the ventricle] performed. Attempts at resuscitation of the heart failed, and cardiopulmonary bypass was continued while the heart was removed in the same manner used for cardiac transplantation. The cardiac prosthesis was placed in the pericardial sac after the atrial cuffs and arterial graft were trimmed and tailored to insure proper fit."[5]

The line between use of the artificial heart as an emergency last-stage procedure in a dying patient and as a purposeful event was a fine one. Many colleagues not directly involved felt that the extensive last-minute preparations implied a prearranged plan. In addition, as the numbers of donors were declining significantly because of the poor results of heart transplantation, Karp had no targeted donor until after his wife's nationwide appeal. While his condition had not obviously deteriorated, sometime before surgery he and his wife gave their permission for the placement of an artificial heart, if necessary, in preparation for a transplant. It was inserted nearly three days later.

Priority for the creation of the pump, as well as the funds for its development, became large issues—particularly since the device implanted at Cooley's institution was built in the Baylor laboratories under contract (like Liotta) with DeBakey's federally funded experimental program. At his presentation of the case during a national meeting a few weeks later (for which he received a standing ovation) and in his subsequent publications describing the event, Cooley confirmed that the device he had implanted into Karp had been produced with Liotta under his aegis. He cited similar work by others but barely acknowledged DeBakey's sustained efforts, even though the drawings of the heart prosthesis he presented were virtually identical to those of the Baylor team.[6] He and Liotta later referred to nine calves (in addition to the seven Liotta had already reported) in which they had tested their device, although specific details were never published.

Ironically, DeBakey heard about the operation while at a conference on artificial hearts in Washington, D.C. Eventually, when he published his final paper on the evolution of the biventricular pump, he and his coauthors took the rather unprecedented step of appending a statement to the title page noting that "this is a true and accurate account of the development and testing of the orthotopic cardiac prosthesis."[7] Because of considerations concerning both its priority and its propriety (as DeBakey pointed out, the patients did no better than the calves), both Baylor and the NHI held formal inquiries. Liotta was eventually suspended from the artificial heart program and his salary withdrawn. Cooley, refusing to submit to institutional guidelines regarding peer review of protocols involving human research, resigned his clinical professorship at Baylor.

The type of human experiment exemplified by the operation on Karp opened up a series of questions within and outside the field. When, for instance, should attempts to salvage the life of a patient slip from the usual, conventional, accepted, or even possible to the extraordinary, heroic, or futile? When should efforts to prolong life merge with those used to prolong death? Important voices even questioned the appropriateness of Karp's heart donor herself, a patient with irreversible brain damage who had not been pronounced dead in Massachusetts before being flown to Texas. Located through Mrs. Karp's highly publicized pleas, she was not declared brain dead until several hours after her arrival in Houston—and then by four physicians who felt that she had suffered a further stroke on the airplane. Desire to save the patient, no matter what the odds, was a prime factor in this complex equation.

Denton Cooley is a charismatic, high-profile, publicly acclaimed figure in Texas. His ambitions, talents, and hard-driving sense of achievement are well recognized. He does not lose patients lightly. He remains a formidable and highly regarded personality in cardiothoracic surgery, recognized internationally for his intellect, technical expertise, and clinical productivity; a professor of surgery at the University of Texas Medical School; and surgeon-in-chief and president of the Texas Heart Institute. One may compare his actions to those of pioneers and innovators in many fields other than medicine and surgery. Such individuals are perhaps so sure of their own abilities that they ignore the need for supporting evidence that more conservative colleagues feel is necessary.

Francis Moore expanded on this theme specifically:

> Desperate measures like the interim substitution of a machine heart, or the implantation of a sheep's heart in man, call up for consideration a special ethical question: Does the presence of a dying patient justify the doctors taking *any* conceivable step regardless of its degree of hopelessness? The answer to this question must be negative . . . There is simply no evidence to suggest that it would be helpful. It raises false hope for the patient and his family, it calls into discredit all of biomedical science, and it gives the impression that physicians and surgeons are adventurers rather than circumspect persons seeking to help the suffering and dying by the use of hopeful measures. The dying person becomes the object of wildly speculative experiments when he is hopeless and helpless rather than the recipient of discriminating measures carried out in his behalf. It is only by work in the laboratory and cautious trial in the living animal that "hopeless desperate measures" can become ones that carry with them some promise of reasonable assistance to the patient. The interim substitution of a mechanical heart in the chest, in the location of the normal heart, had not reached this stage for the simple reason that animal survival had never been attained.[8]

These and similar sentiments brought to a halt much of the work on an artificial heart.

In contrast to the pessimism that permeated society in the United States during the previous two decades, the 1980s were a period of self-confidence and increased expectations. The economy was healthy. Technology was ascendant. Amid a variety of advances and refinements in medicine, surgery, and pharmacology, reconsideration of the artificial heart seemed appropriate to fill a potential need for thousands of patients with end-stage heart failure. This second assault, like the first, was primarily a United States venture, as noted in an essay that commented on its mystique. "[It] is a bit like a star on the 'American' flag, and stopping the artificial heart program would be like picking the star off the flag."[9] For several years the NHI had given high priority to the development of a mechanical circulatory support device. Despite the earlier experience with Haskell Karp, the time appeared right to reexamine the use of such a mechanism in humans.

The continuing vision of Willem Kolff evoked the most productive of these efforts. A persistent and imaginative investigator, he followed his development of the dialysis machine by devising mechanical substitutions for a variety of organs, including the heart. In 1967 he moved to the University of Utah to direct its division of artificial organs. Within a few years he and his team had solved or at least tamed some of the obstacles in mechanics, materials, blood clotting, and infection. The result was a series of pneumatically powered artificial hearts that could sustain calves for progressively longer periods following removal of their native hearts.

Two new individuals joined the group. Robert Jarvik was a medical student when he first went to work in Kolff's laboratory. He studied biomechanics and completed his medical degree before becoming a design engineer on the project. A mercurial and flamboyant entrepreneur, he became a highly visible figure. His picture appeared unexpectedly anywhere from *Playboy* to billboards on which he was portrayed with an eye patch as "the man in the Hathaway shirt." Once, riding up a long escalator in the London underground, I well remember seeing posters of Jarvik's face (and shirt) interspersed again and again among advertisements of the latest plays and museum exhibitions. Unused to such self-promotion among professionals, my emotions flitted rapidly between amusement and incredulity. When Kolff later formed a proprietary company with controversial ties to the university, Jarvik eventually became its president, effectively removing his mentor in the process.[10]

The second new member of the team was William DeVries, who had also worked with Kolff as a medical student, implanting heart devices into sheep (Figure 9.2). Returning to Utah after nine years of

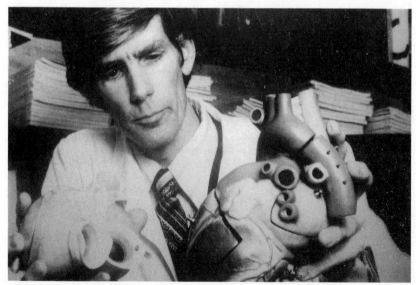

Figure 9.2 William DeVries and an artificial heart (Novartis, with permission)

training in cardiovascular surgery, he became the only surgeon authorized initially by the Food and Drug Administration (FDA) to test the artificial heart in man; his obvious enthusiasm and commitment to the project contributed substantially to its resurgence.

Responsible thinkers from many fields felt that plans for human testing of this new generation of artificial hearts were premature. The results with calves remained problematic, with many becoming infected via the pneumatic tubes that led through the skin from the external power source. Despite these fears, pressures to embark on clinical trials mounted, particularly as investigators perceived that the NHI was losing interest in the subject. And with loss of interest would come loss of research funds. By the early 1980s, twelve goats and calves from university centers in Salt Lake City, Hershey, Berlin, and Tokyo had survived total cardiac replacement for longer than six months. In addition, the artificial heart had been tested in humans. DeVries placed it in cadavers in Utah and at hospitals in Argentina and East Germany. In Philadelphia the device was implanted into five brain-dead patients, sustaining the circulation of two of them for forty-one and seventy-two hours before elective termination. The other three became kidney donors after extended periods on the pump.[11] News that surgeons from the University of Tokyo had placed a mechanical heart in an ill cardiac patient may have increased the sense of urgency.

By the end of 1981 the Human Subjects Committee of the University of Utah and the FDA finally granted permission to test the device clinically. DeVries and his team felt ready. From a carefully screened group of candidates in end-stage cardiac failure, he chose Barney Clark, a 61-year-old retired dentist from Seattle. In December 1982 DeVries and a surgical colleague removed Clark's heart and implanted a "Jarvik-7" artificial heart. Despite careful orchestration by the university and the hospital, media coverage was unremitting. It overwhelmed Clark, his family, the medical staff, and everyone involved. "First there was the press assault . . . Reporters stole Clark's scrapbooks, broke into DeVries' office, sneaked into the intensive care unit in laundry baskets, dated nurses to get access to information, and . . . one prominent reporter who was also a doctor came in a white coat and started making rounds with the radiologists." The patient endured 112 complication-ridden days before dying of multiple organ failure and sepsis. At times he begged to be let go. DeVries later reported, however, that "despite the relatively complicated postoperative course in our patient, the overall experience . . . nonetheless leads to an optimistic appraisal of the future potential for total artificial heart systems."[12]

Perhaps because of this mindset, the young surgeon became increasingly frustrated with the obstacles he felt were being raised against his performing a second procedure. Arguments surfaced within the Human Subjects Committee, dialogue ensued regarding conflicts of interest between the university and Jarvik and between the company and its stockholders (funding had gradually moved from government sources to private capital), while claims were made about priority of invention. Although the FDA approved plans for a second implant in June 1984, within weeks DeVries defected to Louisville, Kentucky, joining the staff of a hospital run by the Humana Corporation, one of the largest of the for-profit health care companies then emerging. Despite its lack of university affiliation, Humana publicly announced its aim to build a major center for cardiovascular disease that would stress excellence in patient care, education, and applied research. Heart transplantation and implantation of artificial hearts were to be priority subjects. For this venture, the company was prepared to spend a great deal of money. DeVries' presence also garnered tremendous publicity: he soon met with President Ronald Reagan, was interviewed by Barbara Walters, and graced the cover of *Time*.

From the plethora of candidates seeking help, DeVries and his team in November 1984 picked William Shroeder as the second patient to receive an artificial heart. Plans for the procedure continued, despite ongoing concerns by some in the press and in the FDA about the rapidity and depth of approval granted by the for-profit institution. Leaders in American medicine also raised doubts about the appropriateness of the program. And as it had with Barney Clark, the media reported and discussed Shroeder's condition after the operation in a stream of daily reports throughout the remainder of his life. He died after 610 complication-full days.

Three months later the team placed a third cardiac implant into Murray Haydon. He endured 488 days of strokes, pulmonary insufficiency, and a variety of serious and ultimately fatal infections. DeVries' final patient, Jack Burcham, survived only ten disastrous days. At about the same time, surgeons in Stockholm implanted an artificial heart in a 53-year-old patient, Lief Stenburg, who recovered quickly but died of multiple strokes seven months later.

Regardless of brave talk from the principals, from Humana, and from the University of Utah, it was apparent that the patients in this second group fared no better than had the calves; the complications were all too predictable. Both enthusiasts and detractors made their views known. Despite protestations of outrage by DeVries, the FDA withdrew its support. He, however, continued to remain positive: "The TAH [total artificial heart] is feasible, practical, and durable and offers life to those who would not otherwise be able to continue living. These patients have enjoyed their families, births of grandchildren, marriages of their children, fishing excursions, and even participated in parades, none of which would have been possible without the TAH. It is extremely rare—if ever—that clinical research has been so dramatically successful for the initial subjects."[13]

Others felt differently. "DeVries . . . define[d] the serious problems that have cast a dark shadow on the currently available pneumatic heart . . . The suggested solutions to these problems . . . seem unlikely to reduce substantially the incidence of complications. Accordingly, adding patients to this series would serve only to document further the magnitude of the complications rather than to demonstrate an acceptable lifestyle in the recipient."[14]

DeVries entered private practice in Louisville; Jarvik and his company continue to develop and refine a series of prototype devices. No further procedures were attempted.

In spite of the failure of the *total* artificial heart, worldwide enthusiasm for the use of *bridge* hearts increased. Between 1985 and 1990, surgeons in several countries placed over three hundred such devices in patients with intractable heart failure. At the same time, critics evoked the possibility that these individuals would be given priority over others awaiting transplantation, or that the presence of the mechanical hearts would make subsequent grafting impossible. Emphasis shifted to temporary use of ventricular assist devices to allow a failing heart time to recover, and to the design of improved versions with better pumps and power sources. Although in a 1988 editorial the *New York Times* described the artificial heart as a "Dracula of Modern Technology, sucking 240 billion out of the National Heart, Lung and Blood Institute," ever more successful efforts with ever improving technologies have become available.[15]

As the twenty-first century opens, effective implantable assist devices are used in many cardiac units and have supported some failing hearts for over seven hundred days. Wearable, increasingly compact, and powered by small batteries placed internally, they are superior to medical management in certain cardiac patients who are not acceptable for transplantation. They are increasingly analogous to the support of renal failure patients by chronic dialysis. In addition, the first of a new-generation TAH was placed in a patient in the summer of 2001, again in Louisville. He did well for several months until a series of strokes caused his death. Several more individuals have recently been added to the experience. Four have died, but often after months of relatively satisfactory existence. Others have had strokes. Although the outcomes are considerably improved over earlier implantations, problems remain. It is expected, however, that as the technology advances, artificial hearts may eventually become so effective that they will reduce the overall need for cardiac transplantation.

IO

The Abdominal Viscera

THE DESIRE TO GRAFT ABDOMINAL ORGANS OTHER than the kidney arose as a natural extension of Joseph Murray's first successful transplant between identical twins in 1954. Within months, attempts to replace the liver in dogs were initiated; in less than a decade, the first patient received a hepatic allograft. Earlier forays into pancreatic transplantation were reexamined, refined, carried out in animals, and then in occasional patients. Small bowel and other viscera in combination were grafted. All attempts were unsuccessful. During the years that followed, a handful of single-minded surgical-scientists labored to wrest the technically demanding transplantation of these complex organs from the realm of total failure. In contrast to the surge of peer recognition after the first kidney grafts, however, and the explosion of excitement following the first heart replacement, relative silence greeted the transfer of abdominal organs.

The successful replacement of a failing liver with a healthy, functioning organ from another individual can resurrect a dying patient. Judge Vincent Ragosta, for example, a respected and otherwise healthy 72-year-old jurist in the Rhode Island Superior Court, first noted blood in his stools in 1994.[1] He was diagnosed as bleeding from veins in his esophagus, which had enlarged under high pressure from his liver, heavily scarred from unknown cause. Despite consistently normal hepatic function tests, his first symptoms of severe cirrhosis arose two years later. At that point he developed increasing mental confusion and coma because of the accumulation of metabolic toxins in his circulation, which his increasingly compromised liver was unable to destroy. He continued his court work by controlling his condition with diet and medications, although his abdomen progressively filled with fluid. After three years of precarious and worsening health, he received a new liver in January 2000. Within two months he had returned to court full time feeling well and continuing all his previous activities. At this writing the liver graft continues to function normally. The gold medal in acrobatic skiing won in the 2002 Olympic Games by a liver recipient is another striking example of the efficacy of this transplant.

Long enigmatic and poorly understood, the liver and its functioning took centuries to define. Zeus punished Prometheus for bringing fire to man by ordering an eagle to feast daily upon his liver, a mythological affirmation of its remarkable regenerative powers. Emotional status has been attached to the liver throughout the ages; the words *choleric* and *melancholy* refer to disturbances within that organ. Although mental decline, jaundice, and coma were recognized to result from liver disease, both Hippocrates and Galen considered the healthy organ to be the center of the bodily spirits and body heat, as well as the source of blood. In Imperial Rome, spectators would occasionally snatch a piece of the liver of dead gladiators. Taken nine times, the tissue reputedly cured epilepsy.

The exalted view of its functions was dashed in the seventeenth century by the discovery that chyle, a milky fluid composed of lymph and digested fat from the intestine, did not enter the liver as the ancients had taught, but emptied directly into the circulation via the great lymphatics. The responsibility of the organ in the formation of blood and the production of body heat also proved erroneous. A disenchanted anatomist of the time wryly summarized existing knowledge by noting in Latin that the liver "was good for nothing but making bile, considering how the world looked upon this bitter fluid and the gloomy persons who had too much of it . . . Any shred of virtue the liver possessed [was taken away]."[2]

In the early nineteenth century, experimental biologists found that the major vein to the organ, the portal vein, carried products of food digested in the intestine to the liver and, later, that the organ stored glycogen, a starch that can be converted to sugar as necessary for energy. At the same time, the hepatic artery supplied the liver cells with oxygen-rich blood. By 1877 Nikolai Eck in Russia had defined the importance of the liver in metabolism by rerouting the portal vein into the inferior vena cava of dogs, a vascular rearrangement that excluded the energy-rich blood of the gut from its destination in the liver. Bypassing normal protein breakdown by hepatic cells, he quickly demonstrated the deleterious effects on brain function of high blood levels of proteins. His observation also explained Shakespeare's description centuries before of the effects of liver disease in the persistently drunken Sir Andrew Aguecheek in *Twelfth Night*: "I am a great eater of beef, and I do believe it does harm to my wit."[3] Whether the bibulous Sir Andrew had cirrhosis cannot be determined, although the opinion of one of his drinking companions that "if he were opened and you would find so much blood in his liver as will clog the foot of a flea, I'll eat the rest of the anatomy" provides a compelling description of the fibrotic, underperfused, and poorly functioning organ of the long-term alcoholic. An additional function of the organ, later described, is that particular cells within the hepatic substance make up a specific part of the body's defenses against bacteria and other hazards.

With its dual blood supply carrying about half of the body's circulation through the organ each minute—as well as its size, character, and consistency—the liver remained outside the surgical purview until well after World War II. Then, an interest in its transplantation encouraged attempts to perform complex surgical operations on the actual substance of the liver itself, including removal of the hepatic lobes and other isolated segments. In 1955 the first experimental auxiliary graft of a liver was placed in parallel with the existing organ.[4] Enthused by the possibility of placement of a new liver into its native site in a recipient, both Francis Moore at the Brigham and Thomas Starzl, then at Northwestern, attempted the procedure. They quickly found that clamping both the inferior vena cava and the portal vein of a dog during removal of the native liver and substitution of a new one almost invariably produced acute venous congestion of the intestine. The procedure also decreased cardiac output because of impaired venous return from the lower half of the body. All these factors culminated in death from shock.

Although the initial mortality of the animals undergoing the procedures was virtually total, technical improvements slowly increased the number of short-term successes. By 1960 the Brigham group was able to report seven of thirty-one transplanted but nonimmunosuppressed dogs surviving over four days, one for twelve days. Starzl's experience with more than eighty animals emphasized the importance of normal portal blood flow for sustained hepatic function. Eighteen of his dogs lived for more than four days, several significantly longer.[5]

The subject broadened quickly. Moving to the University of Colorado in 1962, Starzl was able to attain three-month survival of canine recipients of kidneys and livers treated with azathioprine and steroids, results that only increased his desire to try the technique in a human. He transplanted the first of his five patients, a 3-year-old child with congenital narrowing of the bile ducts, in early 1963 and the remainder shortly thereafter. All died within days. About the same time, Moore and his team grafted a 54-year-old man, who died of infection on day 11. Three subsequent patients also died. An attempt in Paris failed as well. While several of the livers looked relatively normal at postmortem examination, the surgeons called a halt to further clinical procedures until operative techniques, nuances of care, and more appropriate immunosuppression could be perfected. Clinical activity was slowly reactivated, with over thirty teams worldwide reporting 130 cases of replaced or auxiliary liver transplants by the mid-1970s. When the data were published in 1976, however, only twelve patients were still alive.[6]

With these marginal results, the majority of transplant centers showed little enthusiasm for initiation of liver programs. Starzl, for instance, was invited to consider surgical chairmanships in several university departments—as long as he did not undertake clinical liver transplantation (Figure 10.1). Indeed, virtually all procedures worldwide were carried out in only two centers, Starzl's in Denver and that of Roy Calne and his colleagues in a Cambridge-London unit. The drive and dedication of these two individuals alone kept the entire field going. Because of the enormity of the operative undertaking, the vast physiological changes to be overcome during placement of the organ, the functional complexity of the liver, and the persistently unsatisfactory results, little enthusiasm was manifested until others became convinced and joined the effort.

As the investigators discovered quickly in dogs and confirmed all

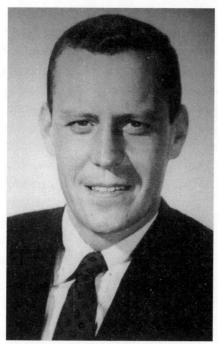

Figure 10.1 Thomas Starzl (Novartis, with permission)

too strikingly in man, the most fearsome acute complications included uncontrollable bleeding, clotting, and infection. In human patients, intraoperative hemorrhage was even more common, for the underlying liver disease severely compromised their coagulation mechanisms. In addition, factors were released into the circulation after reconstruction of the vessels of ischemic organs that had been without blood supply during much of the operation. These caused existing clots on raw surfaces to dissolve with resultant hemorrhage from previously sealed vascular suture lines. Curiously, clots often formed simultaneously within the plastic external bypass tubing or even on newly created sites where vessels were joined, causing local obstruction or even migration of the clot to the lungs. Infection was a common threat, developing not infrequently within the substance of the newly grafted organ itself and stemming from bile leaks, compromised biliary drainage, or obstruction. These enduring problems required a series of innovations and refinements in surgery, operative care, and immunosuppression, and still remain appreciable risk factors for post-operative complications.

But some advances encouraged continuation of the clinical attempts. The addition of antilymphocyte globulin to existing suppressive regimens, though not of obvious benefit in experimental animals, decreased the incidence of rejection of hepatic grafts in patients. The development of a device to store and preserve human livers for several hours by perfusing them with cooled blood under high pressure in special chambers was helpful, based on a protocol for preservation of dog kidneys that Christiaan Barnard had previously devised.[7] Although heavy and cumbersome, the apparatus allowed increased time to plan and carry out the transplant procedure, as well as broadening the geographic area of potential donation.

As with the kidney, these early protocols and techniques, including more effective preservation solutions, improved incrementally over the years. Another source of encouragement was Paul Terasaki's controversial data showing the relative lack of effect of tissue typing on kidney-graft survival. Omitting the test shortened the time considerably before a liver could be transplanted. And as the human experience increased, additional peculiarities of the organ became evident, including the unexpected findings that ABO blood-group compatibility and antibody cross-match were not always necessary.

In contrast to the knowledge gleaned from laboratory experiments that presaged the clinical transplantation of kidneys, understanding of the biology of liver-graft behavior lagged behind the development of surgical techniques. The short survival times of most early dogs, which had died primarily of operative complications, made comprehensive examination of immunological rejection of the transplanted livers difficult. The events were not defined more formally until relatively large numbers of immunosuppressed recipients of cooled livers had survived for weeks or months. Some results were not anticipated. Starzl found that substances in the portal blood that promoted liver growth were necessary to sustain the graft. French workers described the advantages of the pig over the dog as an experimental subject, particularly noting its tolerance to cross-clamping of the inferior vena cava. Using pigs, several investigators realized that not only were many nonimmunosuppressed recipients sustained for prolonged periods by their liver grafts, but that rejection was often weak and easily reversible. Indeed, some animals never experienced a rejection episode at all, while the acute process in others appeared to resolve spontaneously.

Having switched from the dog to the pig as an experimental model, Calne and his colleagues made the intriguing observation that although kidneys and skin transplanted between normal pigs were rejected acutely, they were protected and rarely rejected when grafted together with the donor's liver.[8] The data suggested that an immunomodulatory or immunoprotective effect mediated by the liver may produce a type of specific host tolerance. These unexpected experimental findings were supported when Calne's group showed that transplants of kidneys and other organs often performed better in human patients who also received livers.

Starzl later hypothesized that donor leukocytes from a hepatic graft, residing in the lymphoid tissues of the host for years after transplantation, were responsible for this effect. The ability to graft livers between inbred rats and even mice using microsurgical techniques allowed further opportunity to study these phenomena. Like pigs, rats sustained by functioning liver transplants become tolerant to skin and heart grafts from the same, but not third-party, donors. Finally, the resistance of the liver to hyperacute rejection, in which it appears to convert a state of host sensitization into one of unresponsiveness, has been a fertile field of investigation. The relatively aberrant response of the recipient to the transplanted liver (compared to other organs) remains undefined but has allowed remarkable success in liver transplantation to patients.

Clinical progress increased gradually, particularly after Cyclosporin A became available in the early 1980s. The indications for the procedure have slowly broadened as results have improved. Patients with primary bile-duct disease or liver failure from unknown cause fare best, with about two thirds surviving over eight years. Those whose original disease was hepatitis do somewhat less well, often because of viral reinfection of their transplant. Patients requiring hepatic grafts secondary to alcoholic cirrhosis or liver cancer have relatively mediocre results over the long term. Yet overall, the ability to salvage and sustain a large proportion of appropriate patients with liver trans-plants—with over 80 percent of recipients surviving at one year—has been a remarkable achievement.[9]

Transplantation of the pancreas into diabetic recipients has only re-cently become relatively successful. A gland hidden deep in the upper abdomen, the role of the pancreas in digestion by exocrine secretion of enzymes into the intestine via the pancreatic duct, has long been recog-nized. The discovery of its relationship to diabetes via its endocrine activity, the secretion of hormones directly into the bloodstream, did not occur until much later. Although the ancient Egyptians described some of the manifestations of this condition, the subject lay dormant until 1889, when German investigators produced fatal diabetes in dogs by removing the pancreas. The importance of the gland in carbohy-drate metabolism was then linked to abnormalities of the islets of Langerhans, small collections of specialized cells scattered throughout its tissue.

In contrast to the often milder form of diabetes that affects older persons, the juvenile form of the disease is particularly serious, as nonfunctioning or poorly functioning islets are unable to produce insulin. The resultant elevations of blood sugar, uncontrolled because of lack of the hormone, are associated with severe metabolic derange-ments, coma, and sometimes death. Formidable means to regulate the acute condition, with stringent dietary controls that approached star-vation, were developed early in the twentieth century. These increased the expected survival of afflicted children and adolescents from only two years after onset to eight years.

In 1922 physicians caring for such unfortunate patients gathered in Toronto to learn about a pancreatic extract that could normalize high blood-sugar levels and allow survival of diabetic dogs from which the pancreas had been removed. One of the attendees, Elliot Joslin, re-turned to Boston, where he administered the material to his first pa-tient, a nurse. During the previous five years of "undernutrition" treat-ment, her weight had dropped from 155 to 69 pounds. She was weak and virtually chair ridden. But once the new agent, insulin, moderated her blood sugar, she improved dramatically. Energy, weight, and quality of life improved.[10] Other patients, moribund and without hope, benefited in similar miraculous fashion.

Treatment with insulin heralded a revolution in the care of those afflicted with diabetes. At least one previous surgical investigator who used gland extract in dogs after excision of their pancreas had suggested the potential significance of the islets. But it was left to University of Toronto surgeon Frederick Banting and medical student Charles Best to demonstrate conclusively that material isolated from these cells could lower high levels of blood sugar in diabetic dogs to normal. Despite a series of discouraging failures, they persisted. Insulin treatment kept Marjorie, their first canine success, alive for seventy days. But even this crucial discovery was clouded with controversy when the 1923 Nobel Prize for Medicine and Physiology was awarded to Banting and J. R. MacLeod, a physiologist not directly involved with the work but in whose laboratory it had been carried out. The 23-year-old Best was not included because of his youth. Others claimed credit for their less definitive efforts. Indeed, Nicolas Paulesco, an experimentalist from Romania, had previously reported similar results but in French. While Banting and Best had referenced his work, they had mistranslated the conclusions to suggest that the extract had no effect.[11] It could be argued that if Paulesco's paper or its summary had been in English, the Nobel award might have turned out differently.

The pharmaceutical company Eli Lilly soon took over Banting and Best's successful extraction methods and began to produce large amounts of animal insulin for the hundreds of patients clamoring for it. By 1926 crystalline insulin was isolated. Four decades later, synthesis of the molecule opened the way for genetic engineering of human insulin. In short, the definition and routine use of this hormone by diabetic patients has been a medical milestone of the twentieth century.

Although the life span of insulin-controlled diabetics could be prolonged and the relatively acute lethal disease transformed into a chronic one, unexpected long-term complications arose in many treated patients, often after many years. Blindness not infrequently occurred. Kidney failure developed. Susceptibility to infection increased. Arterial insufficiency and gangrene of the toes or feet often led to amputation. In seeking at least transient reprieve for the afflicted individuals, occasional surgeons sought means to replace the nonfunctioning islets by implanting pancreatic tissue slices, fragments, or mechanically disrupted portions of the gland at various sites in the body.

The first to have considered this maneuver was an English surgeon who treated a severely diabetic child in 1893 by placing three pieces of fresh sheep pancreas in the subcutaneous tissues. Banting and Best later discussed this approach. In the mid-1930s a few research workers unsuccessfully buried cultured pancreatic fragments in skin pockets in pancreatectomized dogs; two decades later, several others placed such tissue allografts in anatomical areas less prone to rejection (such as the cheek pouch of the hamster or the eye of the rat). During the 1970s investigators improved diabetes substantially in rodents after administration of islet-rich pancreatic fragments. As a single disrupted gland could not produce adequate numbers of islets, various digestive techniques were devised to increase the yield of these insulin-producing cells from the pancreas of several donors, particularly animal fetuses.[12] While enthusiasm for the potential of islet transplantation increased during this period even as the results of grafting the whole gland became more discouraging, a series of trials in large animals and in humans were unsuccessful.

Experimentalists also tried to bypass the problem of rejection by grafting islets taken from the pancreas, then returning them to the original donor. Preparations of islets isolated from normal pancreases and transplanted into rats produced normal levels of blood sugar. Islet autografts dissociated from chronically inflamed glands that had produced unremitting pain in fifty patients were given back intravenously. One third of these individuals no longer required insulin for prolonged periods. Unfortunately, the diabetes invariably recurred as the cells gradually ceased to function.[13]

As a corollary to these studies, development of an artificial pancreas became a persistent subject for research. Investigators attempted to inhibit rejection by physically separating the allogeneic islets from the host immune responses by placing them in a filter device connected to the circulation. The semipermeable membrane prevented migration of host leukocytes to the enclosed islets but allowed exchange of soluble factors, including serum glucose from the patient diffusing into the chamber and insulin from the islets entering the bloodstream. Cells cultured in artificial capillaries were used subsequently to achieve the same end. More recent refinements of this technique, tried both in pigs and in patients, have not met with success.

Despite the relative lack of substantive progress, those in the field hope that as the transplantation of these cells eventually becomes possible, they can be grafted before the devastating sequelae of the diabetic process can escalate. Although the supply of human islets remains a critical limiting factor, an experienced Canadian group has reported the successful grafting of allogeneic islets in several individuals, with complete reversal of their diabetes for many months.[14] Their protocol of transferring large numbers of islets plus effective immunosuppression of the patients appears to be a crucial step forward. And if the hurdle of xenografts can be conquered, the use of pig islets may go far toward prevention, attenuation, and/or treatment of the disease.

With interest in the transplantation of vascularized whole organs increasing during the 1960s, reversal of diabetes by replacement of the entire pancreas appeared to be another reasonable course to follow. There was some precedent for such a concept. After World War I, German and French investigators noted transient normalization of blood sugar after revascularized pancreas grafts were placed in diabetic dogs. In 1936, a French research worker reported the seven-day survival of a pancreas grafted to the neck vessels of a dog, although he did not document its function. In the 1950s, investigators transplanted partial or entire pancreases to the lower abdominal vessels of dogs and occasional patients by direct vascular anastomosis. These initial attempts were unsuccessful, however, as the vessels clotted or acute inflammation developed.

Attempts to drain the powerful digestive enzymes to the outside via a plastic tube or to destroy the secretory function by radiation did not stop autodigestion of the isolated pancreas. The pancreatic duct was also led directly through a hole made in the skin for external drainage. Other groups tied off the duct, exploiting the earlier observation of Banting and Best that islet cell function was not altered by occluding exocrine drainage.[15] However, progressive scarring of both the gland substance and the islets themselves discouraged further use of this manuever. Operative techniques gradually improved, however, so that by the late 1960s, transplantation of the pancreas led to graft survival of 169 days in one dog and prolonged function in others. It was time, several investigators felt, to move on to humans.

Richard Lillehei and his surgical colleagues at the University of Minnesota were responsible for much of the early history of clinical pancreas transplantation. Based on extensive prior experience in dogs, in 1966 they grafted a kidney plus the pancreas of a cadaver donor into a 28-year-old diabetic woman. They ligated the pancreatic duct. Although dying of rejection and infection after two months, the patient sustained normal blood-sugar values and was insulin independent.[16]

This team performed pancreas transplants in thirteen more patients over the next seven years, nine of whom received concomitant renal grafts. The majority of the procedures involved placement of the whole gland and anastomosis of the adjacent duodenum surrounding the duct to the recipient small bowel. The return of the blood sugar to normal in several patients allowed reduction or cessation of the dose of insulin for periods of varying lengths. One graft functioned for a year. By 1977 data had accumulated on fifty-seven grafts placed in fifty-five patients. Of these, only a single individual survived long term.[17]

With this dismal record as background, and particularly when insulin could be given to temper the acute metabolic perturbations of diabetes, it was little wonder that transplantation of the pancreas was accepted more slowly than that of other organs. Other reasons for the relative lack of enthusiasm for the pancreatic procedure were obvious. The late sequelae of the disease often ravaged the potential recipients. The potential mortality from the transplant operation and its attendant treatment were of evident concern. Inflammation commonly developed in the new graft. Ductal leaks led to infection. Rejection was difficult to diagnose and control. Several of the immunosuppressive drugs worsened the existing diabetes. And in the same department of surgery as Lillehei, John Najarian and his associates were showing convincingly that renal transplantation in insulin-controlled diabetics could be carried out with reasonable success and that complete control of blood sugar was not necessary for satisfactory kidney function. As a result, many physicians were unwilling to substitute the hazards of transplantation and immunosuppression for the more predictable dangers of insulin replacement.

Improved means of handling the duct and preventing duct-related complications soon provided encouragement to those struggling in the field. In 1978 a young urologist from Lyon (one of Murray's former research fellows in Boston) devised a novel solution to the problem of leakage of pancreatic juice, presumably based on ductal obstruction experiments carried out by French workers in the previous century. J. M. Dubernard and colleagues showed in dogs and then in patients that exocrine drainage could be completely blocked by filling the entire ductal system of the isolated gland with sterile neoprene or other synthetic polymers. Their initial results with ten pancreas recipients who survived between eight and eleven months with no or low doses of insulin were unprecedented, even though the islets gradually lost function as the gland substance scarred over time.[18] Many pancreatic transplanters used this safe and convenient method in the 1980s, particularly after the introduction of Cyclosporin A.

Ever imaginative, Dubernard continues to direct a highly successful kidney and pancreas transplant program in Lyon. He led the team that performed the first transplantation of a hand allograft in 1998, and became a member of the French Parliament and vice-mayor of his city. Subsequent technical improvements have included effective means to drain the exocrine secretions into the recipient bladder or small bowel. As a result, the surgical complications long associated with this complex transplant have markedly diminished.

By the mid-1990s seven thousand pancreas transplants had been performed in 170 centers throughout the world.[19] About 80 percent of the grafts were placed in diabetic recipients, either together with renal allografts or as a separate procedure. Single organs constituted the remainder. About three quarters of those receiving simultaneous grafts achieved insulin independence for more than a year, half when the pancreas was implanted alone. The use of pancreas segments from living-related donors was also introduced, although many clinicians consider such procedures on normal individuals too hazardous for general application. The substantially improved quality of life experienced by many of the patients has been striking, particularly among those receiving both pancreas and kidney grafts who not only can discontinue their insulin but may also stop dialysis.

Despite the increasingly satisfactory results, the overall impact of pancreas transplantation on the treatment of diabetes is ambiguous. In the United States alone, about twelve thousand persons develop juvenile-onset diabetes annually; about half will experience later complications of the disease. At the same time, as the increasing incidence of the adult-onset disease associated with obesity is a growing public health problem, the three hundred to four hundred pancreatic transplants and about nine hundred combined kidney-pancreas grafts performed yearly produce relatively minimal societal effect. The ability of a successful transplant to reverse the complications of long-standing diabetes is also debatable. Neuropathy and early renal dysfunction may stabilize or improve after several years of normal levels of blood sugar, but vascular changes in the eyes are little affected. As physicians and surgeons are faced with individual patients seeking help, this type of transplant will continue, encouraged by the improvements in the best recipients. As with islets, the eventual hope is to graft diabetics earlier in their disease so as to prevent the devastating later effects.

The number of patients requiring replacement of the small intestine to survive is limited to a few thousand per year. Many of these are infants whose bowel twists, loses its blood supply, and dies. Thrombosis of the major nutrient artery more commonly causes necrosis of the adult gut. Progressive improvement in long-term intravenous nutritional management of such individuals has reduced the need for intestinal transplantation. Nutritional treatment, however, imposes severe restrictions on daily activities, may cost as much as $200,000 per year, and may produce life-threatening complications. A successful bowel transplant may be an important alternative for those unable to receive or tolerate total parenteral nutrition. Seventy to eighty intestinal grafts are performed annually in the United States, with a few additional cases in Europe. Use of this procedure and its variations remains quite restricted.

Surgery of the intestine evolved primarily from efforts to correct obstructions resulting from incarcerated or strangulated hernias, adhesions, or tumors. Left uncorrected, the condition was ultimately fatal.

Treatments of bowel obstruction over the ages have included upside-down suspension of the patient, opium, purges, electricity, the administration of water, air, or mercury by mouth, and direct puncture of the dilated bowel with small needles or indwelling trocars (to establish a fistula for release of the contents).[20] Hippocrates treated obstructive symptoms "with enemas and inflation of the rectum by . . . a bladder attached to a pipe." In about 300 B.C., Praxagoras of Cos drained a bowel blocked in a groin hernia by direct incision. Sushruta and the later Arab physicians advocated the use of cautery. William Saliceto, a thirteenth-century Italian surgeon, opened an obstructed bowel segment, excised the gangrenous portion, then placed a piece of animal intestine as an internal stent and closed the bowel over it. Others used the trachea as a splint over which the viable bowel ends were joined. Based on prior suggestions, a French surgeon entered the abdomen of an unanesthetized young woman in 1701, removed several feet of gangrenous bowel, and created an artificial anus on her abdominal wall. She recovered. Emboldened, a few French and British surgeons began to excise dead portions of bowel, exteriorizing the viable ends. Some of the fistulae closed spontaneously or after revision. During the nineteenth century a few surgical innovators gradually perfected means to join bowel together by direct suture or by using a button that passed spontaneously after healing. But not until the 1930s and 1940s—when anesthesia and asepsis had become routine, the intestine could be decompressed by the new technique of external gastric drainage, and fluid and salt management were better understood—did the results of surgical intervention improve and the overwhelming mortality rates drop to acceptable levels.

Although Carrel has been credited with the first intestinal transplant, his papers do not mention this organ specifically. In fact, Emerich Ullmann in 1901 had already described the autografting of small pieces of stomach, small bowel, and colon in piglets, but only as free, nonvascularized patches. For the next half century, the small intestine was transplanted to only a few experimental animals and humans. Lillehei first undertook the procedure in connection with his efforts at canine pancreas transplantation during the late 1950s—initially with autografts, later with allografts. Despite the distant prospects of clinical applicability, he and his colleagues devised methods to remove the small bowel, cool it as long as five hours, reconstruct the vessels, and replace the entire tissue mass in the original host. Some of the surviving animals regained normal intestinal function, but only after a relative delay for regrowth of the nerve supply.[21]

The behavior of allografts was dramatically different from that of autografts, as the recipients invariably died after six to nine days. Acute rejection in the unmodified host was all too predictable, with bleeding and sloughing of the mucosal lining cells, an intense lymphocytic presence, and thickening, inflammation, and perforation of the bowel wall. As the actual cause of death was often not obvious, GVHD was implicated because of the large amount of lymphoid tissue in the transplanted bowel and mesentery.[22] Indeed, later experiments with rats confirmed that both host immunological rejection of the allogeneic bowel and GVHD are integral to the destruction. GVHD appears to be less important in human bowel transplantation.

During the following years, investigators gradually defined the functional, physiological, and immunological changes involved in bowel transplants in pigs and other experimental models, perfecting technical aspects of the operation, examining ways to pretreat the graft to reduce its immunogenicity, and testing more effective means of storage. With the advent of immunosuppression, survival increased to several weeks; a bowel allograft sustained one dog in an early series for six months. The availability of Cyclosporin A improved the results, although the drug could be administered only by injection and not by mouth because of diminished absorption by the new intestine. Even in the longest-surviving dogs, the bowel allografts never regained physiological normalcy, in contrast to the other organs which usually functioned promptly after revascularization. An additional problem was how to biopsy the bowel to assess the morphological changes of rejection. In many instances the solution was to exteriorize a segment for convenient access. More than two decades after Lillehei's original experiments, the remark of his surgical chairman that intestinal transplantation was "an adventure in search of adversity" still held true.[23]

Despite the unpromising experimental results, the early clinical experience with immunosuppression in kidney recipients encouraged the transplantation of small bowel in occasional patients. In 1964 maternal intestinal segments were placed in two children, although details were not presented nor was publication forthcoming. Three years later Lillehei grafted both small and large intestine into a 46-year-old woman who had lost her entire bowel after thrombosis of its arteries. She died twelve hours later of multiple emboli.[24]

Five more intestinal transplants were performed from cadavers and living-related donors—two in the United States, two in Brazil, and one in France. All died between twelve hours and four weeks after surgery, with the exception of a 37-year-old patient who had received a seg- mental graft from her genetically close sister. Although she died on day 79, she had tolerated food for several weeks. Even the benefits of Cyclosporin A for other organs could not be duplicated in bowel grafts. Of sixteen operations carried out in seven centers, over half in Paris, only one could be considered a success: a 42-year-old recipient of a bowel segment grafted between sisters in Germany in 1988. This patient sustained bowel function for more than four years before her death.[25]

An even more extravagant version of this heroic surgery was the trans- plantation of virtually all abdominal organs at once. Thomas Starzl, intent on pushing past established norms, had attempted multivisceral transplantation in dogs in the late 1950s, including liver, pancreas, and bowel. His peers at the time were not ready for such a radical depar- ture, as he recalled when describing the reaction subsequent to the presentation of his data at a national conference. "William P. Longmire of UCLA [a major figure in surgery at the time] deflated any illusions I might have had about the importance of the contribution. He asked wryly if, rather than performing this complex operation, it might be easier to simply anesthetize the dog and have a laboratory assistant carry the animal from one table to another. The ripple of laughter from the audience completed my humiliation."[26] As Longmire implied and Starzl realized full well, such a technical exercise, remarkable and un- precedented as it was, remained irrelevant as long as immunosuppres- sive means to control rejection were inadequate.

The picture improved gradually with the availability of newer agents in the 1980s and 1990s. Starzl undertook nine multivisceral transplants using Cyclosporin A, transferring all organs together in three patients in a "cluster" operation that included liver, pancreas, stomach, kidneys, and large and small bowel, and other organ combinations in the remaining six. The results of these cases plus several others from the United States, Canada, and Europe were marginal. Several combination liver–small bowel transplants were carried out. Although the first patient of an important Canadian series lived several years with a functioning intestine, additional combined grafts were less successful.

The relative effectiveness of FK506, a powerful Japanese immunosuppressive drug that became available in the early 1990s, encouraged a resurgence in the grafting of small bowel, liver plus small bowel, and multiple viscera together. By 1997 the overall data included 273 such grafts in 260 patients performed at 24 transplant centers; 41 percent were of small bowel alone, 48 percent were combined liver–small bowel transplants. A handful of patients received several organs. The one-year results were encouraging: 69 percent of bowel recipients, 66 percent of liver plus bowel, and 63 percent of those with several organs survived. Substantative data at three years are not yet available, although these numbers are expected to decline. Most of the survivors were able to discontinue intravenous nutrition, at least over the short term.[27] The many complications of these huge procedures included a significant incidence of renal failure and diabetes secondary to drug toxicity; still, the experience represents a step forward in an extremely difficult field.

II

A Modern Minotaur

THE RECIPIENT OF AN ANIMAL ORGAN WHO RE-
ceived the most public attention over the years was Baby Fae, a child
born prematurely in Los Angeles in 1984. Weighing just over a pound
and in cardiac distress, she quickly came under the care of Dr. Leonard
Bailey, an experienced pediatric cardiothoracic surgeon. Her diagnosis
was hypoplastic left heart syndrome, an invariably fatal congenital
anomaly characterized by an underdeveloped left ventricle unable to
pump adequate amounts of blood to supply the body's needs. With life
support becoming necessary within days, surgical options were considered. The family ruled out any temporizing procedures, so the
question arose of transplanting a baboon heart. Bailey had gained laboratory experience with xenografts in newborns by placing the hearts
of lambs into fourteen baby goats; ten of these animals had survived an
average of 72 days, one as long as 165 days.

With this background and faced with Baby Fae's critical situation,
he dismissed the notion of waiting for an appropriate human heart as
"impractical." Several baboons were available as potential donors.
ABO blood matching between animal and human was equivocal,
tissue-typing differences and a cross-match relatively weak. When the
infant was thirteen days old, she received the heart of the least-reactive
donor. After initial improvement, inexorable rejection developed and
she died a week later despite intensive immunosuppression. Although
cellular activity was minimal, the heart showed changes secondary to a
progressive humoral immune response, with inflammation and clotting of the small coronary vessels and destruction of the heart muscle.[1]

The handling of this patient inevitably provoked much public attention. Ethicists debated, physicians shook their heads, editorialists gave mixed opinions, and media excitement grew. Questions were asked about why an allograft could not have been found, particularly as Bailey had waited for nearly two weeks after the infant's birth. Doubts were raised by some about the efficacy of the procedure; enthusiasm for the future of cross-species transplants grew in others. An ethical conundrum, certainly. A scientific advance, perhaps. A surgical adventure, indeed. This case and the few others that are comparable continue to stimulate discourse about the transfer of organs between animals and humans.

The concept of xenotransplantation had its origins in lore and myth. Humans with bestial attributes, and animals bearing the features of other animals and birds, have been consistent topics in literature and the arts throughout history, with cross-species examples ranging from the whimsical to the serious, from the sacred to the profane. Imagining the phantasmagorical, however, is always easier than producing the reality. Practical efforts continue to be met with failure, even with current immunosuppressive regimens and sophisticated donor-altering techniques. In fact, the subject has been described as having "a long and undistinguished history."[2]

Regardless of the continuing disappointments, a few surgical investigators have persisted, initially attempting blood transfusion between species, then grafts of skin or teeth, and more recently xenogeneic cells, tissues, and organs. Both patient hopes and professional efforts have intensified over the past few years with the goal of applying such strategies to those in organ failure. Investigators have been stimulated in part by new departures in research, in part by increased industrial interest and support, and most important by the ever more critical shortage of donor organs. The subject remains an intriguing intellectual challenge to scientists and clinicians alike.

Like organ transplantation in general, interest in xenografts evolved over three eras: initial strivings, the middle period of the 1960s, and rapid subsequent events, particularly during the 1990s. Several of the early experimentalists, including Giuseppe Baronio and John Hunter, had occasionally grafted skin and other tissues between species. Even

Gasparo Tagliacozzi had considered the use of xenografts in nasal repair but concluded that the effectiveness of such a venture was highly improbable. By the late nineteenth century, surgeons in Edinburgh and Brooklyn reported independently that grafts of skin from puppies, kittens, frogs, and rabbits aided the healing of cutaneous ulcers of human patients. A few years later, a country practitioner from Red Bluff, Colorado, transplanted skin from Mexican hairless puppies to humans, suggesting that the immaturity of the donor contributed to its alleged acceptance. One zealot claimed to have transplanted skin from frogs, chickens, pigs, and even a water lizard to the foot of an Italian "with a fair measure of success." Leg ulcers were covered with pieces of pigskin, a technique resurrected in the 1970s when both fresh and freeze-dried preparations came into vogue as a biological dressing for burns or skin defects in patients.[3] These enthusiastic and uncritical anecdotes by the early clinical skin xenografters contrasted sharply with detailed documentation of the inevitable and rapid destruction of thyroid glands, skin, and other tissues grafted between a variety of animal species by biologists before World War I.

The modest experience of German and French surgeons with kidney xenografts during the optimistic prewar era, 1900–1914, was bleak. Emerich Ullmann has been credited with performing the first cross-species kidney transplant between goat and dog; however, no description of this experiment appears in his writings. He did later note that "the hopes which we entertained 15 years ago regarding . . . auto-transplantation have been partially fulfilled; in heteroplastic [xeno] transplantation it appears that the obstacle to success lies in anaphylaxis."[4] After his earlier experience with human kidneys sutured to the arm vessels of two patients, Mathieu Jaboulay in Lyon transplanted pig kidneys to two additional individuals, noting that they were rapidly destroyed and giving possibly the first formal description of the fulminating and rapid rejection response that occurs in organ xenografts.

Embolded by the newly characterized close relationship between monkeys and humans, Ernst Unger in Berlin grafted the kidney of a macaque monkey into a 21-year-old seamstress dying of kidney failure, although the unsuccessful outcome forced him to conclude that this surgical departure should be undertaken "with great care." His extensive laboratory experience in transplantation within and between animal species included the placement of kidneys between pig and dog, dog and goat, cat and dog, and stillborn infant and baboon. Investigators all described the prompt and universal failure of kidneys transferred across species, including those in an occasional human. Perhaps as important was the subsequent observation that the tempo of rejection and extent of graft destruction related to the apparent closeness or disparity of donor and recipient, confirming Ullmann's observation that "the cell protoplasm specific for each organism varies with the individual."[5]

A flurry of interest in the immunological behavior of xenografts resurfaced after World War II, based on earlier studies of tumors and the observation that some human tumors could become established in immunocompromised animal hosts. These results stimulated additional investigations examining the influence on xenogeneic tumor growth of cortisone, ALS, removal of the thymus, and x-radiation with and without bone-marrow replacement. Several groups later described the establishment of human colon carcinoma and other cancers implanted in "nude" mice, a genetic variant introduced in 1962. These immunodeficient animals, bred without a thymus and, as a result, lacking T lymphocytes, were unable to reject foreign tissue.[6] Other research workers reported prolonged tumor survival in some models of tolerance. Although relatively unappreciated by many of the early organ transplanters, these experiments provided retrospective hints that xenogeneic tissues could survive in appropriately manipulated hosts.

One meaningful corollary to the critical question of whether an organ could be accepted by a cross-species recipient was whether it could function appropriately. The liver provoked the most obvious concern because it was not known if its complex array of activities, which ranged between the degradation of metabolic waste products to the production of proteins and clotting factors, could be duplicated by an organ from a different species—or even to what species the proteins would belong. Initial studies from the United States and South Africa in the 1960s and early 1970s addressed these uncertainties by perfusing with human blood livers isolated from a variety of large animals including pigs, baboons, monkeys, and cows, then instituting a series of cross-circulation experiments between patients in coma from hepatic failure and pig livers, or between such individuals and living baboons.[7] Despite synthesis of their own species' proteins and other factors by the animal livers, many of the patients awoke, neurological abnormalities improved, and toxic cell breakdown products diminished. Indeed, about 20 percent of the fifty patients undergoing these procedures recovered and survived. The use of an isolated animal liver or even an animal itself as a bridge device for those with serious but potentially reversible hepatic failure is still under investigation; improvements in these and related techniques may allow the native organ to survive its acute insult and obviate, at least in some cases, the need for actual replacement.

One of my earliest and more unforgettable experiences as a surgical resident in the mid-1960s involved cross-circulation. I was called in the middle of the night to our rather rudimentary intensive-care unit to aid an individual in liver failure. He lay in bed, in coma. Next to him on a stretcher, arms outstretched on a cross-like restraint, was a sedated baboon. My job was to help connect the groin vessels of the patient to those of the animal so that blood filled with metabolic toxins from the patient's dysfunctional liver would flow continuously from his artery to the vein of the baboon, enter the healthy liver, and be detoxified. The cleared blood would then return from animal to man. When apprised of the plan, I remember wondering what kind of institution I had come to for training. Remarkably, however, during the cross-circulation the patient awoke and became lucid; the baboon remained unaffected. In fact, despite his sedation the monkey seemed displeased with the entire proceedings.

After several hours we disconnected the tubing and repaired the vessels. The baboon, still on his cross, was carried out by the young surgeon who had brought him from another hospital across the city. Placed in the back seat, the animal made such an unusual silhouette that a suspicious policeman stopped the car during the return journey. He asked the surgeon, a rather brash research fellow from Rhodesia, to step outside the automobile to be searched. The physician objected. The policeman insisted, wanting to know exactly what the crucifixion-like figure was. The officer was invited to put his head in the window and see for himself. The baboon snapped; the policeman recoiled, losing his cap, his nerve, and his demeanor. So flustered was he that he insisted on leading the surgeon's car back to the hospital at full speed, with siren blaring. Unhappily, the effect of the treatment was only transient and the patient lapsed back into ultimately fatal coma.

The increasing experience and occasional successes with organ allografts after the introduction of chemical immunosuppression emboldened a few surgeons to transplant xenogeneic organs into human recipients. A spate of attempts in 1963–1964 included twenty kidneys grafted directly between nonhuman primates and patients by four surgical groups in North America, one in Italy, and three in France. A Minnesota team transplanted a cadaver kidney into a 65-year-old diabetic woman with renal failure from chronic infection. As this was quickly rejected, team members substituted a kidney from a baboon. Although the organ functioned for three days, the patient died of massive gastrointestinal hemorrhage.[8]

At about the same time in New Orleans, Keith Reemstma performed thirteen kidney xenotransplants in humans, the first from a rhesus monkey donor, the remainder from chimpanzees. Despite intense immunosuppression, most of the organs failed within a few weeks, showing primarily inflammation and clotting of small vessels. Remarkably, one chimpanzee kidney continued to function for nearly nine months, possibly an example of transplantation between a "concordant" combination—a term later coined by Roy Calne to describe genetically close species in which graft rejection may be delayed and attenuated. Thomas Starzl and a few other investigators then reported somewhat prolonged function of baboon kidneys in patients, but only under maximal immunosuppression.[9] A gradation of results between nonhuman primate donor species and man became apparent, with organs from chimpanzees surviving the longest, followed by those of baboons, then those of various monkeys. In retrospect, this finding may not be too surprising because only 2 percent of the genetic makeup of chimpanzees differs from that of humans. It also appeared that xenogeneic donor-recipient combinations with some ABO blood-group compatibilities performed better than combinations with different blood types.

In contrast to the relatively extensive laboratory experience that

James Hardy had accrued before attempting lung and heart xenotransplantation in his two patients, the renal cases were carried out with less
substantial experimental background data. Even over the next decade,
the biologic information on grafts placed across species increased only
minimally. Occasional descriptions of the often violent destruction of
xenografted kidneys in animals were apparently ignored. A report of
the dramatic ninety-minute rejection of a goat kidney grafted into a
dog by Calne in 1961, for instance, received little attention before the
clinical transplants were carried out.[10]

As information from animal models slowly broadened and the few
human cases were analyzed and considered, it became clear that existing immunosuppressants such as azathioprine, which primarily depressed lymphocyte-mediated alloimmunity, were relatively ineffectual in prolonging the survival of whole organs grafted across species.
No alternative chemical means were available to modulate the powerful host responses to xenogeneic organs, because the process is mainly
humoral. Indeed, the events orchestrating destruction of a xenograft
are strikingly parallel to those occurring with hyperacute rejection of
allografts in presensitized recipients or in patients with specific anti-
donor antibodies in their circulation. With rejection of the cross-
species organ, xenoreactive "natural" antibodies react almost instantaneously with carbohydrate antigens on the organ's vessels. These
preformed natural antibodies are present in the serum of all vertebrates, and even of primitive fish, reptiles, and amphibians. As they
may respond to many antigens without evidence of previous exposure,
their presence may indicate an early host defense mechanism that
comes into play before more specific antibody formation can occur.
Upon revascularization of the graft, the entire inflammatory cascade is
rapidly activated. The resulting complex of acute-phase proteins includes the complement system, a plethora of inflammatory and vaso-
active substances, adhesion molecules, and clotting factors. Platelets
and white blood cells aggregate on vessel walls, filling and obstructing
them. Capillaries become increasingly permeable as their lining cells
are destroyed. Inflamed larger vessels clot. Within a strikingly brief
period, the organ is dead.

With the exception of chimpanzee livers transplanted to three patients by Starzl between 1969 and 1973, no more clinical activity oc-

curred until Christiaan Barnard used nonhuman primate hearts as temporary assist devices in two patients in Cape Town, and Leonard Bailey placed a baboon heart into Baby Fae in Los Angeles a decade later. An unsuccessful pig-to-human cardiac transplant was performed in Poland in 1992. Starzl transplanted baboon livers into two patients in 1993. In one of these, an individual with viral hepatitis and AIDS, he used the baboon specifically as a donor because its liver is not susceptible to the virus. Under primary immunosuppression with FK506, the hepatic graft remained relatively undamaged and produced baboon proteins, including clotting factors. The recipient became dialysis dependent from the toxic effects of the drugs, however, and died of infection after seventy days.[11] No further attempts have been forthcoming.

A variety of technological, biological, commercial, and social forces have fueled the tempo of discourse, argument, and activity in xenografting. Relevant clinical experience has slowly accumulated from the transplantation of xenogeneic cells, including pig pancreatic tissue and pig islets to diabetic patients in Stockholm, baboon bone marrow to an immunodeficient individual in Pittsburgh, placement of cells from fetal pigs into the brains of those with Parkinson's or Huntington's disease in several centers, and the grafting of cow adrenal cells in patients with severe pain. One trial is planned for cross-circulation between isolated pig livers and patients with end-stage hepatic failure, and another is being considered in which pig liver cells placed in a chamber will be tested to provide support for patients during episodes of liver failure. Regardless of the type of tissue transplanted, the problem of controlling the host responses not only remains unsolved but continues to generate substantial controversy. Still, investigations persist. Many years ago when asked about the ethics of the procedure, Peter Medawar dismissed doubts about heart allografting by remarking: "One can be as philosophical as you like about the ethics of transplantation. The fact of the matter is, people would rather be alive than dead."[12] This opinion may also serve as a motto for xenotransplantation.

Regardless of these occasionally optimistic hints, public and professional criticism has colored the entire experience since the burst of animal-to-human xenografts in the mid-1960s. Brent summarized the reaction of many toward what was generally considered an overly publicized, controversial departure from standard treatment. "Looking back at this year [1964], it seems as if some sort of collective madness had taken over in the United States, where the [most] attempts were made, for despite the introduction of azathioprine and steroids in the treatment of patients who had been given renal allografts, the omen certainly could not have been good." And after Baby Fae had received her baboon heart, a prominent ethicist also decried the trend: "Only when it is clear to the medical community, or regulatory bodies . . . and the general public that both researchers and their subject . . . fully understand that clinical trials involving xenografts have as their primary goal the acquisition of generalizable knowledge should further research be undertaken." In other words, given the state of knowledge at the time, the patients had been used only as vehicles to increase scientific information without realistic hope of success.[13]

Although xenotransplantation of solid organs into patients has not again been attempted over much of the last decade, ongoing advances in the laboratory continue to provoke discussions of practicalities, immune mechanisms, the potential transmission of known and unknown infections between animals and man, and the ethics of animal use. The rapid and irreversible rejection orchestrated by host natural xenoreactive antibodies and complement has been largely uncontrollable, specifically because of major genetic differences between human complement, a powerful inflammatory mediator in the serum, and complement-regulatory proteins on pig tissues. However, several investigative approaches are beginning to challenge this almost inevitable rejection. Plasmaphoresis, an established dialysis-like technique that physically removes antibodies from the circulation, has been attempted clinically in sensitized human allograft recipients and experimentally in xenograft models. While the onset of the accelerated rejection process can be delayed, the influence of the method is usually transient. There are fewer data on the ability of other means to inhibit complement or to block or remove antibody. In general, these strategies are temporary, probably incomplete, and require stringent ongoing immunosuppression to prolong graft survival.

An alternative approach increasingly in vogue has been the transplantation of organs from genetically altered or transgenic pigs that bear human complement or similar regulatory proteins, thus bypassing the initial phase of hyperacute rejection after grafting. These pigs are produced by the microinjection into fertilized pig eggs of clones bearing the desired human genes. Appropriate offspring are taken for organ donors. Although such a concept is exciting in theory, the animals are difficult and expensive to generate. Relatively few live to adulthood. Their development has also engendered serious arguments between individual investigators and industry over intellectual property rights, and over accountability and responsibility for premature publicity. Such disagreements have done much to dampen enthusiasm on both sides.

Even though the hyperacute rejection of the transgenic organs can often be averted, a later type of graft destruction, a process termed delayed xenograft rejection, may occur. Although some hearts and kidneys from transgenic animals transplanted into heavily immuno-suppressed nonhuman primates have functioned for days or occasionally for weeks, they have been ultimately destroyed by the immune system of the host. Graft deterioration and failure from chronic rejection or other attenuated host processes occurring over time may, at least theoretically, be an even more important specter in xenotransplantation than in allotransplantation.

Beyond the difficulties with the feasibility and practicality of xenotransplantation, ongoing debate is concerned with the use of animals for such a purpose. Although chimpanzees are an attractive potential donor population owing to their genetic closeness to humankind, their numbers are few, their intelligence high, and their overall similarity to humans so obvious that public outcry has virtually stopped such experiments. As comparable arguments apply to other apes and monkeys, the pig has become the donor of choice. This animal is plentiful, breeds prolifically, is raised in large quantities for meat and leather, and has organs of a size appropriate to humans. There are physiological and functional similarities between pig and patient. The use of porcine heart valves and porcine insulin has long been established. Once transgenic techniques are perfected, donor animals can presumably be raised in adequate numbers. Most feel that specially bred animals are ethically acceptable as organ donors, an opinion driven primarily by clinical need.

A compelling issue of greater potential consequence is the risk of

zoonoses, infections transmitted from the animal donor to the immunosuppressed recipient via the transplanted organ and even, once established, to the general population. As knowledge of the immunocompromised state has increased (whether secondary to anticancer
agents or from viral infestation such as AIDS), the possible effects of as
yet unrecognized or mutating pathogens have gained attention. What
is to prevent, for example, viral precursors that reside silently in a
foreign species from changing into forms such as HIV that may potentially harm humans? Indeed, investigators have shown that viruses in
normal pig tissue may infect human cells in the test tube.[14]

While no such instance has occurred in transplantation, the possibilities of an epidemic of disease from a recognized or unrecognized
virus remains frightening to many. These concerns have increased with
the devastating outbreaks of the monkey-borne ebola virus in Africa,
the presence of mad cow disease in Britain and other European countries where more than a hundred people became infected and died, the
mortality from a severe viral pulmonary disease (hantavirus) in the
United States, and the death of a laboratory worker from a monkey
virus. The AIDS epidemic, possibly triggered a relatively few years ago
by monkey-to-man contact, has been devastating. Communicable-
disease experts evoke the specter of the 1918 epidemic of influenza
from a swine flu virus, which caused millions of deaths worldwide.
The recent instances of anthrax in the postal system have accentuated
these fears. To inflame the public imagination further, a cluster of
novels and television fiction on the subject has arisen. Although actual
evidence for such a threat from xenotransplantation of organs is minimal, the issue raises persistent questions. Efforts have therefore been
stepped up toward careful animal selection and testing of herds of
transgeneic pigs, and investigations into obscure viruses and viral
forms continue.

Overall anxiety about the subject and its ramifications has been
enough to evoke discussions on the national level. In 1995 a committee
in the United Kingdom assessed social and ethical issues of xenotransplantation, concluding that primate use would be unacceptable, but
that pig organs could be potentially satisfactory for human trials. A
year afterward, a clinical moratorium, later supported by the Council
of Europe, was passed—even though the importance of gaining new

experimental knowledge was stressed. In the United States the Institute of Medicine suggested that "the potential benefit will outweigh
the risks." Various federal bodies have expressed concern but have not
produced requirements. Despite all the debate, pursuit of the subject
continues.[15]

While considerably more difficult and complex to undertake than
allotransplantation, our body of knowledge about xenotransplantation
is expanding. In 2002 two research groups successfully cloned piglets
lacking a gene that stimulates the human immune system to reject
transplanted pig organs.[16] The impetus from such an advance, and from
others to come, will continue to drive the subject and give hope to all
involved. Unfortunately, the overall pace of progress—particularly in a
culture attuned to instant gratification and in a climate that demands
finite medical answers to complex problems—has been discouraging.
Research has been slowed further by the withdrawal of significant
funding by one of the field's principal and most generous corporate
sponsors. Norman Shumway, a man who did so much to bring cardiac
allotransplantation to the mainstream, has been heard to quip in public
lectures that "xenotransplantation has a great future . . . and always will
have!" Roy Calne echoes these sentiments: "Success in xenografting is
just around the corner—but it's an awfully long corner!"

Coming of Age

12

CLINICAL TRANSPLANTATION EXPANDED SUB-stantially during the 1970s, becoming more visible as a potential treatment option for the swelling roster of patients seeking help. As hospitals in the United States in particular approached what was later to become a maelstrom of marketing forces, competition between institutions was fueled by incentives to provide "full-service" care with all current diagnostic technologies and treatment modalities. Tragically, some of the advances were limited to those who could pay. But after federal reimbursement of the expenses of individuals with renal failure became available under Medicare in 1972, adequate medical coverage for this population at least was assured. The relative improvements in kidney transplantation and dialysis, the occasional provocative replacement of other organs, and the new revelations of the biologists were driving the imagination of the enlarging pool of young professionals who were joining this innovative field. As a result, more surgeons were performing more transplants in more centers all around the world.

The spectrum of achievements during the 1960s had ranged from substantial gains in scientific and clinical knowledge to instances of apparent medical adventurism. The 1970s were generally a time of retrenchment and consolidation. In this relatively stable period in the experimental laboratories, investigations shifted from definition of principles to the unraveling of precise immunological mechanisms. Several of the important early figures started to direct their energies into new areas. Peter Medawar and Michael Woodruff, for example, were increasingly involved with cancer biology. Joseph Murray returned full-time to plastic surgery, where he became a major innovator in the new field of craniofacial repair of children and adults with severe disfigurements. Rupert Billingham examined the immunology of gestation and birth. The clinical results of transplantation plateaued despite strenuous efforts by many investigators to devise and exploit novel immunosuppressive strategies.

At the same time, the prevalent philosophy that the addition of ever more steroids could inevitably reverse what was often an irreversible rejection process produced a high incidence of complications and death from oversuppression. Indeed, the data derived from many centers through 1974 showed that 14 percent of patients bearing kidneys from living-related donors died within the first year, as did 28 percent of those who had received organs from cadavers.[1] The surgeons and physicians most directly involved remained enthusiastic, and the occasional successes were striking. Still, it is little wonder that the mediocre results persuaded many that the risks, particularly of cadaver donor transplantation, were unacceptable.

With increasing clinical experience and appreciation of the hazards of immunosuppression, innovations and refinements of existing treatment were undertaken to reduce the dangers. Our group at the Brigham were among the first to call attention to the excessive fatality rate and suggest means to ameliorate it.[2] Through judicious use of antibiotics and limitation of steroid doses, we were able to reduce substantially the incidence of infection. The new radiologic technique of ultrasound became an accurate tool for identifying accumulations of urine, blood, and lymph around the kidney. Prompt surgical evacuation of these substances reduced substantially the incidence of abscesses and their complications, which included disruption of vascular suture lines, spread of infection throughout the body, or even death of the recipient. Expeditious correction of mechanical abnormalities of the transplant procedure itself (such as urine leakage or obstruction) became routine. When we saw irreversible changes of rejection on biopsy specimens under the microscope, we discontinued the immunosuppression and quickly removed the graft. This rather aggressive surgical approach to serious complications not only reduced mortality in transplant recipients but in the dialysis population as well.

In essence, those responsible for patients lowered their threshold for acceptance of failure, replacing the previous atmosphere of zealotry to retain a graft at all costs with more sensible clinical judgment. The death rate within the first year after transplantation fell to 2 and 5 percent among recipients of kidneys from living-related and cadaver donors, respectively. A comparable but less dramatic pattern of declining mortality for recipients of other organs followed. The stage was set for new advances.

In the November 1978 issue of the British medical journal *Lancet*, two short papers appeared that radically changed the complexion of clinical transplantation. In the first, a group in London showed that treatment with a new immunosuppressive drug, Cyclosporin A, substantially diminished the incidence and severity of GVHD in recipients of foreign bone marrow. In the second, Roy Calne and his Cambridge associates reported that the same agent had been strikingly effective in several patients with kidney grafts (Figure 12.1). One year later they described in detail their results with thirty-four recipients of thirty-six organ allografts, all treated with Cyclosporin A. Twenty-six of the thirty-two kidneys continued to support their hosts, as did two pancreases and two livers. Twenty patients received no adjunctive steroids. No additional chemical agent such as azathioprine was used in fifteen individuals. Compared to the clinical results of the previous fifteen years, these data were unprecedented. The investigators carefully concluded, however, that "safe and effective immunosuppression remains an elusive goal . . . in the foreseeable future . . . Highly selective agents will be required in clinical organ grafting. [Cyclosporin A] is a move in this direction . . . Despite careful assessment in animals, when a drug is first used clinically the patient embarks on an uncertain and possibly hazardous journey. Every effort must be made not to repeat mistakes, and careful review of patients is essential before widespread use of the drug is advocated."[3] As transplantation has evolved further, the truth of these sentiments is increasingly obvious.

Cyclosporin A, today so critical to the field (and later renamed cyclosporine), had a difficult birth. A product of the giant Swiss pharmaceutical house Sandoz, its potential importance and the advisability of further development were debated hotly by those in the company.

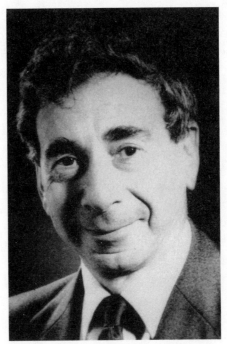

Figure 12.1 Sir Roy Calne in about
1985 (Novartis, with permission)

In 1969–1970, two new strains of fungi were isolated by Sandoz field
botanists from two sites, a bleak highland plateau in Norway called
Hardanger Vidda, and a valley in Wisconsin. Only one of the strains,
Tolypocladium inflatium (Gans), could be grown in submerged culture: a fungal product was isolated from the culture broth. Enough of
the crude extract, eventually characterized chemically as a ring of
eleven protein fragments, became available for biological screening.
Initial analysis was unexciting, although the substance was noted to be
unusually nontoxic to mice.

As such compounds often showed unexpected actions different
from their more usual antifungal activity, Jean Borel, a young scientist
who had joined Sandoz only three years earlier, was assigned to examine the material for other pharmacological properties (Figure 12.2). He
quickly discovered that one of the metabolites isolated from the extract was markedly immunosuppressive. Within months the influence
of this factor, Cyclosporin A, on both cellular and humoral immune

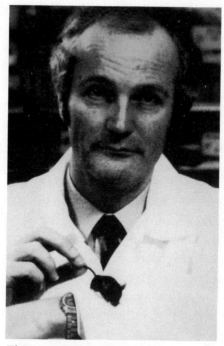

Figure 12.2 Jean Borel in the
mid-1980s (Novartis, with permission)

activity had been established in cultured cells. Its striking effectiveness in treating experimental arthritis and in prolonging survival of
skin grafts in mice was soon piquing the interest of his colleagues.
Impressed by its immunosuppressive abilities combined with its apparent lack of toxicity, Borel and his superiors pushed ahead despite
some opposition within the company. As experimental data accumulated, they found that the new agent reversibly inhibited the function
of T lymphocytes and was nontoxic to several cell populations in a
variety of animal species. Indeed, they were able to report that they
had discovered "a prototype of a new generation of immunosuppressants."[4] The selective interactions of Cyclosporin A with the host
immune responses contrasted to those of the other immunosuppressants then available, which indiscriminately destroyed rapidly dividing
cells throughout the body.

Along with his biological interest in the agent, Borel was well aware of its clinical possibilities. In 1976 he presented his data at a surgical meeting in England. In the audience was a young scientist working in Calne's laboratory at Cambridge University, David White. Excited about the prospects for the material in transplantation, White managed to obtain a small amount to initiate a series of experiments. He asked a Greek research fellow, A. J. Kostakis, to test it in rats that had received heart transplants, a popular experimental model at the time. Fat soluble but not water soluble, Cyclosporin A was absorbed poorly in the intestines of most animal species as well as man. The powdered form, taken by mouth in a gelatin capsule or suspended in alcohol, was ineffectual. Only oil appeared to be a satisfactory vehicle. Part of the lore surrounding this drug involves the concern of Kostakis' mother that her son would not thrive on what she considered to be the relatively bland English fare. Accordingly, she sent him some high-quality Greek olive oil to enliven his diet. The young investigator soon confirmed that, upon heating, the new compound would dissolve readily in the oil. From then on, administration of the oil-based solution to allograft recipients became standard treatment.

Within weeks, Kostakis reported to Calne the unprecedented prolongation of his heart grafts following only brief treatment of the recipients. Skeptical, the professor sent him back to the laboratory to repeat his experiments. His results were the same. Studies of its effects in other transplant models gathered in a rush. Enthusiasm spread, particularly after confirmation of its striking immunosuppressive effects in rabbits receiving kidney transplants, an exceptionally demanding experimental system.[5] Induction of a state of tolerance was even suggested. Investigators in Oxford, in our research laboratory at Harvard, those at the University of Minnesota, and then other groups, soon produced similar data in heart, liver, and pancreas allografts in rats and pigs, skin grafts in several species, and kidneys in dogs and nonhuman primates (Figure 12.3). The results in a few human patients were equally compelling, although both they and the large experimental animals were found to require daily maintenance doses (in rats and rabbits a short initial course of the drug produced indefinite graft survival).

The mechanisms of action of Cyclosporin A were also being unraveled. Borel and others had shown that the agent inhibited the prolif-

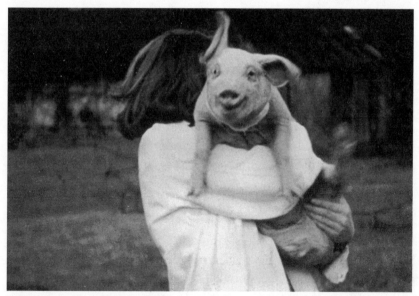

Figure 12.3 One of Roy Calne's early Cyclosporin A–treated heart-transplant recipients, smiling after a successful result (R. Y. Calne, with permission)

erative response of cultured naive lymphocytes of many species, but not if the cells were sensitized against antigen. Primarily directed against T helper cells, Cyclosporin A prevented the elaboration of one of their products, interleukin 2, which promotes clonal expansion of T-cell populations. The compound was eventually found to alter the basic machinery within the lymphocyte by binding calcium-dependent proteins in its cytoplasm, and to prevent the signaling in the cell that was responsible for the production of a variety of immune factors. These immunosuppressive activities were the most selective and specific yet identified.

News of the early laboratory and clinical results traveled rapidly throughout the international transplant community. Only months after a handful of publications had appeared, the halls of the 1978 Transplantation Society Congress in Rome were abuzz with conversation about the new agent. Lecture rooms overflowed during the few presentations on the subject. Four years later Cyclosporin A had become virtually the centerpiece of the 1982 meeting. Extensive discussion of

its actions and characteristics culminated in a report by Calne and
White of one-year actuarial survival of 82 percent of sixty cadaver-
donor kidney grafts in fifty-nine patients, a figure far superior to results ever achieved using older forms of immunosuppression.[6]

Other centers in Europe, the United States, and Australia soon
initiated their own clinical series. Two large controlled trials began to
enroll patients. By 1983, overall results from both multicenter trials
and from individual units, including our own, had shown an approximately 20 percent increase in one-year graft function compared to
conventional therapy, and a 10–15 percent advantage at three and five
years. Liver and heart transplantation also improved substantially.
With these encouraging statistics, patients who would not hitherto
have been considered for transplantation were added to the rolls. The
new agent transformed the field, increasing dramatically the number
of organs grafted and of persons demanding them. In 1976, worldwide,
six scientific papers on the subject had been published; in 1980 there
were 107, and within a few years, there were thousands.[7]

Few effective drugs are without side effects, and Cyclosporin A
was no exception. Calne quickly discovered what was to become a
serious problem: the compound's sometimes-profound ability to inhibit renal function.[8] All of us testing it during that early period unknowingly administered much higher doses than are usually given
today. As a result, kidney toxicity was common. We initially attributed
the initial state of low or no urine output from the new organ to the
ischemic injury the kidney had sustained when it was without blood
flow during the period of storage before transplantation. Although not
evident in any of the experimental animal models, this unexpected
complication in patients manifested itself in three patterns.

The incidence of early delayed graft function was so high that we
limited use of the drug to those recipients diuresing immediately after
surgery, or we postponed administration until renal function had returned. I remember two of our patients vividly. One put out no urine
for one hundred days, the other for fifty-seven days. Repeated biopsies of their transplants showed no rejection, only signs of slowly
resolving changes of ischemia. The two waited on dialysis. All of us
waited for the grafts to function. Finally, in desperation, we substituted azathioprine for Cyclosporin A as maintenance immunosup-

pression, a step that was far from standard practice at the time. Within twenty-four hours, both individuals excreted large amounts of urine. Kidney function returned to normal and the patients were discharged. This unheard-of graft behavior gave us much to think about.

The second pattern of functional deterioration developed after days or weeks, a type of renal toxicity difficult to differentiate from acute rejection, even on biopsy.

Late toxicity, the third pattern, resembled chronic rejection. It appeared after months or years and was characterized by progressively declining graft function associated with increasing scarring and fibrosis of the organ as seen microscopically. These chronic changes developed not only in kidney transplants but in some previously functioning native organs of patients receiving Cyclosporin A for autoimmune conditions or to immunosuppress other types of organ grafts. The incidence of renal failure in heart-transplant recipients, for instance, was surprisingly high. Various strategies initiated to reduce this often serious side effect included dose adjustments, standardization of serum concentrations, examination of drug-interaction influence on its effectiveness and toxicity, and later, substitution of azathioprine.

Other side effects of the agent, all more or less dose related, included neurological complications such as tremor of the hands or numbness of the legs, alterations in liver function, swelling of the gums, growth of facial hair, and hypertension. The most serious complication was the unexpected specter of cancer. In Calne's early series of thirty-four renal allograft recipients, three developed unusual B-cell lymphomas.[9] Cessation of the drug and surgical excision of the tumor were relatively successful, although reports of lymphomas continued to arise.

It took considerable experience on the part of many clinical groups before such adverse effects were generally appreciated and effectively controlled, primarily by progressive reduction of dose and close regulation of levels in the blood. Before accurate chemical assays became available and blood or serum levels of Cyclosporin A were measured or understood, dosages were administered empirically, based primarily on data from the dog experiments.

One of the more ingenious methods of gauging toxicity of the drug was described in a conference by members of a Canadian group in the early 1980s who were testing its immunosuppressive effect in transplanted monkeys. The animals were exceptionally well cared for. Each lived in a large cage equipped with its own television set, which they had learned to operate. The monkeys followed the daily soap operas enthusiastically, taking great pleasure, it appeared, in the endless adventures and crises of the characters. The investigators assured us that they could tell with relative ease when the cumulative dose of Cyclosporin A had become too high and reached toxic levels: the monkeys lost interest in the soaps!

Within a few years of the advent of cyclosporine, as the company (now called Novartis) had renamed it, additional agents were introduced with ever-increasing frequency. By the end of the 1990s, several were well along in clinical trials and becoming generally available. A variety of forces apparently drove this burst of activity. Improving success for the patient was paramount. What could be more discouraging for recipient and physician alike than to be faced with a rejection episode unresponsive to standard therapy and the threat of graft loss, particularly as the relatively low number of available organs often meant years of waiting for a new one? The possibility of more effective drugs encouraged not only clinicians interested in improving results, but also basic scientists who used the compounds as probes to examine the complexities of molecular events occurring in activated cells. Changing dynamics in the increasingly powerful and competitive pharmaceutical industry hastened the development of the new drugs as well. As the breadth of the field increased and immunosuppression was discovered to be potentially big business, the industrialization phase of transplantation commenced.

Three new agents in particular—FK506 (tacrolimus), rapamycin (sirolimus), and mycophenolate mofetil (Cell Cept)—used alone or in combination with cyclosporine, have improved the short-term results of organ transplantation by reducing the incidence of acute rejection. Although the often-serendipitous development of each is interesting, only FK506 will be described here.

In a manner remarkably similar to cyclosporine FK506 was isolated from a soil fungus, *Streptomyces tsukubaensis*, found 100 kilometers north of Tokyo on the slopes of Mount Tsukuba by scientists of the Fujisawa Pharmaceutical Corporation. At the Transplantation Society Congress in 1986, Calne and Starzl were in the audience during a presentation by a young Japanese surgeon, Takenori Ochiai of Chiba University, on the immunosuppressive effectiveness of FK506 in a rat heart-graft model.[10] Calne had already tested the agent and felt that it had little potential, as it was exceptionally toxic to the gastrointestinal tract of dogs and produced significant inflammation of their small blood vessels. He also noted, as had Ochiai, that it was considerably more potent by weight than cyclosporine. Starzl, in contrast, was so enthused by the data that he promptly traveled to Japan, where he was given some material for experimental use. He determined that organ allograft survival was prolonged in treated rat, dog, monkey, and baboon recipients. The biochemical structure of the new agent was subsequently shown to be distinct from that of cyclosporine; it bound to related but not similar protein receptors in the cell and interfered early in the cell activation process. Thus, it blocked generation of various lymphocyte products that mediate rejection.

Although experimental work on FK506 was ongoing in Cambridge, at Chiba University, and at the Fujisawa laboratories, the majority of the early clinical experience emanated from the University of Pittsburgh. Having created a major transplant unit there after his arrival in 1981, and enlivened by funding from the pharmaceutical company to the university, Starzl was almost messianic in his approach. He took on the drug as a cause and controlled its use for months. Having rescued it from virtual oblivion following the initial adverse reports of its toxicity, he persuaded the FDA and the hospital administration to allow him to use FK506 in selected patients. He soon reported that the agent was strikingly effective in human recipients of liver, small bowel, heart, pancreas, and kidneys—perhaps most obviously in its ability to rescue liver grafts failing from rejection episodes resistant to steroids or to anti–T-cell monoclonal antibodies. A company-sponsored satellite meeting to discuss the new agent was arranged and held immediately before the Transplantation Society Congress late in 1989. Twenty-six of the thirty-one papers presented were from Pittsburgh. The remarkably convincing data were embellished by reports that the hospitalized graft recipients who had not received the drug virtually rebelled in their insistence on the treatment.[11] Controlled trials were not considered.

It was a difficult time for Starzl. In addition to the stress of launching FK506 and convincing his colleagues of its efficacy, his group had been under fire for several years because of a series of Pulitzer Prize–winning articles in the *Pittsburgh Press*. They enumerated a series of alleged irregularities that included the transplantation of organs from local cadaver donors into foreign nationals who paid large amounts for the operation and jumped to the head of the line to receive their grafts. The U.S. Department of Justice became involved. The transplant community in general remained frustrated and skeptical about the new drug, for no one could obtain it. As the protocols devised by Fujisawa were not satisfactory to regulatory agencies in the United States and Europe, many transplanters felt that clinical events were streaming from Pittsburgh too rapidly and without adequate control. Overenthusiastic articles in the press competed with ongoing concerns of the Food and Drug Administration about toxicity. A front-page article in the *New York Times* extolling the benefits of FK506, which appeared during the 1989 annual meeting of the American College of Surgeons and before publication of Starzl's first clinical paper on the subject, evoked additional cynicism.[12] Perhaps some of the hyperbole that had dotted the field of transplantation over the previous decades sensitized the clinical investigators of the time against a too-precipitous acceptance of individual claims.

But Starzl was correct. As others began to use FK506 in their patients and data from two later multicenter trials eventually became available, the agent was increasingly accepted. Although the one-year actuarial graft survival differed little from that of cyclosporine-treated hosts, refractory rejection could often be successfully reversed by conversion from cyclosporine to FK506. The new agent also became popular among those caring for pediatric recipients of organ grafts—not only for its effectiveness, but also because of its steroid-sparing properties.

Side effects, however, were significant. FK506 was found to be extremely toxic to kidneys, relegating some heart, liver, and multi-organ recipients to dialysis. As many as 20 percent of liver recipients developed mild central nervous system abnormalities. The onset of diabetes, both acutely and over the short term, was an unexpected and distressing problem, with one third of renal transplant patients in one large study requiring insulin treatment.[13] Despite these adverse reactions, use of FK506 has gradually become more routine, particularly in multiorgan transplantation. Dosage, duration of action, and interactions with other pharmacological agents now are better understood. The data generated by many programs and involving many patients has effectively hastened knowledge of this drug and of those that followed. Markedly effective under some circumstances but markedly toxic in others, FK506 has found a useful niche in the spectrum of current clinical immunosuppression.

The introduction of Cyclosporin A not only changed clinical practice and opened new avenues of research in transplantation, but it also aroused debate among the original European investigators on the justification for a prospective randomized study of its effectiveness in cadaver-donor transplantation. Opponents said that the results of treatment were already so unequivocal compared to historical controls that such a study would be unethical. Roy Calne initially took this position, based in part on his previous experience with azathioprine (which, being unique, had never been subjected to such an examination). Encouraged by the Sandoz company and by several of his colleagues, however, he eventually supported a formal comparison between Cyclosporin A and standard immunosuppression with azathioprine and steroids. The ensuing European multicenter trial and the independently organized Canadian multicenter transplant study group were triumphs of therapeutic investigation in transplantation.[14] Indeed, without the convincing results of these exemplary studies, it is questionable whether Sandoz would have invested so heavily in the agent for worldwide application.

Groups in the United States never agreed to such a venture, feeling that the experience of individual units, and the use of retrospective results, were adequate to assess the new agent. This dislike of (or disregard for) multicenter data was a recurrent theme during the 1980s, not only with regard to immunosuppressive modalities but in many other aspects of medicine as well. By the beginning of the next decade, however, the FDA was demanding randomized multicenter trials of most new drugs, in part because of the efficacy of the large cyclosporine trials and in part because of the professional unrest surrounding the initial experience with FK506. Clearly, the federal agency would seriously delay permission to test FK506 further and block its marketing until other clinical transplant groups developed experience in its use. Eventually two large trials were initiated, one in the United States and one in Europe, with controlled data from these studies and from individual units providing accurate information for a comprehensive evaluation.

These controlled randomized blind or double-blind multicenter clinical trials provided large numbers of patients for exhaustive statistical analysis and introduced a rigor and discipline new to medicine. Previously, statistics in biology had been concerned primarily with measuring differences at a single time point. The subsequent ability to determine the efficacy of various treatments over time has been of enormous clinical importance. Such studies are based on the "null hypothesis" first established in patient-based studies in Britain in 1977: differences between two series of observations within a restricted system are proven either to represent chance or to measure the real effects of a given manipulation or other identifiable variables. In transplantation in particular, such assessments of the value of cyclosporine and subsequent drugs have been critical to their clinical acceptance and success.

While controlled trials have become standard procedure for the testing of new agents in a variety of clinical areas, unanticipated ramifications have appeared. The drugs have, for instance, become crucial marketing ploys by which competing companies achieve enduring name recognition for their products. Frequently updating of results at national and international conferences keep the drugs in the professional consciousness. The 1990s saw not only a large ongoing FK506 versus cyclosporine liver trial, but also three mycophenolate mofetil versus cyclosporine kidney trials. These expensive sustained efforts were underwritten by the companies involved.

Early data on the use of mycophenolate mofetil showed a 50 percent reduction in the incidence of acute rejection episodes as compared to cyclosporine. Simultaneously, with exquisite timing, a new and easily absorbed form of cyclosporine that can be taken by mouth was licensed after yet another Novartis-sponsored trial showed a similar reduction in kidney rejection within the first six months as compared to the standard formulation.[15] This brilliant marketing strategy did much to overcome enthusiasm for the competition. In spite of such commercial machinations, the lasting advantage of such trials has been to produce objective reports on the efficacy of a given agent compared to other drugs, all based on unassailable, statistically significant data.

Although the recent emphasis on clinical trials has been a significant step forward in determining the efficacy of various treatments, it is intriguing to note that a thousand years ago the great physician of Baghdad, Avicinna or Ibn Sina (980–1037), laid out rules for testing drugs that remain completely applicable today: "The drug must be free of any extraneous accidental quality. The drug must be tested on two types of diseases because sometimes a drug cures one disease by its essential qualities and another by its accidental ones. The time of action must be observed, so that the essence and accident are not confused. The effect of the drug must be seen to occur in many cases, for if this does not happen it was an accidental effect. The experimentation must be done with the human body, for testing on a lion or horse might not prove anything about its effect in man."[16] While many aspects of history progress, others do not change.

13

The Industrialization of Transplantation

A FEW CLINICAL INVESTIGATORS, CONFIDENT enough to acknowledge the marginal effectiveness of the new modalities and their substantial hazards to the desperately ill patients willing to accept the risks, tentatively introduced total-body radiation then chemical immunosuppression to recipients of kidney transplants. Perhaps stimulated by the ongoing political and social restlessness of the 1960s, all parties involved may have been more ready than in calmer periods to exploit innovative concepts in science and nonconformist departures in medicine. Although this iconoclastic attitude persisted over the next decade, the majority of clinical scientists, like the population itself, were tiring of disorder and turmoil and were seeking retrenchment and security. As the ongoing societal fluctuations were ebbing, immunosuppressive advances were few, clinical results plateaued, and enthusiasm for the new field was tempered by realism.

The 1980s heralded a different spirit, driven by private and corporate opportunity. The success of cyclosporine substantially changed the scope of transplantation by increasing the number of institutions offering this clinical service, of physicians and surgeons interested in the subject, and of patients seeking more feasible answers to their ills. Despite a progressively inadequate donor supply, enthusiasm for this treatment for end-stage organ failure accelerated throughout the 1990s as newer and more effective immunosuppressive drugs entered the collective consciousness.

In most market economies, commercial forces react directly to supply the demand for a given product or service. After the use of cyclosporine became routine and clinical results improved, why did the events of transplantation continue to evolve? Perhaps less because the subject remained technically, intellectually, and professionally gratifying than because in this new Gilded Age the highly visible prestige and financial rewards became paramount. It was not lost on anyone—from scientists to clinicians, from industrial marketers to hospital administrators, from third-party payers to patients—that the stakes were high. The subject had become a potential monetary and public relations bonanza.

In the United States in particular, the clinical field grew in proportion to the new entrepreneurial spirit. Private hospitals expanded the ranks of traditional university programs by opening their own transplant units, stretching already limited resources, increasing public expectations, and enlarging the pool of those desiring new organs. By the mid-1990s, for instance, over 250 hospitals offered kidney transplantation. One third performed fewer than 30 procedures per year.[1] One hundred fourteen liver transplant units had been started, 70 of which carried out fewer than 20 surgeries a year and not infrequently reported substandard results. The dubious workload of those involved in the grafting of thoracic organs was even more striking. Less than 10 cases per year were undertaken by 58 of the 89 centers that had sprung up. Programs in cardiac transplantation grew precipitously to more than 160 in 1995; yet fewer than 10 hearts a year were grafted in 44 of the units.

It could be argued that the large numbers of hospitals offering a variety of organ transplants not only have engendered an expensive and inefficient duplication of effort, but that by their very availability they have increased the rolls of borderline, inappropriate, and unrealistic patients who demand part of a limited resource and place additional stress on an already inadequate donor pool. Indeed, the very size of the undertaking here seems out of phase with that of many other countries. In Britain, for instance, with about a quarter of the population of the United States, there are thirty-three renal programs and seven experienced cardiothoracic transplant centers—perhaps a more practical centralization of skills. But even there, changes are in place aimed at producing fewer and busier programs.[2] This centralization of specialty resources in most European countries is distinctly different from the laissez-fair attitude of the United States allowing the opening of ever more competing units. And of course, with more programs and more patients, there is more demand for expensive drugs from the pharmaceutical industry.

Despite the tremors, alarms, and diversions that became almost a routine part of late-twentieth-century life and that continue ominously into the new century, most developed countries thrive economically. Their ongoing financial health has encouraged the development of novel technologies in many areas. These in turn have created new markets, revitalized older ones, and have left still others abandoned in their wake. A striking example is the pharmaceutical industry, an ever-enlarging enterprise of multinational corporations (known as Big Pharma). Without its influence and innovations, modern transplantation could not have evolved.

This industry grew rapidly during the middle years of the twentieth century.[3] Until World War I, only a handful of medicaments were available to a public besieged by the claims of charlatans peddling their nostrums. In addition to the surgical advances that resulted from the conflict, however, new medical tools and treatment options began to supplement the relatively few synthetic pharmaceutical agents that were primarily useful in relieving symptoms without affecting the diseases themselves. Although the United States imported many drugs from the highly developed German companies with their extensive experience in aniline dyes and coal tar medicinals, a few visionaries in America began to create an industry based on scientific research. These pharmaceutical manufacturers soon produced their own biologicals and synthetics, not infrequently through licenses from German patents.

Several new compounds arose from collaborations between academic laboratories and commercial companies, particularly in Europe. The cooperation between the university-based scientist Paul Ehrlich of Robert Koch's great school of bacteriology and the Hoechst Company, for instance, set an important precedent by orchestrating the production and distribution of diphtheria antitoxin, and subsequently by examining the therapeutic effects of arsenicals in treating various infections. In Britain, Nobel physiologist Sir Henry Dale left his professorship at Cambridge to head the new laboratories of the Wellcome

Company. Many in the United States entertained such relationships in a less kindly fashion; medical faculties were generally forbidden to step outside their institutions. The American Society for Pharmacology and Experimental Therapeutics ruled, for instance, that "entrance into the permanent employ of a drug firm shall constitute forfeiture of membership."[4] In a literary example of this antipathy, Sinclair Lewis described the moral and intellectual failure of his idealistic scientist-hero, Martin Arrowsmith, who joined industry after years in private practice and research.

Regardless of these differences in attitude, increasing numbers of relatively effective medications became available between the wars. Companies in the United States introduced several sulfanilamide derivatives, the parent compound having been synthesized previously by the German firm of I. G. Farben. Other agents followed quickly, including diuretics, antitubercular drugs, and early nonsteroidal anti-inflammatory agents. Insulin, tetanus toxoid, estrogenic hormones, and adrenal and pituitary extracts entered clinical use. The first effective treatment for pernicious anemia was initiated. Vitamins were synthesized. A vaccine against yellow fever was created.

By World War II, pharmaceutical research had expanded dramatically. The polio virus had been cultured, and a vaccine produced to control this scourge with its selective tragedy to the young and its ghastly sequelae of paralysis, leg braces, iron lungs, and sometimes death. Other vaccines against childhood diseases followed, making safer this hitherto vulnerable period of life. Stimulated by the acute needs of wartime, industrial money poured into the development of antibiotics. Penicillin was discovered by Alexander Fleming in London in 1929. Methods to concentrate it were formulated and its clinical significance demonstrated by Howard Florey and Ernst Chain in Oxford a decade later. Companies in the United States produced this "wonder drug" in bulk for the armed services toward the end of the war, and later for civilian use. Selman Waksman identified streptomycin at Rutgers University in 1944. (In this instance, the relationship between university and industry, never completely smooth, broke down with a series of lawsuits concerning priorities of discovery.) Chloramphenicol and the tetracyclines soon became available. In the 1950s E. P. Abraham in Florey's Oxford department introduced the cephalosporins, important drugs that are effective against a variety of bacterial infections and that became especially useful in transplant recipients.

War-related research involved the corticosteroids too. In response to an erroneous rumor that the Germans had developed an adrenal hormone that could increase the performance of soldiers beyond their normal limitations of fatigue and stress, E. C. Kendall at the Mayo Clinic, then workers at the Merck and Upjohn companies, identified and subsequently produced a series of steroid hormones. One of these, progesterone, was found to be abundant in a Mexican yam; cortisol could be easily synthesized from it. Based on the action of this and similar agents, the birth control pill was created and tested clinically, a pharmacological departure that changed the mores of an entire people. This class of compounds also became critical in transplantation, as first suggested by George Thorn and his collegues at the Brigham and by René Küss and associates in Paris. Thomas Starzl in Denver later demonstrated their effects conclusively. Other drugs germane to transplantation and produced by the growing American and European pharmaceutical companies included the anticoagulant heparin, the thiazide group of diuretics, and a variety of antihypertensive agents. Anticancer drugs were also forthcoming—both alkylating agents derived from the feared nitrogen mustard gas of World War I, and antimetabolites that included the first chemical immunosuppressant, 6-mercaptopurine.

Stimulated by more frequent successes in the identification, development, and production of various active compounds and through effective collaborations with university laboratories and federal research institutes, a new philosophy dominates the modern pharmaceutical industry. With advances in medicine providing understanding of various disease states on increasingly intricate levels, the potential for drugs of many capacities and functions to combat these ills appears almost without limit. Drug research, drug discovery, and drug design have grown in parallel with the knowledge provided by the cellular and molecular biologists. Indeed, as molecular biology becomes increasingly better understood, subcellular definition of the activities of specific drugs has opened entirely new areas for examination of cell physiology and pharmacologic interactions. These efforts have been embellished and hastened by the tools now available to define molecules and their specific activities within the cellular machinery.[5] Technologies including x-ray crystallography, nuclear magnetic resonance spectroscopy, molecular modeling and computer sequencing, computational chemistry, and enzymology have become influential enterprises unto themselves. Even routes for administering the new agents are topics for development. A drug that can only be given intravenously, for instance, can hardly compete with one that can be taken as a pill. A seemingly unimportant subject such as method of delivery may make the difference between loss and profit for a company.

Having developed from small drug houses producing and selling patent medicines into a vast, lucrative, and multifaceted global industry, Big Pharma currently serves an ever-expanding market. But success has brought a variety of pressures. Hundreds of thousands of compounds undergo testing at tremendous cost. Only a few substances (cyclosporine, for instance) exhibit novel activity, in contrast to the customary refinement of existing themes.[6] Of all these compounds, the FDA ultimately approves about thirty each year. In-house scientists are pressured by company, stockholders, and public alike for new and more effective agents. In addition, external university-based laboratories desire recognition for their contributions. The optimistic economy of the 1990s encouraged venture capitalists and scientific entrepreneurs to create small start-up biomedical companies to develop their own specific molecules, antiviral drugs, inhibitors, or vaccines. In this frenzy of drug development, occasional ventures succeed and are bought by Big Pharma. Most fail.

Provoked by the commercial spirit of the last two decades, competition between companies has intensified. With its obvious financial interest in the profits surrounding a promising agent, Big Pharma can direct massive efforts toward specific goals. If a drug is thought to be potentially significant, vast resources may be provided for its development and marketing. A single successful blockbuster drug may reap enormous dividends. The pressures are intensified by the relatively short lives of many highly profitable drugs, based on expiration of their patents or by new drugs deposing them.

As an example, the patent for cyclosporine expired toward the end of the 1990s after only about fifteen years of general distribution and sales. At the same time, a small drug house in California received permission from the FDA to provide a generic, less expensive derivative. Other newly introduced immunosuppressives, or variations on existing themes, compete strenuously not only with cyclosporine but with one another for a significant market share, enhanced by the encouraging and repeatedly publicized results of individual clinical trials. Activity in advertising and public relations has accelerated.

The increasing rivalry between already huge companies has begotten national and international mergers in Europe and the United States. To solidify their positions, individual organizations may form strategic partnerships with others. Some of these maneuverings are for efficiency, some to combine resources, others to solidify markets, and some to invest in outside expertise. Even governments have become involved, driven by lobbyists to target research monies toward specific medical goals and particular diseases. The war on cancer, active throughout the administrations of Presidents Nixon, Ford, and Carter, was an early example. The push to create a vaccine for AIDS is currently under way.

Several of the smaller drug houses in Japan are expanding, fueled not only by imported technology but also by the progressive sophistication of their science. Indeed, the Japanese government has made the exportation of pharmaceutical products a national priority. The domestic market is becoming saturated in a culture where doctors own their own pharmacies, and prescribe and sell medications to an aging and long-lived population that takes many prescription drugs. The globalization of FK506 by the Fujisawa Company is an obvious example of this change in strategy.

The association between academe and industry, always uneasy, has grown closer in recent years.[7] Much of this cooperation is based on expediency. Research is expensive and the competition for grant money intense, with only about 15 percent of applicants for NIH funding actually receiving awards. It is little wonder that university-based investigators turn to private industry for help, encouraged increasingly by federal funding bodies and by their own institutions. The aims of the two groups have been traditionally different. Immersed in their subject, academic scientists are all too cognizant of what publications, presentations, and peer recognition of their investigations produce for them in research support, promotion, tenure, and prestige—and sometimes power and prizes. Those in industry work on specific company interests, keeping relevant information from competitors in other companies until a new process can be patented, proprietary advantage can be protected, or a given agent is introduced to the market.

These differences in philosophy and culture have led to problems such as the potential loss of investigator objectivity and loyalty secondary to promises of research support and other monetary advantages of company affiliation. Authors of articles in medical journals on the efficacy of drugs, as well as editorial writers discussing the findings, may have financial ties to drug companies—a relationship that is anathema to most editors. Investigators may act as consultants, enjoy a variety of extramural benefits, and be included as authors of articles ghostwritten by company functionaries. An even more problematic aspect of such arrangements is that research workers with ties to pharmaceutical companies may report results more favorable to a given product than those without such relationships. Negative data may be underreported.[8]

The growing emphasis on money in university-initiated science may disquiet the academic parent institutions, traditionally dedicated to scholarship, free exchange of ideas, unlimited inquiry, and knowledge for its own sake. In addition, as the relationships between commercial enterprises and institutions of learning grow stronger, so do questions of intellectual property rights and ownership of data. There have been a few episodes where university-based clinical scientists involved in drug trials have been threatened or even sued by the companies when they publicly voiced concern about a particular agent. Publications showing adverse results have been withdrawn from journals because of corporate pressure.

With at least some entrepreneurial faculty members raising capital, forming companies, offering stock, and extolling the profit motive based on their research results, the rules of academe have had to change. University patent offices are more proactive; lawyers and managers insert themselves into professional collaborations; technology transfer agreements between basic-science laboratories and the marketplace are common. And it all adds up. At Yale University, for instance, the annual income from royalties and licenses for university-developed projects in 1996 was $3 million. Two years later, this figure had reached $38 million.[9] Other large research universities have accrued similar dividends. As early as 1963, Ernst Chain had extolled the potential of this ecumenical spirit, speaking of his experience with penicillin at Oxford: "Notwithstanding the many important contributions from university laboratories, drug research and development without the active participation of the pharmaceutical industry is impossible . . . The best results in the field [have] been obtained by close collaboration between industrial and academic laboratories."[10] Despite the potential problems, the increasing cooperation between the two groups has yielded ever more effective drugs for a variety of diseases, as well as vastly increased influence of Big Pharma in medical care.

The field of transplantation has been no exception to these dynamics. The few university-based clinician-scientists working in the early days had little background knowledge about immunosuppression, a word thought to have been coined by Francis Moore in the 1960s. Data on the few available agents produced by a handful of pharmaceutical companies came primarily from animal experiments and their use in individuals with cancer. Dosage, scheduling, utility, and short- and long-term side effects all had to be defined. Company scientists and program directors encouraged the investigators to go ahead and use the products in the laboratory and in patients, donating them in exchange for information. Financial obligation either to answer specific research questions or to support the fledgling clinical efforts was modest at best. The few early investigators received relatively small stipends, which often supplemented monies from the NIH, the medical research councils, and other government agencies to carry out studies designed to understand activity and efficacy of the agents in controlled experimental settings. This early relationship between the drug houses and the clinical scientists was exemplary and is still one of the best models of disinterested cooperation.

The interaction between the program directors at Sandoz and those of us initially testing Cyclosporin A remains a sterling example. Yet the relationship did not always run smoothly. I recall an acrimonious meeting at the Brigham in the early 1970s between the transplant team and senior members of a pharmaceutical company that produced and supplied antilymphocyte globulin. As one of our patients had recently died from anaphylaxis after receiving the agent, the clinicians refused to continue its use in the program. They were accused of wanting to undermine the company!

With the heightened visibility of organ transplantation since the 1980s, the need for improved immunosuppressive agents has increasingly captured the interest of Big Pharma. Those in the companies realize full well that actual recipients of these agents are relatively few compared to the vast numbers of individuals taking antihypertensives, antidepressants, anti-inflammatories, histamine blockers, cholesterol-lowering drugs, and the other highly profitable classes of medicaments apparently necessary in the modern Western world. In the case of transplantation, not only has the field itself become prestigious and visible, but the associated medications may also be relevant to a potentially much larger patient population with autoimmune disorders that include diabetes, rheumatoid arthritis, psoriasis, and lupus. This relationship has not been lost on the companies that produce the medications. In addition, the possibilities of more effective, specific, nontoxic agents concern not just the afflicted patients, their doctors, and biologists, but those in insurance companies, public policy, and health care administration as well. The cost of these drugs is particularly startling: the annual overall expenditure in the United States alone for immunosuppressive medication, for instance, is well in excess of $900 million.[11]

No one in the field has been immune from the revolution in the pharmaceutical industry. With the advent of Cyclosporin A, striking changes have evolved in the relationship between those participating in organ transplantation and what was at the time becoming Big Pharma. Announcements of favorable company-generated data, public relations maneuverings, and corporate rivalries intensified during the 1990s with the gathering numbers of useful drugs seeking a share in the international market. In the increasingly competitive and overmanaged profession of medicine, significant numbers of transplant physicians and surgeons, although still primarily university affiliated, have moved from their prior interests in basic biology toward involvement in multicenter clinical trials with specific agents. They work closely with particular companies and their representatives toward the primary goal of "market penetration." Inasmuch as the use of a particular immunosuppressant in a trial precludes the investigators and their teams from testing other competing drugs at the same time, the clinicians and their patients have in essence been captured by the parent company. The overall impetus is difficult to control, as industry today generates $6 billion for clinical trials worldwide—$3.3 billion for investigations in the United States alone.

Big Pharma has also begun to devote entire international congresses to discussions of its new products, under the guise of basic science. Attendees are often flown in from all over the world to present their own data and hear the results of others. Such sessions, beautifully crafted and held in attractive locales, seem more like infomercials than educational sessions, with the sponsors apparently more interested in selling their products than in basic research. Indeed, it took many of us who were invited to participate some time to understand the motives behind the conferences, as the corporate presence was a subtle one. With this change in direction of a subject driven from its inception by scientific advances to one that industry seems increasingly to direct or influence, have come potential conflicts between clinician-scientists and company aims. Not unique to transplantation, such conflicts are occurring throughout many commercially sponsored or underwritten areas of medicine.

A related contention has been the industrial promotion of xenografting. A topic examined by only a few investigators since the 1960s, interest in the use of organs from various animal sources, especially the pig, has gained impetus over the last decade—particularly as the demand for scarce donor organs has increased so dramatically. Powerful pharmaceutical companies, often with a long and beneficial history of innovation and support for allotransplantation, have sponsored handsomely a few established, high-profile xenograft investigators, their laboratories, their research, their travel, and other conveniences. These same companies have become financially active in projects initiated in small biotechnology research institutes that involve expensive genetically altered donor animals designed to avoid devastating hyperacute rejections. Some companies are even considering specific university-based sites for eventual clinical application. One small trial transplanting pig islets into diabetic children has been already carried out in Mexico. Another is planned in New Zealand.[12]

This development proceeds regardless of lack of scientific understanding of the complexities of the host responses to the tissues of other species, a consistent dirth of significant success in experimental models, minimal and often confusing clinical anecdotes, and enduring fear of the possibility of transmission of zoonoses. Even with recent calls for a moratorium to balance medical, social, scientific, and ethical aspects of xenotransplantation before the onset of human trials, some clinicians remain eager to try; as noted, they have engrafted a handful of patients with animal tissues. Although companies appear ready to encourage these advances, they well understand that they must carefully balance their responsibility to their stockholders with modulation of their interests. Appropriate caution can only help the long-term progress of both the transplantation and the commercial communities.

In transplantation, as in many other areas of medicine, the once informal relationship between industry and academe, each dedicated to the health of the public, is shifting. Obvious advantages accrue to the field, particularly the enhancement of drug development and the support and organization of multicenter drug trials. Less disinterested motives are also involved, though: increased networking among nonobjective and prejudiced clinicians, businessmen, administrators, and managers via industry-sponsored conferences; prolonged clinical trials; secrecy; and reward. Pressures on researchers for improved results have increased, originating from the desire for enhanced public and professional recognition by the companies who want to sell their products, and from the patients, their doctors, and those who pay. Some of these changes have been significantly influenced by the rush toward managed care in the United States, with its reputed cost containment but relative lack of concern with the humanitarian traditions of medicine. The commercialization and industrialization of transplantation during the past two decades, as of many other medical specialties, is a product of its own success and is significantly altering the course of the entire field.

Many of us are increasingly concerned with these developments, believing that they threaten intellectual independence and may subvert the integrity of faculty research. Further, they may reduce pressure on government agencies to fund basic and applied investigations and seduce researchers away from "curiosity-driven science."[13] We have suggested strategies to emphasize the best parts of the relationship between Big Pharma and academic investigators and minimize the least favorable:

> 1. The formation of dispassionate committees comprising independent academics and professionals, with responsibility to organize and appraise clinical trials via institutional clinical research offices. Pharmaceutical interests would contribute to planning and analysis of the trials, but not to their control or direction.
> 2. Industrial support for national and international conferences could be placed under the aegis of objective central program-organizing committees.
> 3. Company funding for relevant associated research would be handled via a central foundation organized by the professional societies and distributed via peer-reviewed grant applications.
> 4. Agreements regarding ownership of data and objective reporting of results should be formalized between industry and academe before starting a study or a trial. The arrangement must emphasize freedom of publication and specify dissemination of adverse results.

While such recommendations may be construed as idealistic, they might well serve to restore professional autonomy and integrity, increase the credibility of industry, and reduce drug costs through decreased promotional spending and unnecessary or overlapping clinical trials.[14]

Unexpected Specters

14

MODERN TRANSPLANTATION CURRENTLY PRO-
vides new lives for about forty thousand patients who receive organs
each year throughout the world, and new hope for tens of thousands
who await them. But the very success of the subject has opened a variety
of challenges ranging from the logistical to the ethical. Clinical research
is increasingly driven by industries devoted to the developing and
marketing of immunosuppressive drugs, sometimes to the detriment of
objectivity. Basic investigations are shifting from those potentially applicable to patient care to less immediately relevant studies in molecular
biology and genomics. Most significant is the divergence between the
ever-increasing numbers of potential recipients and the consistently
inadequate organs becoming available. With transplant professionals,
the public, and responsible government agencies progressively frustrated with this situation, the entire field is beginning to suffer.

Several factors have contributed to the dichotomy between demand
and supply. The relatively satisfactory results of organ transplantation,
more effective immunosuppression, and improvements in care have all
made this treatment a realistic option for a greater proportion of individuals desiring help. More and more, these include older persons and
other groups at high risk. Kidney and heart transplants are now offered to those with significant preexisting medical conditions. Potential recipients positive for hepatitis C antigen, ex-alcoholics, and even
those with primary hepatic tumors receive livers. And because of the
deterioration of their primary graft due to chronic rejection or other

processes, the number of persons seeking *re*transplantation has burgeoned. At the present time, the largest patient group entering the
dialysis rolls is made up of those whose original kidney transplants
have failed.[1]

A recent episode on the television program *Sixty Minutes* examined the priority transplantation of a heart to a prison inmate in terminal cardiac failure. California state law mandates the provision of total
health care to all convicts; hence the operation. This case (and others
like it) raises not only its own issues about societal fairness but unresolved questions about whether organs should be provided to repeated
felons or to muderers on death row. Ethical dilemmas apply increasingly as more and more individuals swell the transplant lists.

Certain groups too are more visible than in earlier years: African
Americans are the most obvious example. Constituting about 13 percent of people in the United States, their high incidence of renal disease
secondary to hypertension and diabetes results in a disproportionate
segment on dialysis (more than 30 percent of the total) and awaiting an
organ. Not only is the time spent on the waiting list for renal transplants longer than it is for whites, but overall the results are less satisfactory. Immunological considerations are part of the equation. Variations in blood groups, distribution of tissue antigens of wide genetic
diversity, and a high proportion of positive cross-matches put blacks at
a disadvantage. And societal causes add substantially to the discrepancy. This population often has less ready access to sophisticated
health care. The rate of organ donation is lower than in other racial
groups. The generally lower socioeconomic status of African Americans has been correlated with diminished compliance but may be more
often caused by the inability of individual recipients to afford the
considerable expenses of maintenance immunosuppression.[2]

For much of its existence, Medicare coverage would inexplicably
cease three years after a successful kidney allograft, but continue for as
long as a patient remained on chronic dialysis. With no additional
private insurance, and even with federal help, the yearly cost for medications, reaching many thousands of dollars, often became so unrealistic that some recipients were forced to discontinue their drugs. As a
result, their grafts failed and they reappeared on transplant lists for a
second or third kidney, increasing the already disproportionate num-

bers awaiting transplantation. With the annual cost of dialysis considerably higher than for those with a stable transplant (1995–1999 Medicare payments per patient per year are $54,021 for dialysis and $17,091 for transplants), such a decision by federal planners is not easy to understand.[3] Since 2000, however, the rules have been altered so that graft recipients may receive Medicare funds for their medication *as long as they remain disabled*. Since the objective of organ transplantation is to return afflicted individuals to a relatively normal life, the administrative thinking behind this change is also murky. Those with private insurance, however, may obtain relatively reasonable coverage for their drugs, despite intermittent threats of withdrawal by the insurance companies.

A variety of causes for the inadequate donor supply have been identified. Safer automobiles, use of seat belts, more stringent gun laws, distrust of the medical establishment, apathy, fear of AIDS, and occasional negative publicity in the popular press or on television all contribute to the inadequate numbers and have kept the rate of donation relatively static. Although 50–60 percent of patients with renal failure have been estimated to benefit from a kidney graft, only about 10 percent currently receive an organ each year. To compound the problem, the percentage of living donors, regardless of genetic relationship to the recipient, remains relatively small in many countries. It should be noted, however, that the number of living donors has increased substantially in the United States—from 5 percent of the total donors in 1991 to 22 percent in 2000. Overall, the proportion of living donors doubled during this period, whereas that of cadaver donors increased minimally.[4]

In other regions, cadaver donors are not used for cultural or religious reasons. The teachings of Islam, for instance, stress that the body should remain whole after death. Although some rabbis support donation, orthodox Jewish beliefs define death as the cessation of function of the heart, not the brain. The concept of brain death is unacceptable throughout much of Asia. In Japan specifically, death is not considered to occur at a particular moment but is a continuum that may not be complete for many days. As conversion of a dead person into an ancestor may take an extended period, the body must remain whole. A dead relative whose body is incomplete before burial or cremation is associated with misfortune, as suffering in the other world never ceases. As a result, cadaver renal transplantation is rare, and heart donation is essentially not an option. Indeed, despite legal recognition of the state of brain death by the Japanese in 1997, by 2000 there had been only nine kidney donors. (A tenth could not be used.)

In most Western countries, the rate of actual donation also remains low despite ongoing media campaigns to highlight transplantation, and the public's acceptance of the concept of brain death. One critic suggests that the "unwillingness to donate organs reflects an underlying antipathy to science and a fear of artificially creating life." Another suggests less kindly that "Americans are unaccustomed to sharing resources of any kind when it comes to medicine. Since they refuse to care for each other in life—as witness the debacle of National Health Service—why would they do so in death. Receiving help is one thing, giving it is another."[5] Whether such remarks are fair or not, relatively few options are open for many patients with failing organs.

Thoughtful people have made stringent efforts to increase donor numbers and to distribute organs in the way that is biologically most effective and socially most equitable. Physicians, nurses, organ-bank personnel, social workers, and patient groups have persistently informed, cajoled, and reminded hospital administrators, neurosurgeons, and emergency room staff about organ donation. Programs in the media have enhanced public education. Politicians have spoken in favor. There is documentation of intent to donate on drivers' licenses, advertisement on bumper stickers, and dissemination of relevant information in open gatherings. Despite everything, the number of donors worldwide has increased but marginally. The exceptions are Spain, where highly motivated transplant coordinators virtually live in hospitals and are constantly visible to the rest of the staff; Belgium, which has a required law of "presumed consent," stating that unless specifically declined any patient dying in or near a hospital is a potential donor; and Austria, where autopsy (therefore donation) can be performed without family request based on an eighteenth-century law created by Empress Marie-Therese. But even the results of these highly successful efforts may be leveling off.

The demographics of the donor pool is also changing over the world, with increasing acceptance of "marginal" or "extended" donors to make up the deficit. Although not fully defined, these include individuals in the older (over 55 years) or younger (under 5 years) age groups, persons with hypertension, diabetes mellitus, vascular disease, brain-dead patients in shock or with circulatory instability at the time of organ removal, or persons who have died of stroke. Between 1988 and 1994 in the United States, for instance, the number of cadaver kidney donors under 49 years of age remained relatively stable, whereas those older than 49 years increased 168 percent, about 25 percent per year.[6] Unfortunately, organs from such individuals may not perform well over either the short term or the long term. The inverse association between donor age and graft survival is greatest (78 percent at three years) when the donors were between 20 and 24 years old and lowest (57 percent) when the donors were over 65 years. Similar data have accrued when other donor-associated risk factors are examined.

Although less than ideal donors are used secondary to strenuous attempts to gain more organs, eventually the results may not justify the efforts. More radical measures have been suggested and undertaken to increase the cadaver donor supply. Instead of indiscriminately pairing organs and recipients based on tissue matching, as has been standard procedure, some urge that the most favorable organs be reserved for the healthiest patients with the best prognosis. Conversely, they feel, organs from older donors or other high-risk groups should go to older recipients whose life expectancy may be relatively short. "Swapping" has been suggested. The kidney from a living donor could be placed in a well-matched stranger, while the original recipient designee, who could not use the organ because of a positive cross-match or other factor, would be placed first on the list for an appropriate unrelated living-donor kidney. Additional suggested measures include age limitations on potential transplant recipients, the awarding of only one organ per patient, and formal rationing or strict prioritization. For a time, the state of Oregon withheld funds for the relatively less successful transplantation procedures such as liver and bone marrow, feeling that state monies could be spent more effectively on basic health care for the general population rather than for imperfect treatment for a few.[7] Because of public protest, however, this plan was curtailed. Presumed consent laws have been successful in some European countries but not in others.

At the end of the 1990s, a brouhaha arose in the United States concerning a proposal by the Secretary of Health and Human Services that organ allocation policies should be based on equity, not utility. The status of individual patients on a national transplant list would depend on uniform countrywide criteria, not as traditionally on their evaluation by physicians in individual transplant centers. Livers, in particular, would be assigned to individuals with the highest medical urgency regardless of geographic locale. Similar criteria for the distribution of other solid organs would be applied in subsequent years. The plan evoked intense reactions among the transplant community and its professional organizations that ranged from grudging agreement to vituperative contention. Many clinicians strongly disagreed with these premises, feeling that the inclusion of patients hitherto denied transplants because they failed minimal acceptance criteria would only increase the mortality rate, worsen the results, and waste scarce resources. Shipping a given organ farther to a suboptimal recipient would also add storage time and potentially diminish the success of the procedure. Particularly inflammatory were strong accusations by the Secretary toward the professionals of "needlessly frightening transplant patients about maintenance of organ waiting lists and distribution" and embarking "on a misleading lobbying campaign that factually misrepresents the Department's intent in issuing the rule and mischaracterizes its provisions."[8] Fortunately, a partial compromise was ultimately reached. Such regulatory mandates, however well meaning, do little to solve the underlying problem of the increasing paucity of donors.

Altruism in organ donation has been the linchpin of transplantation since its inception. The "gift of life" is a concept that comforts many donor families faced with the sudden and often tragic death of a relative and allows them solace by realizing that the organs or tissues of someone they loved may live on in another. The principle of the gift has been equally important in donations from related living individuals such as parents or siblings, as emphasized by the increasing numbers of extrarenal tissues given (liver and lung segments, even portions of the pancreas and small bowel).

As demand for precious organs grows, unexpected categories of donors have emerged, often raising disturbing ethical issues.[9] Although the concept of "altruistic donation" of organs from genetically unrelated spouses, friends, and colleagues is slowly becoming acceptable, questions of motivation or coercion inevitably arise. These concerns overlap with another category of living donation, termed *rewarding gifting*, in which the donor receives monetary or material compensation for the sacrifice. A final classification, *rampant commercialism*, that involves the actual buying and selling of organs has surfaced most visibly over the past decade and has attracted increasing public attention.

In the face of ever-expanding numbers of patients tired of waiting and willing to pay for a transplantable organ, the three categories of living donors have become progressively blurred. Many of the changing circumstances are based on expediency; a desperate individual with end-stage disease must obtain an appropriate transplant by any means available or die. Conversely, those faced with crushing financial debt or irrevocable poverty may be willing to sacrifice a body part for recompense. A plethora of proposals calling for financial incentives as a solution to the shortage of organs and tissues arose during the mid-1980s; some persist to the present day. Even the American Medical Association has come out in favor of the concept.

As donation by African Americans has been particularly low for a variety of understandable social reasons, this group has been a specific target for financial compensation schemes to increase the rate. Advocates argue that as inadequately insured medical expenses and/or funeral costs may be burdensome to bereaved relatives, the prospect of compensation might encourage greater participation. Those favoring legal payment for cadaver body parts support the morality of such policies by noting that since other parties involved in transplantation— from procurement organizations to hospitals to surgeons and physicians—make money from the procedure, it should not be illegal for donor families to be similarly compensated. As yet there is little evidence that such schemes have been particularly effective, but money for burial costs is being provided in a few areas. In 1995, for instance, Pennsylvania established funds to pay families of organ donors $1,000 for such expenses.[10]

The argument against such policies is equally persuasive. Programs on a regional or national basis to permit direct or indirect payment for cadaver organs may further reduce any enthusiasm for donation—which would be additionally deleterious to those on a waiting list.[11] Allowing the sale of body parts, the argument suggests, reduces people to objects and turns the body into a commodity to allow more transplants to be performed. As the problems faced by the poor and underrepresented in gaining appropriate health care are all too real, efforts by the medical community to procure organs from the dead of these or any groups by remuneration could be construed as a conflict of interest.

Such an approach may carry special moral significance for African Americans. For centuries, members of this population were bought and sold as chattel. Physicians often used slaves without consent for experimentation and for teaching purposes after death. Indeed, the last time the federal government and private agencies paid funeral expenses for poor blacks was when the bodies of those who died in the notorious Tuskegee syphilis study (a program designed to follow the course of this disease in purposely untreated patients) were sought for autopsy.[12] The attitudes of the black population toward payment for organs and tissues may be substantially influenced by these historical realities. Efforts on the part of transplanters, the states, or the federal government, may therefore be self-defeating.

Other schemes to increase the organ supply have been proposed. Entrepreneurs in the United States have suggested a futures market, defined as "an organized publicly operated future delivery market where an individual can contract for valuable consideration with a government agency for delivery of a specific organ after death."[13] In other words, a patient can receive money during life for the use of his or her organs after death. Even less acceptable proposals were forthcoming. At least one opportunist suggested importing poor donors from the Third World to the United States and paying them for their kidneys. Some transplant professionals and their centers compounded the problem by advertising in other countries for potential recipients with means to pay, guaranteeing prompt and successful transplantation with cadaver organs. Local citizens who believed that the distribution system was equitable were often forced to wait for prolonged periods while affluent foreigners essentially bought their way to the head of the queue. These practices amplified the problem of inadequate donor numbers, at the same time outraging the public. A subsequent decrease in donations was the result.

Similar activities occurred elsewhere, at least for a time; others continue. During the late 1980s in London, several surgeons and physicians in private clinics (some owned by for-profit hospital chains from the United States) transplanted kidneys from destitute Turkish or Indian peasants into rich foreign (often Arab) recipients who claimed that the potential donors were related. Although this behavior attracted highly adverse notoriety and was eventually curtailed by law, comparable practices persist, sometimes with tacit government acceptance. Affluent foreigners still receive cadaver kidneys, and impoverished local donors sell their organs in the United States. Italians travel from a country with the lowest rate of organ donation in Europe to Belgium and Austria, with their relatively high donation rates, for cadaver transplantation. Israelis, also with a low rate of donation, enter rural Turkey and other Eastern European countries with their surgeons to be grafted with kidneys bought from the poor. Patients from Arab Gulf states and Egypt buy organs in India. Citizens of wealthy Asian nations and territories travel to China for kidneys. In 1999 in Canada, dozens of patients obtained kidneys in China via a Canadian broker. Organs are sold in Russia and Iraq. In some South American countries, newspaper advertisements appear from desperate persons desiring to sell a kidney or even an eye for corneal transplantation. And sporadically, transplant clinicians in Western countries receive heartrending appeals from individuals in disadvantaged nations who want to sell a body part to get money for care of a sick relative.[14]

I have been faced with several such entreaties during my own professional career, in particular poignant requests from individuals in poorer countries offering to sell a kidney to improve their financial state or the lot of their families. The most striking query came from high officials in the Philippine government, asking members of our group to travel to Manila and perform a kidney transplant on President Ferdinand Marcos, then on dialysis. The donor was to be chosen from soldiers in the army, depending on the closeness of the tissue match. Although we declined this opportunity because of both the politics of the dictator and the source of the donor, one of our colleagues in a distant city in the United States did undertake the procedure. During the years that Marcos' kidney functioned, a Philippine doctor returned with the surgeon to his center, essentially living at the airport. He acted as a messenger shuttling blood and other specimens from the patient to the transplant laboratory, and communicating back to the Philippines the results and changes in treatment protocols. Unfortunately, with a new government in power after Marcos' death, this individual and one of his colleagues were assassinated upon returning to their country.

To illustrate more graphically the potential exploitation of "the gift," the course of a patient desiring transplantation was documented in a 2001 article in the *New York Times*.

> After four years on dialysis, with no sign that he was nearing the top of the transplant waiting list, Moshe Tati decided to buy a kidney. This was easier than he had imagined. Several months previous, the name and telephone number of an organ broker had been passed, furtively, around his dialysis group. At the time, Moshe did not think he would use the telephone number. He thought he would wait. Then his health began to fail . . .
>
> Moshe lives in Israel, which happens to be one of the more active nations in the international organ-trafficking market. The market, which is completely illegal, is so complex and well organized that a single transaction often crosses three continents: a broker from Los Angeles, say, matches an Italian with kidney failure to a seller in Jordan, for surgery in Istanbul . . .
>
> "I can get you a kidney immediately" said the broker whom Moshe Tati called. "All I need is the money." Then he quoted a price: $145,000, cash, paid in advance. This would cover everything . . . all hospital fees, the payment to the seller, accommodations for accompanying family members and a chartered, round-trip flight to the country where the surgery would take place. The trip would last about five days, he said, and the destination would be kept secret until the time they left.
>
> The broker promised that one of the top transplant surgeons in Israel would be flying with them to perform the operation. . . . "I can guarantee you a living donor," the broker said, "a young, strong man. This won't be a cadaver organ."
>
> Moshe told his broker he'd get the money . . . The broker said they'd meet a week later at the Tel Aviv Hilton, and everything would be arranged . . . Moshe [and his companions] handed over the money, a bank check for $145,000, and were driven to [the] airport, where a chartered plane was waiting. There were no papers to sign. "Everything was done by handshake" . . . Once he was aboard, Moshe learned he'd be going to Turkey.
>
> When Moshe's plane landed in Istanbul, there was no need to clear customs, no asking for passports. "Everything was already taken care of,"

Moshe says. "The organization was like clockwork." Moshe and the other three patients were driven to a hospital . . . The transplant surgeries were performed late at night, when the hospital was on skeleton staff and fewer people could question what was going on . . . Two surgeries were done the night after they landed; two more the following night."

As Moshe awoke from his transplant surgery, the Israeli doctor was at his bedside, grinning . . . "Congratulations, everything's great."[15]

The majority of such kidneys function well. In Moshe's case, however, a postoperative heart attack caused him to lose his organ and return to dialysis.

Such practices have become so large and so successful in several countries that even some of the patients' doctors have reversed their previous antipathy toward commerce in human organs. Michael Fried-laender, Mosha Tati's personal physician,

will tell you that the experience is a perfect example of why kidney sales should finally be legalized. "What's happening now is absurd," Fried-laender says. "Airplanes are leaving every week. In the last few years, I've seen 300 of my patients go abroad and come back with new kidneys. Some are fine, some are not—it's a free-for-all. Instead of turning our backs on this, instead of leaving our patients exposed to unscrupulous treatment by uncontrolled free enterprise, we as physicians must see how this can be legalized and regulated."

[Indeed,] Friedlaender [discovered] that the percentage of illegal transplants still functioning after one year was, in fact, slightly higher than his own hospital's success rate—and that of many U.S. hospitals. The difference, he says, is attributable to the benefits of transplanting kidneys from living donors.

"After I realized that, . . . I softened my stance. Examining those 300 patients brought me down from my high horse of ethics. Now I'm more practical. My patients don't want my opinion on whether or not buying a kidney is moral—they want to know if it's safe. And I have to say that it is. It's as safe as having a transplant at a U.S. hospital. I realized that I had no right to actively stop my patients from going. I realized that it may be harming them not to go. So when they ask, I tell them "Yes, you should go."[16]

Besides being an eloquent commentary on the social inequities of society in general, these examples raise unsettling ethical questions. Commerce in human organs has long been anathema to members of the international transplant community, their patients, and their governments—with the possible exception of Iran. When some of the early proposals and irregularities were uncovered, legal blockades were raised. A 1972 Canadian law made trade of human tissues a crime. In 1978 the Council of Europe resolved that "no substance may be offered for profit." A 1984 law in the United States expressly forbade acquisition or transfer of human organs for "valuable consideration." The World Medical Association resolved subsequently that "the purchase and sale of human organs for transplantation is . . . condemned." The World Health Organization came out with similar guidelines.[17]

Not everyone is convinced. Some feel that "the selling of kidneys . . . finds a negative response in our society unless the recipients are chosen without respect to ability to pay, ie, some form of government subsidy." Others argue that "kidney donation is a good act. The financial incentive to promote such an act is moral and justified." Still others suggest that families who agree to donate should be rewarded, either monetarily, as has occurred in the United States, or publicly, as in Saudi Arabia, where such individuals receive the King Abdulaziz Medal, grade 3. A few suggest that Western opposition to organ trade targets developing nations in a paternalistic manner, and that informed consent and free choice by potential willing donors should be honored. After all, the argument runs, if blood and sperm can be sold and surrogate mothers are paid to produce babies for others, why not organs? An obvious answer, as most lawmakers agree, is that these constitute nonrenewable tissues.[18]

A laissez-faire, free-enterprise system in which virtually anything can be bought or sold has become virtually a shibboleth of the late twentieth century in many countries. Then should the rules for obtaining and distributing scarce commodities such as organs be different? Examples of exploitation of the weak by the powerful abound in all aspects of life. In well-publicized examples relating to transplantation in the United States, livers have become available promptly to the influential and important, to those with connections in politics or the media, and to those who go public with their needs. The ill-advised replacement of the cancerous liver of baseball idol Mickey Mantle is an obvious example. In some nations, organs can be purchased from those willing to sell. In others, the organs of prisoners can be bought. Differences in social and cultural pressures may be significant. It is often difficult for individuals living under Western traditions to appreciate or even understand the circumstances faced by those in less developed countries. There the pressures from the ill combined with the prestige surrounding a medically sophisticated transplant program appear to transcend more equitable distribution of health-associated resources. By 1990, for instance, kidneys were being transplanted in nine countries in the Middle East, six in South America, and four on the African continent.[19]

Simple need remains the most compelling argument. India may be the most striking example. About a hundred thousand people in that country develop renal failure each year. Dialysis is scarce. Patients must pay for each treatment to sustain their lives. As the average per-capita yearly income of the population of 900 million is about 9,500 rupees (about $300 U.S.), only a relative few can afford renal replacement therapy. Despite recent laws prohibiting the sale of human organs, many individuals in desperate financial straits are willing to sell an organ to increase their resources, pay back debts, or finance a dowry. Thus, middle-class Indians and foreign nationals from nearby Arab states where cadaver organs are virtually unobtainable take advantage of kidneys offered for sale by impoverished donors in several cities. Hundreds of such renal transplants are performed annually in these "kidney belts." In addition to the individuals receiving the organs, a large coterie of middlemen, brokers, and physicians benefit substantially. Despite the $1,000 or so that the donor receives for a kidney, such individuals (usually women, "low paid domestic workers with husbands in trouble or in debt") have found that the sale only improves their lives for a time. "The money was soon swallowed by the usurious interest charged by the local money lenders, and the families were in debt again."[20]

This one-way traffic in organs from poor to rich is believed by many to be exploitative and an abuse of human rights. To compound the philosophical objections of those decrying such practices, significant practical problems abound. Blood products are often contaminated with HIV, and 70 percent of regular plasma donors are positive for the virus—presumably the same donors willing to sell their organs. Endemic hepatitis poses an additional hazard. Despite the objections and dangers, similar practices have arisen in Malaysia and

Singapore, and large profits accrue to brokers in the Philippines who arrange transplantation between poor local donors and affluent Japanese recipients.[21]

The sale of body parts from executed prisoners in China is perhaps the most extreme example of commercial trade in organs, a situation increasingly brought to public attention by concerned individuals, human rights organizations, and occasional television features. An incident in New York City in 1998 in which two Chinese businessmen were arrested for attempting to sell corneas, livers, lungs, and kidneys from executed prisoners on order and for large fees attracted much publicity. It has been estimated that the majority of the ten thousand or more kidneys transplanted in China were obtained from the four thousand to six thousand prisoners executed each year. These organs are grafted predominantly into recipients from Singapore, Hong Kong, Korea, Japan, and Taiwan, as well as occasional Westerners who travel to China for the elective procedure. In spite of a law enacted in 1984, "Rules Concerning the Utilization of Corpses or Organs from the Corpses of Executed Prisoners," which allows organs to be used if no one claims the body or if the condemned individual volunteers and if the family agrees, permission is rarely obtained, as neither prisoner nor family is informed of the impending donation. Allegedly, a blood sample is taken before execution for blood-group and HLA matching and for a lymphocyte cross-match. Driven to the countryside on the final day, the prisoner kneels and is killed by a bullet to the back of the head if the organs are to be used, or to the chest if only the corneas are to be saved. The body is transferred to a mobile operating room on site. The organs are quickly removed and sent to appropriate hospitals, where the arranged recipients await them. I have personally seen a video, smuggled out of China, of the executions and removal of the bodies to the van. It is a shocking and repugnant scene.[22]

This trade remains a clandestine operation, as the law goes on to imply that "the use of the corpses or organs of executed criminals must be kept strictly secret, and attention must be paid to avoiding negative repercussions . . . A surgical vehicle from the Health Department may be permitted to drive onto the execution grounds to remove the organs, but it is not permitted to use a vehicle bearing Health Department insignia or to wear white clothing. Guards must remain posted around the execution grounds while the operation for organ removals is going on." Such arrangements produce substantial financial rewards for hospitals and officials alike. The fee for a kidney transplant in China was about $30,000 in 1992 and it has undoubtedly increased since then, so such programs not only generate income but the hospitals involved also profit from superior ratings and greater prestige. This lucrative practice, denied by the Chinese authorities, has turned into a small industry.[23]

Variations on such practices have not been limited to China. Similar activity allegedly occurred in Taiwan between 1987 and 1994 before the practice was legally terminated. In the United States, kidneys from consenting prison inmates were used in the 1960s, a practice of living donation that may still continue in some states. In general, the engraftment of organs from executed prisoners, despite the early use of those from guillotined criminals in France, was never considered seriously until the availability of cyclosporine made transplantation a relatively successful proposition.

Discussions of this subject still arise intermittently. A 1977 Geneva Convention amendment banned the use of organs and tissues from prisoners of war, but accepted blood transfusions and skin for grafting if offered voluntarily and based on combat need. The Transplantation Society has twice published guidelines decrying such practices. A declaration by the World Medical Association in 1994 condemned the practice of using organs from executed prisoners, but left open the possibility if supported by informed consent. Not quite comparable, but perhaps as distasteful to many, was the introduction of a bill ("life for a life") in the Missouri state legislature in 1998, which would allow a death-row prison inmate to exchange a kidney or bone marrow cells for a sentence of life without parole. In discussing this idea, a prominent ethicist noted, "In China, they kill you to get your organs; here we kill you unless you give your organs."[24] With the continuation of such practices, organ donation has strayed a long way from its founding principle of altruism.

Although the majority of instances of buying and selling organs are well documented, other irregularities are less tangible. One of the most highly publicized examples, never proven, involves the organs of children. Along with increasing media attention in the mid-1980s to the benefits and successes of transplantation and the negative reports of adventurism and greed came several reports of the use of organs from kidnapped and murdered children, primarily from countries in Central and South America. These allegations were not only publicized in newspapers and television around the world, but also embellished by various government sources. The European Parliament stated that "organized trafficking in organs exists in the same way as trafficking in drugs . . . It involves killing people to remove organs which can be sold at profit." A United Nations publication, "On the Sale of Children," was circulated. The BBC produced a program entitled "Baby Parts." In 1987 and 1988 the Russian newspapers *Pravda* and *Tass*, as well as various Soviet groups, publicized reports about such occurrences in Honduras. At the same time, accounts appeared in the world press of abductions, disappearances, and political assassinations by military regimes in Chile and Argentina; of mass murders of street children in cities in Brazil; and of paramilitary decimation of villages in Central American nations. Perhaps based on these real events, local peasants remain convinced that "they or their children are at risk of being mutilated and murdered. Stories are often told of foreigners who arrive in a village, kidnap and murder several children, remove their organs for sale abroad, and leave the dissected corpses exposed in the graveyard."[25]

Many of the rumors about child donors were apparently exaggerated from reports of atrocities occurring between warring factions or among villagers caught between opposing military and political forces. Other tales were thought to have been generated via a formal disinformation campaign initiated by various pro-Soviet groups, the Cubans, and other anti-Western cabals. The pressure on transplant organizations and governments alike was enough to provoke lengthy investigations and ultimate rebuttals by officials from the U.S. Information Agency, the European Parliament and the Geneva-based Defense for Children International, the United Network for Organ Sharing, the FBI and Interpol, as well as by officials in Guatemala, Honduras, and Columbia. Despite lengthy investigations, no such examples have ever been substantiated, although allegations of Egyptian orphans killed for their body parts have recently appeared—a practice reputedly involving large sums of money with "the collaboration of powerful figures."[26] The subject does not disappear.

Some of these accounts may have been perpetuated through oral and written stories that have recurred in each succeeding generation, stories of kidnapping and murder in folklore, in children's fairy tales, and in fantasy fiction. These have ancient roots. Human sacrifice in the Mayan culture is well known. Ritualized murder by the Christians was reported in ancient Rome. Similar fabrications involved Jews in the Middle Ages. Other examples abound. Despite all the denials, such devastating publicity has affected donations and has influenced public opinion about transplantation in general. Not only does it take time for such rumors to ebb, but they keep resurfacing with distressing regularity. The public thrives on such fodder, and the media can always use "the public needs to know" mandate to sell their material. Yet this type of information or disinformation does the entire subject a grave disservice.

A less obvious but equally disquieting example of irregularities involves "an unregulated, international, multi-million dollar business in tissue and body parts." Although the human body has been used for slave and sex labor throughout history, only with advancing technology from the mid-twentieth century have body parts gained commercial value.[27] Since the perfection of blood-banking techniques around the time of World War II, blood and blood products have been bought by the United States, often from individuals in Third World countries. Canada and most European countries, in contrast, rely primarily on voluntary donation. Commerce in other human products is also prevalent: eggs, sperm, fetal cells, and tissues. As businesses have sprung up to meet the demand, the conditions of "giving" such materials are not always clear.

Some private biotech companies buy bodily structures and turn them into commercial products. Human skin, for instance, can be processed for implantation or injection into the face to reduce wrinkles or enlarge the lips. Fragments or paste made from cadaver long bones are used in orthopedics to fill in large bony defects following massive trauma or surgical removal of tumors. In some Third World countries, heart valves and other tissues are removed from the dead without consent and sent to European companies for processing and sale to the medical marketplace. On a positive note, at least some of the profit may go back to the original country to fund technical expertise or laboratories. Although donor families throughout the United States think of their "gift" as fully altruistic, some of the tissues of their loved one, unbeknownst to them, may be sold through organ banks to companies for commercial gain. Such use of human tissues as market commodities has been described by one knowledgeable critic as "neo-cannibalism."[28]

As these unexpected aspects of transplantation become recognized, they are generating increasing disquiet. Some ethicists see a rapid decline in the humanist values intrinsic to the traditional purpose of medicine. In their place are arising new and unwelcome relations between patient care and financial incentives, between those seeking help and those paying for it, and difficulties in appropriate access among social groups. Exacerbation of the ancient divide between those who have and those who do not has spawned a bizarre market for organs and other body parts. Race, class, and gender all play a role. The flow follows that of capital: from south to north, from Third World to First World, from female to male, and from nonwhite to white. In the worst instances, this unfortunate niche market has led some to the self-serving belief that they have property rights over the spare parts of the poor.

The most obvious of these variations from accepted ethical principles has been movingly summarized in poetry, with particular reference to the practices in China.

Harvesting

Chinese whispers
pass from cell to cell

as doctors walk their rounds
examining the inmates,
taking samples, making notes.
Harvesters among them
boost their meager earnings
organizing. . . .

A chance encounter
with a foreigner in need
sows seeds, a scheme
to combat shortage,
nurture dollars.
Secret meetings mulched with bribes.

Autumn plucking:
Surreptitiously the harvesters
reap local prisons,
specimens for typing,
mix-and-matching dissidents
awaiting execution.

At death, excisions.
Harvesters transport each prisoner
in pieces, trade their gleanings—
kidneys, liver, lungs, corneas, pancreas, and skin
for transplantation.

Selling.
Walls of silence[29]

Future Prospects

THE TRANSPLANTATION OF SOLID ORGANS AND
its biology have advanced remarkably in the half century since the first
successful kidney graft. Clinical conditions were primitive when I first
became involved four decades ago, shortly after the introduction of
chemical immunosuppression. At that time in our hospital, individuals
dying with uremia were cared for in the general wards. If hemodialysis
could be offered at all, it was performed not infrequently using the
same dialysis bath for two different patients. As a result, hepatitis was
rife—not only among those dialyzed but also among nurses, residents,
and consultant staff. One of the dialysis nurses died in liver failure.
Several surgeons were sick for months. Vascular access was rudimentary. Glass cannulae used for separate treatments were eventually exchanged for reusable plastic shunts, most of which had relatively short
functional life spans. Indeed, the gradual lack of suitable access sites
often forced cessation of dialysis with the subsequent death of many
patients. Complications associated with a transplant operation were all
too common and greatly prolonged the hospital stay. With the overuse
of immunosuppressive drugs, recipient mortality was prohibitive.
Even those with functioning grafts often became seriously debilitated
from the long-term sequelae of their original disease, uremia, and the
side effects of the antirejection medications, particularly steroids.

Because medical insurance did not cover their devastating kidney
failure, the economic condition of the survivors frequently became
tenuous; some were destroyed financially. On the other hand, the enthusiasm and hope inherent in the new treatment—and most particu-

larly the courage, endurance, and will to survive that the patients showed—tempered and relieved many negative aspects of the experience. It was an extraordinary and rather rudimentary beginning of a subject that has evolved to its present state through cooperation and communication among imaginative scientific investigators, enthusiastic clinicians, and willing patients.

Modern transplantation came of age with the introduction of Cyclosporin A and the immunosuppressive drugs that have followed. Results have improved significantly throughout much of the world, as tabulated by registries and databases from the United States, the United Kingdom, Canada, Europe, Australia and New Zealand, Japan, and other sources. By the end of 2001, representative information had been collected on more than 110,000 renal transplants performed in the United States over ten years, with comparable numbers available from other reporting regions.[1] The functional survival of cadaver kidney grafts has risen to about 90 percent at one year, over 80 percent at three years, and more than 40 percent at ten years. Survival of grafts from living donors is even more favorable. Almost forty thousand livers were grafted over the last decade, with similar numbers accruing from other geographic areas. The overall survival rate of adult recipients is about 86 percent at one year and 76 percent at three years; that of children is higher yet. Transplantation of the pancreas, and kidney and pancreas in combination, remains less common, with about ten thousand cases reported from the United States and three thousand from Europe. Curiously, the 80 percent functional success of simultaneous pancreas and kidney transplantation at one year is better than that of patients who receive a pancreas after a kidney transplant or pancreas alone (approximately 60 percent). Approximately thirty thousand thoracic organs, particularly the heart, have been transplanted in the United States, and about twenty thousand in Europe. About 85 percent of cardiac recipients survive at one year, 77 percent at five years. Results of lung and heart-lung transplants remain lower, although the numbers are expected to improve with more effective immunosuppressive strategies.

Clearly, today's patients with organ failure who undergo transplantation can be relatively optimistic about their future, particularly over the relatively short term. In addition, long-term sequelae of chronic immunosuppression are becoming less severe and debilitating with ever more effective and selective agents. Considering the short history of the subject, its complexities, our still-imperfect knowledge about the breadth and sophistication of host responses, and the incompletely defined positive and negative manifestations of the powerful medications needed to sustain the grafts, the current record is striking.

The future of the field may be even more interesting than its past. The induction of immunological tolerance remains a principal topic of investigation, stimulated by encouraging results of several novel experimental treatments, at both the cellular and molecular levels. While biologic research to create tolerance for solid organ grafts continues apace, selective immunologic manipulation of the recipient is not yet ready for general clinical testing, despite early trials to combat GVHD and psoriasis.

The practical possibilities of xenotransplantation are more problematic. It is unlikely that substantial successes with this strategy are imminent, although bridge techniques to support failing organs for finite periods are improving. Transient maintenance of those in hepatic failure by external perfusion through allogeneic or even xenogeneic livers is under investigation, for instance, although the threat of cross-species viral infection is always present. In some instances, external support of this sort will allow the organs to recover adequate function so that transplantation may be avoided and others in need may receive the available livers. Mechanical ventricular assist devices are used with increasing regularity in patients with heart failure, some over prolonged periods.[2] The more basic possibilities of gene transfer to control development of the original organ diseases are under investigation but so far are rarely applicable.

The inadequate number of organs to meet the increasing demands continues to be the major limiting factor to clinical transplantation. Numbers of cadaver donors will probably remain relatively static, although the low numbers of living donors are rising. Indeed, the increasingly popular technique of laparoscopy for kidney removal from living donors is catching public attention and is encouraging this type of donation. The method is far less invasive than the formal operation, shortening considerably the time in hospital and the period of recovery. Portions of liver, pancreas, and lung from living sources are used increasingly. Cadaver-donor livers can be divided for transplantation into two recipients.

An interesting alternative approach to overcoming the apparently insurmountable difficulties of inadequate donor supply may be to use relevant functioning cells that could expand and regenerate into an organ. This concept is particularly pertinent to the relatively homogeneous liver. Healthy cells can be isolated from a portion of the tissue uninvolved with disease, for instance, allowed to proliferate in appropriate culture medium in a test tube, then returned to the host. As specific immunogenic cell populations become more precisely identified, their removal from allogeneic cultures may inhibit host immunity and decrease or obviate the need for immunosuppression.

Engineered tissues are under intense investigation. Cultured cartilage and bone are already used effectively in patients. Interest is growing in the treatment of Parkinson's disease and other neurological disorders by the implantation of fetal cells into the brain. Experimental successes with this strategy are intriguing, and occasional reports of striking benefit in a few patients are encouraging. "Artificial skin" increasingly covers large burns. Appropriate skin cells either from the patient or from a third-party donor may be cultured on a synthetic polymer framework. Sheets of the material are then placed on open burn sites. With healing, new growth of host connective tissue and blood vessels eventually replaces the polymer, producing a satisfactory cutaneous layer. Engineered preparations of pancreatic islets have been transplanted into various models with some success, although inadequate numbers of these cells limit their general use. Fragments of small bowel, cells from the urinary tract, and vascular cells, all grown on absorbable tubular scaffolds, may form surgically usable pieces of appropriately organized tissues. The delivery of large numbers of cultured liver cells on biodegradable templates is perhaps closer to practical reality. This arrangement provides enough space for the cells to regenerate and reorganize into functioning units. Under the proper circumstances they may ultimately form an organ. The experimental success of these techniques in several stringent animal models makes them potentially relevant for human use.

The possibility that manipulation or bioengineering of stem cells

may replenish a variety of tissues or even create new organs has provoked intense interest and fervent discussion. These progenitor cells
arising early in embryonic life are capable of differentiating into cell
types representative of each and every developing tissue or organ in
the body. Successful bone marrow transplants between histocompat-
ible infants and their siblings with leukemia have increased enthusiasm
for this treatment strategy. Over fifteen hundred such procedures have
been carried out worldwide, using stem cells from umbilical-cord
blood.[3] A few couples have deliberately created a baby as a potential
HLA-identical bone-marrow and stem-cell donor for an older sibling.

Alternatively, the selection of a compatible embryo as a source of
appropriate cells, and the discard of noncompatible embryos produced by in vitro fertilization, is engendering a great deal of public
debate, political posturing, and media exposure. Because of social and
emotional issues surrounding the use of fetal cells, the potential for
adult stem cells has gained increasing attention. In general, these cells
differentiate in a narrower range than embryonic cells and have been
less satisfactory in experimental systems, although investigations are
still at an early stage. However, if adult cells could be used, new advances would quickly accumulate.

Despite considerable progress in the bioengineering of skin, cartilage, bone, and liver using mature cells, the generation of anatomically
more complex organs would probably require more sophisticated manipulations. Increasingly appreciated is the unexpected importance of
scaffolding, a fine mesh of either natural proteins or synthetic polymers on which the cells can be grown. This scaffolding not only sup-
ports normal cells but also can direct them to differentiate into the
desired tissue or tissue components by altering gene expression and
changing their function.[4] A myocardial muscle "patch" is currently
being developed, with eventual plans to produce an entire heart. Blood
vessels can be made. Growth factors embedded in the scaffolding may
allow the formation of livers. The kidney, in contrast, may be struc-
turally too complex to create because of the precise arrangement of
cells of distinct types and functions, and perhaps the necessity for
pulsatile blood flow during the period of growth. Tiny embryonic
kidneys implanted in adult hosts, however, do grow to form normal
organs. These exciting experiments may be of future importance for

clinical application and ultimately may do much to obviate the necessity for at least some cadaver organs.

In virtually every aspect of human endeavor, a simple idea, the desire to improve, an actual advance or a departure from existing beliefs, methods, or everyday behavior almost invariably becomes more complicated than initially visualized. Particularly over the past few decades, the accelerating pace of scientific and medical knowledge has broadened established fields of exploration and treatment. At the same time, the new areas that have opened pose questions and conundrums ranging from the theoretical to the practical to the ethical. Observers have emphasized the benefits of modern technology, computerized data gathering, the rapidity of global communication, the unprecedented opportunities for those with imagination, and the potential for products of all sorts—material to intellectual—to be disseminated everywhere for the benefit of all. But others remain skeptical, pointing out that the gap between rich and poor, educated and undereducated, skilled and unskilled, those who receive adequate health care and those who do not, is greater than ever, and that sophisticated technologies have only created more arcane and less solvable problems.

Doubts are also being raised about the role of the new biologies and their relation to patient care. Despite remarkable successes since World War II, the increasingly research-directed, technology-based, and pharmaceutically oriented thrust of medicine has, in the minds of many patients and physicians alike, replaced clinically structured, humanitarian, and individualized care. As high-tech medicine is also very expensive, the well-publicized administrative changes designed to hold down costs are perceived as evoking the less socially conscious ethics of business; the fear is that the doctor-patient relationship and the art of medicine are becoming transformed into an impersonal interaction between "provider" and "client." It may be years before the more benevolent side of medicine will transcend market forces and regain its prior role.

Organ transplantation has not emerged unscathed from these two cultures. Initiated by a few surgeons desperately attempting to rescue their patients, the subject has become an accepted medical specialty. Indeed, the relatively infrequent failure of an organ or death of a recipient at the present time is a subject of angst and soul searching among the clinical team. Despite the remarkable scientific and clinical evolution of the field, however, there is growing concern that all is not well. Insufficient numbers of organs, too many disappointed patients, and the importance of the "bottom line" are taking their toll.

Even those entering the field may be declining in numbers, interest, or breadth of commitment. Recruitment of new transplant surgeons in the United Kingdom, for instance, is becoming difficult. Although the numbers remain steady in the United States, many young surgeons are interested only in the highly technical engraftment of organs such as the liver. An increasing coterie of such individuals, trained in transplantation but frustrated by the inability to pursue parallel research careers because of unrelenting clinical pressures, are joining other specialties. Voices describe with alarm the decline in the number of physicians active in the laboratory setting, fearing the loss of one or more generations of investigators both committed to basic research and trained to translate the innovations of science into the practical treatment of human disease. In partial response to these pressures, in 2000 the research budget for the NIH was raised to $17 billion. Yet even this sizable inducement may not retain academic clinicians interested in applied research; currently, the surgeon-scientist seems most at risk.[5] The number of principal investigators involved with clinical research is also decreasing, partially as a result of the huge loans, often averaging more than $100,000, that each student carries upon leaving medical school. Another element is the lack of funding for young or midcareer clinical investigators. The major reason, however, appears to be the impact of managed care on reducing the time available to those in clinical research to carry out their research projects; augmenting patient "through-put" is emphasized instead.

The situation is comparable among internists caring for the ever-increasing numbers of dialysis patients.[6] Their numbers are declining because of the aging and retirement of the original dialyzing nephrologists, and there is little incentive among newly trained physicians to enter the field because they basically can do no more than sustain and not cure individuals with chronic renal failure. Perhaps as sinister for idealistic new doctors is that the progressively industrialized and incorporated dialysis enterprise appears to emphasize stockholder dividends over actual health care. Capitated reimbursements for treatment have changed little since the 1970s for those responsible for the patient. Nevertheless, the appeal of investment by companies and their share-holders in dialysis facilities has been strengthened by far-flung oppor-tunities in the delivery of pharmaceuticals, the sale of dialysis-related equipment and associated technologies, and the services of company-based, salaried nurses and technicians. It is interesting that the number of approved dialysis facilities in the United States climbed from two thousand in 1995 to more than three thousand in 1999. While the number of units owned by nonprofit hospitals and independent non-profit facilities dropped dramatically to approximately 25 percent of the whole, ownership of for-profit facilities climbed strikingly. At the same time, emerging data show that patient mortality is increased, and placement of individuals with chronic renal failure on transplant wait-ing lists is reduced, when for-profit dialysis facilities are compared to those that are not for profit.[7]

The potential hazards of this situation have been described in a broader economic context. "Few trends could so thoroughly under-mine the very foundation of our free society as the acceptance by corporate officials of no social responsibility other than to make as much money for the stockholders as possible."[8] Such a transformation of responsible health care to care controlled by Wall Street has already created difficulties at many levels. The now-intimate relationship of industry and health care, both in academic centers and in the private sector, will have to be seriously addressed in the future.

These changes in emphasis throughout the transplant field have sev-eral causes. The intellectual challenge inherent in a new subject has been largely replaced by a mood that is tempered by overwork, over-regulation, micromanagement, and dullness of the routine. Clinical transplantation, particularly among surgeons trying to solve difficult patient-related problems, inherently carries a high emergency work-load and antisocial hours. These physicians perform long and complex operations, then confront unscheduled periods spent in organ re-trieval, repair of dialysis access, acute changes in patient status, and the like. The emotional toll generated by the extremely ill, the relative youth of many with organ failure, the inevitable complications, infec-tions, and drug toxicities frequently drain the caregivers. The pro-gressive industrialization of the practice of medicine, and the single-minded institutional emphasis on increased practice revenues and cost containment, have provoked almost universal professional discouragement. And as a result of growing financial constraints, time spent previously on research and other intellectual pursuits has too often diminished to unsupportable levels.

Despite these caveats, many talented individuals remain intensely interested in organ transplantation. The biology continues to be captivating, fast moving, and stimulating. Novel scientific advances of potential relevance to patients appear at an accelerating pace. More effective immunosuppressive strategies are being found. Results progressively improve. Fascinating to biologists, engineers, pharmacologists, and physicians alike, organ transplantation and its multiple ramifications continue to hold great promise. Overall, the successful replacement of failing organs with healthy ones has changed the face of scientific research and clinical medicine in one of the most remarkable adventures of the last half century. With the current unfolding of cellular and molecular biology, the fascination of genetic manipulation and the potential for reconstruction of failing organs, the future of this remarkable field will continue to challenge those who enter it.

Finally, the patients. Any annoyances, frustrations, or challenges the doctors endure are magnified a hundredfold by those the patients experience. Generally healthy except for the dysfunction or failure of a single organ system, often young, with a family, and in their most productive years, they must feel—like Job—that fate has singled them out unfairly. Smitten with a potentially fatal disease that they must deal with for the rest of their lives, they seek whatever help is available. Some receive an organ transplant. Others wait and hope. Still others die. Many of us who deal with these individuals get caught up in their difficulties and strive urgently to temper them. Indeed, our most rewarding moments come when recipients visit us several years or even decades after transplantation, and we find that they continue to live relatively normal lives.

As transplant surgeons and physicians, our thrust is twofold: day-to-day care and follow-up, and taking the clinical puzzles our patients pose to the laboratory, where we try to solve them. This dichotomy of effort has reaped huge dividends throughout the history of organ transplantation. It will continue to improve the lot of patients in the future, probably in ways we cannot yet visualize.

Time Line*

Organic Transplantation

Experimental

1900–1914	Organ autografts, allografts, and xenografts in dogs
1920s	Kidney allografts in dogs
1940s	Kidney preservation by cooling
	Extrarenal transplants in dogs
1950s	Kidney transplants in dogs
1952	Determination of immunosuppressive effects of antilymphocyte serum
1953	Reversal of acute rejection of canine kidney allografts with cortisone
1957	Immunosuppression with total-body x-radiation in animals
	Identification of drugs that depress immune responses
1959	Drug-induced immunologic tolerance
1959–1960	Use of chemical immunosuppression in animals
1960s	Liver transplants in dogs and pigs
	Pancreas transplants in dogs, and monkeys
	Heart and lung transplants in dogs
1970s	Organ transplants in rats and mice by microsurgery
	Islet transplantation in rats and mice

*Adapted from L. Brent, *A History of Transplantation Immunology* (San Diego: Academic Press, 1997)

1975	Identification of immunosuppressive properties of Cyclosporin A
1977	Determination of effectiveness of Cyclosporin A in transplant models
1980s	Heart-lung transplants in monkeys
1990s	Novel immunosuppressive strategies

Clinical

1906	Human kidney allograft
1950–1953	Kidney transplantation in nonimmunosuppressed hosts
1954	First successful identical-twin kidney transplant
1959–1961	Kidney transplants in irradiated hosts
1960–1963	Clinical use of chemical immunosuppression
1962–1964	Attempts at liver, pancreas, small bowel transplantation
1963	First lung transplant
1964	Addition of steroids to reverse acute rejection
1967	First heart transplant
1978	First clinical reports of Cyclosporin A in organ transplantation
1980	Selective therapy with monoclonal antibodies
1986	Introduction of FK 506 (tacrolimus)
1995	Clinical introduction of mycophenolate mofetil
1999	Rapamycin (sirolimus) trials

Associated Refinements

1940s	Introduction of hemodialysis
1958	Definition of human leukocyte antigens (HLA)
1959	Description of coma dépassé
1960	Description of dialysis shunt
1967	Cross-match
	Organ preservation
1968	Definition of brain death
1970s	Tissue typing, organ banks, organ sharing
	Reduction in patient mortality

Xenografts

1906–1914	Kidney xenografts in humans
1963–1964	Chimpanzee kidneys, lungs, and heart to humans
1970s	Chimpanzee livers to humans
1984	Baboon heart to Baby Fae
1992	Pig-to-human heart transplant
1993	Baboon livers to humans

Transplantation Biology

Humoral

1907	Identification of blood group antigens A, B, O
	Delineation of antigen-antibody reactions
1937	Identification of major histocompatibility locus (H2) of mouse
1939	Separation of antibodies into classes
1950	Determination of humoral components of acute rejection
1956	Immunological function of the bursa of Fabricius
1957	Clonal selection theory of acquired immunity
1959	Elucidation of antibody structure
1966	Cell cooperation in antibody production
1970	Concept of T-cell "help" in antibody production

Cellular

1916	Description of free-martin cattle
1924	Destruction of human maternal skin grafts
1942	Identification of behavior differences of human isografts and allografts
1943	Skin-graft rejection in humans
1944	Determination of immunological basis of skin-graft rejection in rabbits
1945	Chimerism in cattle twins
1949	Derivation of concepts of "self" and "nonself"
1951	Acceptance of skin grafts by chimeric cattle twins
1953	Acquired immunological tolerance
	Cellular transfer of sensitivity
	Biology of acute rejection of kidney allografts in dogs
1957	Recirculation of the lymphocyte

1958	Definition of graft-versus-host disease (GVHD)
	Recognition of lymphocyte as an immunologically competent cell
1961	Determination of immunological function of thymus
1969	Definition of T and B lymphocytes
1970s	Antigen-presenting cells in induction of immunity
	First understanding of cytokines and their receptors
1973	Involvement of major histocompatibility complex (MHC) in T-cell recognition of viruses appreciated
1975	Elaboration of T-cell subclasses
	Monoclonal antibodies
1987	Definition of MHC as antigen-presenting molecules by crystal structure of HLA
1990s	Definition of T-cell receptor—MHC antigenic peptide interaction
	Transplantation of fetal cells
2000	Stem cells and construction of organs

Notes

Chapter 1. Legends, Possibilities, and Disasters

1. J. E. Murray, ed., "Human kidney transplant conference," *Transplantation* (1964), 2:147.

2. F. D. Moore, *A Miracle, A Privilege* (Washington, D.C.: Joseph Henry Press, 1995), 186.

3. R. Küss and P. Bourget, *An Illustrated History of Organ Transplantation* (Rueil-Malmaison, France: Laboratoires Sandoz, 1992), 8–23; J. B. deCM. Saunders, "A conceptual history of transplantation," in J. S. Najarian and R. L. Simmons, eds., *Transplantation* (Philadelphia: Lea and Febiger, 1972), 3.

4. B. Teratti, "Transplantation and reimplantation in the arts," *Surgery* (1974), 75:389; D. K. C. Cooper, "Introduction," in D. K. C. Cooper, E. Kemp, et al., eds., *Xenotransplantation* (Berlin: Springer-Verlag, 1991), vii.

5. Ezek. 11:19.

6. J. Dewhurst, "Cosmos and Damian, patron saints of doctors," *Lancet* (1988), 2:1479.

7. *The Works of Mr. Francis Rabelais* (privately printed, London: Navarre Society, 1921), 295.

8. G. Majno, *The Healing Hand: Man and Wound in the Ancient World* (Cambridge, Mass.: Harvard University Press, 1975), 292–293.

9. R. M. Goldwyn, "Historical introduction," in G. Baronio, *Degli innesti animali* (On grafting in animals), 1804 (Boston: Boston Medical Library, 1985), 17.

10. R. Fludd, "Answer to M. Foster: On the squeezing of Parson Foster's sponge ordained by him for the washing away of the weapon salve" (London: Butterworth, 1631), cited in T. J. S. Patterson, "Experimental skin grafts in Britain," *British Journal of Plastic Surgery* (1969), 22:384; S. Butler, *Hudibras* (London: H. Brown, 1761), 21.

11. J. P. Bennett, "Aspects of the history of plastic surgery since the 16th century," *Journal of the Royal Society of Medicine* (1983), 76:152.

12. Hindu method cited in C. M. Balch and F. A. Marzoni, "Skin transplantation during the pre-Reverdin era, 1804–1869," *Surgery, Gynecology and Obstetrics* (1977), 144:766; Royal Society minutes in T. J. S. Patterson, "Experimental skin grafts in England," *British Journal of Plastic Surgery* (1969), 22:384.

13. Balch and Marzoni, "Skin transplantation," 769.

14. J. F. Dieffenbach, "Surgical observations on the restoration of the nose," trans., with additional notes, John Bushman (London: Highley Publishers, 1833); cited in Balch and Marzoni, "Skin transplantation," 771.

15. E. Lexer, "Free transplantation," *Annals of Surgery* (1914), 60:166; G. Schone, "*Die Heteroplastische und Homoplastische Transplantation* (Berlin: Springer-Verlag, 1912); H. L. Underwood, "Anaphylaxis following skin grafting for burns," *Journal of the American Medical Association* (1914), 63:775; E. Holman, "Protein sensitization in iso-skin grafting. Is the latter of practical value?" *Surgery, Gynecology and Obstetrics* (1924), 38:100.

16. J. B. Brown and F. McDowell, "Epithelial healing and the transplantation of skin," *Annals of Surgery* (1942), 115: 1166; Loeb cited in J. E. Murray, "Reflections on the first successful kidney transplantation," *World Journal of Surgery* (1982), 6:372.

17. R. Lower, "Tractatus de corde," 191–192, cited in A. R. Hall, "Medicine and the Royal Society," in A. G. Debus, ed., *Medicine in Seventeenth Century England* (Berkeley: University of California Press, 1974), 439.

18. S. Pepys, *Diary and Correspondence of Samuel Pepys, Esq., FRS*, November 18, 1666, vol. 4 (London: Bickers and Son, 1877), 161; Hall, "Medicine," 439.

19. J. Kobler, *The Reluctant Surgeon: The Life of John Hunter* (London: Heinemann, 1960), 141.

20. Cited in R. Richardson, "Transplanting teeth," *Lancet* (1999), 354:1740.

21. Ibid.; Kobler, *Reluctant Surgeon*, 142.

22. F. D. Moore, "Surgery," in J. Z. Bowers and E. F. Purcell, eds., *Advances in American Medicine: Essays at the Bicentennial* (Baltimore: Port City Press, 1976), 614–684.

23. D'A. Power, "Robert Liston (1794–1847)," *Dictionary of National Biography* (1909), 11:1236; O. H. Wangensteen and S. D. Wagensteen, *The Rise of Surgery: From Empiric Craft to Scientific Discipline* (Minneapolis: University of Minnesota Press, 1978), 37.

24. G. Williams, *The Age of Miracles in Medicine and Surgery in the Nineteenth Century* (London: Constable, 1981), 45.

25. D. N. H. Hamilton, *The Monkey Gland Affair* (London: Chatto and Windus, 1986); quotation from J. F. Palmer, *The Complete Works of John Hunter*, vol. 3 (Philadelphia: Haswell Barrington and Haswell, 1841), 273.

26. Cited in D. N. H. Hamilton, *Monkey Gland Affair*, 12; R. Tattersall and B. Turner, "Brown-Séquard and his syndrome," *Lancet* (2000), 356:61.

27. *Thyroid Glands*, words and music by R. P. Weston and B. Lee (© London 1921, cited by permission of Frances Day and Hunter, London).

28. Cited in Hamilton, *Monkey Gland Affair*, 28.

29. "Virginia expresses regret for past sterilizations," *New York Times*, September 15, 2001.

30. E. Harris, "Forty-four years of correspondence between Eugen Steinach and Harry Benjamin," *Bulletin of the New York Academy of Medicine* (1969), 45:761.

31. F. Lydston, "Sex gland implantation: Additional cases and conclusions to date," *Journal of the American Medical Association* (1916), 66:1540; Hamilton, *Monkey Gland Affair*, 26.

32. *New York Times*, July 1, 1924.

33. "Testicular transplantation" (editorial), *Boston Medical and Surgical Journal* (1924), 191:1045.

34. C. Moore, "Physiologic effects of non-living testis grafts," *Journal of the American Medical Association* (1930), 94:1912.

35. D. Greenburg, "Oh, bury me not at Clinique la Prairie," in D. Cooper, ed., *Chris Barnard by Those Who Know Him* (Vlaeberg, South Africa: Vlaeberg Publishers, 1992), 175.

Chapter 2. Attempts and Failures

1. T. Stark, *Knife to the Heart: The Story of Transplant Surgery* (London: Macmillan, 1996), 7–8.

2. G. Majno, *The Healing Hand: Man and Wound in the Ancient World* (Cambridge, Mass.: Harvard University Press, 1975), 29–68.

3. A. Paré, *The Works of That Famous Chirurgeon, Ambrose Paré*, trans. Thomas Johnson (1634), 459–633.

4. "Valentine Mott," *Lancet* (1865), 1:553.

5. W. A. Dale, "The beginnings of vascular surgery," *Surgery* (1974), 76:849.

6. E. Ullmann, "Tissue and organ transplantation," *Annals of Surgery* (1914), 60:195; N. Floresco, "Recherches sur la transplantation du rein," *Journal of Physiological and Pathological Genetics* (1905), 7:47; A. Carrel, "La Technique opératoire des anastomoses vasculaires et la transplantation des viscères," *Lyon Médecine* (1902), 98:859.

7. S. P. Harbison, "Origins of vascular surgery: The Carrel-Guthrie letters," *Surgery* (1962), 32:406, 418.

8. A. Carrel, "The ultimate result of a double nephrectomy and the replantation of one kidney," *Journal of Experimental Medicine* (1911), 14:124; potential attempt in man cited in R. Küss and P. Bourget, *An Illustrated History of Organ Transplantation* (Rueil-Malmaison, France: Laboratoires Sandoz, 1992), 30; *New*

York Times cited in D. N. H. Hamilton, *The Monkey Gland Affair* (London: Chatto and Windus, 1986), 9.

9. A. Carrel, "The transplantation of organs," *New York Medical Journal* (1914), 99:839; W. Myer, "Contributions to the analysis of tissue growth. XI. Autoplastic and homeoplastic transplantations of kidney tissue," *Archiv für Entwicklungs-Mechanik* (1913), 38:1.

10. M. Jaboulay, "Greffe du reins au pli du conde par soudres arterielles et veineuses," *Lyon Médecine* (1906), 107:575.

11. A. Carrel, *Man, the Unknown* (1933), cited in W. S. Edwards and P. D. Edwards, *Alexis Carrel, Visionary Surgeon* (Springfield, Ill.: Charles C Thomas, 1974), 98.

12. D. N. H. Hamilton and W. A. Reid, "Yu Yu Voronoy and the first human kidney allograft," *Surgery, Gynecology and Obstetrics* (1984), 159:289; M. B. Mirskili, "The Soviet surgeon Yu Yu Voronoy, pioneer of allotransplantation of the cadaveric kidney in the clinic," *Klincheskaya Zhurnalya* (1973), 5:76.

13. Yu Yu Voronoy, "Transplantation of a conserved cadaveric kidney as a method of biostimulation in severe nephritides," *Vrachebnoe Dyel* (1950), 9:813.

14. R. Bright, "Cases and observations illustrative of renal disease accompanied with the secretion of albuminous urine," *Guys Hospital Reports* (1836), 1:338.

15. R. H. Lawler, J. W. West, et al., "Homotransplantation of the kidney in the human," *Journal of the American Medical Association* (1950), 144:844; *Newsweek*, July 3, 1950.

16. Cited in Stark, *Knife to the Heart*, 29; "Foreign letter–kidney transplantation," *Journal of the American Medical Association* (1951), 146:393.

17. C. Dubost, N. Oeconomos, et al., "Note préliminaire sur l'étude des fonctions rénales de reins greffes chez l'homme," *Bulletin et Mémoires de la Société des Médecins et Hôpitaliers de Paris* (1951), 67:105; M. Servelle, P. Soulié, et al., "La greffe du rein," *Revue de Chirurgie de Paris* (1951), 70:186.

18. R. Küss, J. Teinturier, and P. Milliez, "Quelques essais de greffe de rein chez l'homme," *Mémoires de l'Académie Chirurgique* (1951), 77:755; J. Hamburger, "Past, present and future of transplantation," *Transplantation Proceedings* (1981), 13:41.

19. G. W. Thorn, "A 50th anniversary celebration," *Transplantation Proceedings* (1981), 13:24.

20. A. Blalock and S. E. Levy, "Studies on the etiology of renal hypertension," *Annals of Surgery* (1936), 106:826.

21. E. G. L. Bywaters, "Ischemic muscle necrosis. Crushing injury, traumatic edema, the crush syndrome, traumatic anuria, compression syndrome: A type of injury seen in air raid casualties following burial beneath debris," *Journal of the American Medical Association* (1944), 134:1103; G. W. Thorn, "Physiologic considerations in the treatment of nephritis," *New England Journal of Medicine* (1943), 229:33.

22. F. D. Moore, *Give and Take: The Development of Tissue Transplantation* (Philadelphia: W. B. Saunders, 1964), 55.

23. J. P. Merrill, "The use of an artificial kidney. I. Technique; II. Clinical experience," *Journal of Clinical Investigation* (1950), 29:423; Thorn, "50th anniversary celebration."

24. Cited in Moore, *Give and Take*, 14.

25. D. M. Hume, J. P. Merrill, et al., "Experiences with renal homotransplantation in the human: Report of nine cases," *Journal of Clinical Investigation* (1955), 34:327; D. M. Hume, J. P. Merrill, and B. F. Miller, "Homologous transplantation of human kidneys," *Journal of Clinical Investigation* (1952), 31:640.

26. G. Murray and R. Holden, "Transplantation of kidneys, experimentally and in human cases," *American Journal of Surgery* (1954), 87:508.

27. R. Küss, in Küss and Bourget, *Illustrated History*, 44; Küss, Teinturier, and Milliez, "Quelques essais."

Chapter 3. Hopes and Occasional Successes

1. J. E. Murray, "Reflections on the first successful kidney transplantation," *World Journal of Surgery* (1982), 6:372.

2. J. E. Murray, "Remembrances of the early days of renal transplantation," *Transplantation Proceedings* (1981), 13:9.

3. Murray, "Reflections"; J. H. Harrison and N. L. Tilney, "Renal transplantation: Part I," in *Perspectives in Urology* (American Urological Association and Hoffman-LaRoche, 1980).

4. Murray, "Reflections"; J. P. Merrill, J. E. Murray, et al., "Successful homotransplantation of the human kidney between identical twins," *Journal of the American Medical Association* (1956), 160:277.

5. N. L. Tilney, "Renal transplantation between identical twins: A review," *World Journal of Surgery* (1986), 10:381.

6. N. K. Hollenberg and N. L. Tilney, "Renal transplantation: Donor selection and surgical aspects," in B. M. Brenner and F. C. Rector Jr., eds., *The Kidney* (Philadelphia: W. B. Saunders, 1981), 2599; Murray, "Remembrances."

7. W. J. Curran, "A problem of consent: Kidney transplantation in minors," *New York University Law Review* (1959), 5:891; Hollenberg and Tilney, "Renal transplantation."

8. N. Fost, "Children as renal donors," *New England Journal of Medicine* (1977), 296:363.

9. T. E. Starzl, "The landmark identical twin case," *Journal of the American Medical Association* (1984), 251:2572.

10. "Landmarks: Murray JE et al.: Study on transplantation immunity after total body irradiation in clinical and experimental investigation," *Journal of the National Institutes of Health Research* (1993), 5:69.

11. L. Hektoen, "The influence of x-ray in the production of antibodies," *Journal of Infectious Diseases* (1915), 17:415.

12. R. E. Billingham, L. Brent, and P. B. Medawar, "Actively acquired tolerance of foreign cells," *Nature* (1953), 172:603.

13. W. J. Dempster, B. Lennox, and J. W. Boag, "Prolongation of survival of skin homotransplants in the rabbit by irradiation of the host," *British Journal of Experimental Pathology* (1950), 31:670; J. E. Murray, J. P. Merrill, et al., "Study on transplantation immunity after total body irradiation: Clinical and experimental investigations," *Surgery* (1960), 48:272; J. A. Mannick, H. L. Lochte, Jr., et al., "A functioning kidney homotransplant in the dog," *Surgery* (1959), 46:821.

14. E. D. Thomas, H. L. Lochte, Jr., et al., "Sublethal whole body irradiation and isologous marrow transplantation in man," *Journal of Clinical Investigation* (1959), 38:1709.

15. "Landmarks," 65.

16. J. E. Murray and J. H. Harrison, "Surgical management of fifty patients with kidney transplants including eighteen pairs of twins," *American Journal of Surgery* (1963), 105:205.

17. B. O. Rogers, "Genetics of skin homotransplantation in humans," *Annals of the New York Academy of Science* (1957), 64:741.

18. Cited in J. E. Murray, *Surgery of the Soul: Reflections on a Curious Career* (Canton, Mass.: Science History Publications/USA, 2001), 99.

19. T. E. Starzl, in "Landmarks," 71; J. Hamburger, J. Vaysse, et al., "Transplantation d'un rein entre non-monozygotes après irradiation du recouver," *Presse Médicale* (1959), 67:1771.

20. T. E. Starzl, "The French heritage in clinical kidney transplantation," *Transplantation Reviews* (1993), 7:65.

21. Murray, "Remembrances."

22. R. Schwartz and W. Damashek, "Drug induced immunological tolerance," *Nature* (1959), 183:1682.

23. R. Y. Calne, "Recollections from the laboratory to the clinic," in P. I. Terasaki, ed., *History of Transplantation: Thirty-five Recollections* (Los Angeles: UCLA Tissue Typing Laboratory, 1991), 227–241.

24. G. B. Elion and G. H. Hitchings, *The Chemistry and Biology of Purines* (Boston: Little Brown, 1957).

25. Murray, "Remembrances."

26. J. E. Murray, A. G. R. Sheil, et al., "Analysis of mechanisms of immunosuppressive drugs in renal homotransplantation," *Annals of Surgery* (1964), 160:449.

27. Starzl, "French heritage."

28. J. P. Merrill, J. E. Murray, and F. Takats, "Successful transplantation of kidney from a human cadaver," *Journal of the American Medical Association* (1963), 185:347.

29. J. E. Murray, J. P. Merrill, et al., "Prolonged survival of human-kidney homografts by immunosuppressive drug therapy," *New England Journal of Medicine* (1963), 268:1315; Calne, "Recollections from the laboratory to the clinic."

30. J. E. Murray, ed., "Human kidney transplant conference," *Transplantation* (1964), 2:147; D. M. Hume, J. H. Magee, et al., "Renal homotransplantation in man in modified recipients," *Annals of Surgery* (1963), 158:608.

31. T. E. Starzl, T. L. Marchioro, and W. R. Waddell, "The reversal of rejection in human renal homografts with subsequent development of homograft tolerance," *Surgery, Gynecology and Obstetrics* (1963), 117:385.

32. T. E. Starzl, *The Puzzle People: Memoirs of a Transplant Surgeon* (Pittsburgh: University of Pittsburgh Press, 1993), 109.

33. *Le Quotidien du Médecine*, October 10, 1990; *Le Monde*, October 10, 1990, cited in T. Stark, *Knife to the Heart: The Story of Transplant Surgery* (London: Macmillan, 1996), 52.

Chapter 4. Host Defenses and Immunity

1. Cited in G. Williams, *The Age of Agony* (London: Constable, 1975), 69.

2. A. E. Housman, "Terence, this is stupid stuff," in *A Shropshire Lad* (London: Ballantyne Press, 1903); with permission, Bartleby.com.

3. F. M. Voltaire (1727) in *Lettres philosophiques*, 3rd ed. (Paris: G. Lanson, 1924), 130–151.

4. F. D. Moore, "Surgery," in J. Z. Bowers and E. F. Purcell, eds., *Advances in American Medicine: Essays at the Bicentennial* (New York, Joshiah Macy, Jr., Foundation, 1976), 614–684.

5. J. Hunter, letter to Edward Jenner, August 2, 1775.

6. R. J. Dubois, *Louis Pasteur: Free Lance of Science* (Boston: Little, Brown, 1950), 116–358.

7. T. D. Brock, *Robert Koch: A Life in Medicine and Bacteriology* (Washington, D.C.: ASM Press, 1999), 169–177.

8. J. Kobler, *The Reluctant Surgeon: The Life of John Hunter* (London: Heinemann, 1960), 108; H. W. Florey, *General Pathology* (Philadelphia: W. B. Saunders, 1970), 23.

9. E. Metchnikoff, *Lectures on the Comparative Pathology of Inflammation, 1891* (Mineola, N.Y.: Dover Publications, 1968).

10. D. J. Dibel, *Milestones in Immunity: A Historical Exploration* (Madison, Wis.: Springer-Verlag, 1988), 117.

11. L. Colebrook, *Almroth Wright* (London: Heinemann, 1954), 30–46.

12. L. Brent, *A History of Transplantation Immunology* (San Diego: Academic Press, 1997), 63; P. Ehrlich, "Experimentelle Karzinomstudien an Mäusen," *Der Arbeiten aus dem Königlichen Institut für Experimental Therapie Frankfurt* (1906), 1:85.

13. A. Carrel, "The transplantation of organs," *New York Medical Journal* (1914), 99:839; H. D. Taylor and J. B. Murphy, "The lymphocyte in natural and induced resistance to transplanted cancer," *Journal of Experimental Medicine* (1918), 28:1; A. R. Rich, "Inflammation in resistance to infection," *Archives of Pathology* (1936), 22:228.

14. J. L. Gowans, "The lymphocyte—a disgraceful gap in medical knowledge," *Immunology Today* (1996), 17:288.

15. Ibid.

16. F. M. Burnet, *The Clonal Selection Theory of Acquired Immunity* (Nashville: Vanderbilt University Press, 1959), 102; H. W. Florey, *General Pathology* (Philadelphia: W. B. Saunders, 1964), 176.

17. P. B. Medawar, "The immunology of transplantation," *Harvey Lectures* (New York: Academic Press, 1958), 52:144.

18. J. F. A. P. Miller, "Immunological function of the thymus," *Lancet* (1961), 2:748.

19. B. Glick, T. S. Chang, and R. G. Jaap, "The bursa of Fabricius and antibody production," *Poultry Science* (1956), 35:224.

20. P. A. Gorer, "The genetic and antigenic basis of tumor transplantation," *Journal of Pathology and Bacteriology* (1937), 44:691.

21. M. C. Raff, "Theta isoantigens marker of thymus-derived lymphocytes in mice," *Nature* (1969), 224:378.

22. P. B. Medawar, *Memoir of a Thinking Radish: An Autobiography* (Oxford: Oxford University Press, 1986), 135.

23. G. P. J. Alexandre, "From the early days of human kidney allo-transplantation to prospective xenotransplantation," in P. I. Terasaki, ed., *History of Transplantation: Thirty-five Recollections* (Los Angeles: UCLA Tissue Typing Laboratory, 1991), 340; P. S. Russell, "Some personal recollections on the development of transplantation," in Terasaki, *History of Transplantation*, 309.

24. P. L. Starr, *The Social Transformation of American Medicine* (New York: Basic Books, 1982), 343.

25. P. B. Medawar, *The Art of the Soluble* (Harmondsworth: Penguin Books, 1969), 148; idem, *The Threat and the Glory: Reflections on Science and Scientists* (Oxford: Oxford University Press, 1991), 82.

26. T. Friedmann, "Human gene therapy—an immature genie, but certainly out of the bottle," *Nature Medicine* (1996), 2:144.

27. J. Hixon, *The Patchwork Mouse* (New York: Anchor Press, 1976); T. Stark, *Knife to the Heart: The Story of Transplant Surgery* (London: Macmillan, 1996), 114–126.

28. Medawar, *The Threat and the Glory*, 74, 82.

29. K. J. Lafferty, M. A. Cooley, et al., "Thyroid allograft immunogenicity is reduced after a period in organ culture," *Science* (1975), 188:259; W. L. Elkins and R. D. Guttmann, "Pathogenesis of a local graft versus host reaction. Immunogenicity of circulating host leukocytes," *Science* (1968), 159:1250.

Chapter 5. Peter Medawar and Transplantation Biology

1. J. Medawar, *A Very Decided Preference: Life with Peter Medawar* (New York: W. W. Norton, 1990), 51.

2. P. B. Medawar, *Memoir of a Thinking Radish: An Autobiography* (Oxford: Oxford University Press, 1986), 77.

3. T. Gibson and P. B. Medawar, "The fate of skin homografts in man," *Journal of Anatomy* (1943), 77:299.

4. P. B. Medawar, "The behavior and fate of skin autografts and skin homografts in rabbits," *Journal of Anatomy* (1944), 78:176.

5. W. J. Dempster, "Problems involved in the homotransplantation of tissues with particular reference to skin," *British Medical Journal* (1951), ii:1041.

6. M. Simonsen, J. Buemann, et al., "Biological incompatibility in kidney transplantation in dogs. I. Morphological investigations," *Acta Pathologica et Microbiologica Scandinavica* (1953), 32:1.

7. P. B. Medawar, "Transplantation of tissues and organs," *British Medical Bulletin* (1965), 21:97; idem, "The behavior and fate of skin autografts."

8. B. C. Rogers, "Guide and bibliography for research into the skin homograft problem," *Plastic and Reconstructive Surgery* (1951), 7:169.

9. Dempster, "Problems involved"; G. Murray and R. Holden, "Transplantation of the kidney, experimentally and in human cases," *American Journal of Surgery* (1959), 87:508.

10. Cited in J. E. Murray, *Surgery of the Soul: Reflection on a Curious Career* (Canton, Mass.: Science History Publications/USA, 2001) 91; F. R. Lillie, "The theory of the free-martin," *Science* (1916), 43:611; R. D. Owen, "Immunogenetic consequences of vascular anastomoses between bovine twins," *Science* (1945), 102:400.

11. F. M. Burnet and F. Fenner, *The Production of Antibodies* (Melbourne, Australia: Macmillan, 1949).

12. C. H. Danforth and F. Foster, "Skin transplantation as a means of studying genetics and endocrine factors in the fowl," *Journal of Experimental Zoology* (1929), 52:443; J. A. Cannon and W. P. Longmire, Jr., "Studies of successful skin homografts in the chicken. Description of a method of grafting and its application as a technique of investigation," *Annals of Surgery* (1952), 135:60.

13. M. Hašek and T. Hraba "Immunological effects of experimental embryonic parabiosis," *Nature* (1955) 175:764; P. B. Medawar and J. S. Medawar, *Aristotle to Zoos: A Philosophical Dictionary of Biology* (Cambridge, Mass.: Harvard University Press, 1983), 176.

14. Medawar, *Memoir*, 11.

15. R. E. Billingham, L. Brent, and P. B. Medawar, "Actively acquired tolerance of foreign cells," *Nature* (1953), 172:603.

16. A. M. Silverstein, *A History of Immunology* (New York: Academic Press, 1989), 284.

17. R. E. Billingham, "Reminiscences of a transplanter," *Transplantation Proceedings* (1974), 6:5.

18. R. D. French, *Anti-vivisection and Medical Science in Victorian Society* (Princeton: Princeton University Press, 1975).

19. Cited in French, *Anti-vivisection*, 23; M. Shelley, *Frankenstein* (New York: Penguin Books, 1963), 53.

20. S. Johnson, *The Idler*, XVII (August 5, 1758); quoted in French, *Anti-vivisection*, 16.

21. J. Turney, *Frankenstein's Footsteps: Science, Genetics and Popular Culture* (New Haven: Yale University Press, 1998).

22. H. G. Wells, *The Island of Dr. Moreau* (Harmondsworth: Penguin, 1896), 78.

23. Quoted in S. Benison, A. C. Barger, and E. L. Wolfe, *Walter B. Cannon: The Life and Times of a Young Scientist* (Cambridge, Mass.: Harvard University Press, 1987), 172.

24. Ibid., 281–282.

25. F. H. Bach, J. A. Fishman, et al., "Uncertainty in xenotransplantation: Individual benefit versus collective risk," *Nature Medicine* (1998), 4:141–144.

Chapter 6. Innovation and the Struggle for Legitimacy

1. T. E. Starzl, "Inaugural: Presidential address, American Society of Transplant Surgeons," *Surgery* (1976), 79:129.

2. F. T. Rappaport, "The life and times of a transplant immunosurgeon," in P. I. Terasaki, ed., *History of Transplantation: Thirty-five Recollections* (Los Angeles: UCLA Tissue Typing Laboratory, 1991), 363.

3. "The tenth report of the human renal transplant registry," *Journal of the American Medical Association* (1972), 221:1495; T. E. Starzl, "The French heritage in clinical kidney transplantation," *Transplantation Reviews* (1993), 7:65.

4. M. J. Whitelaw, "Physiologic reaction to pituitary adrenocorticotropic hormone in severe burns," *Journal of the American Medical Association* (1951), 145:85.

5. W. J. Dempster, "The effect of cortisone on the transplant kidney," *Archives of International Pharmacodynamics* (1953), 95:253.

6. T. E. Starzl, *The Puzzle People: Memoirs of a Transplant Surgeon* (Pittsburgh: University of Pittsburgh Press, 1993), 114.

7. L. Brent, *A History of Transplantation Immunology* (San Diego: Academic Press, 1997), 247–257; E. Metchnikoff, *Résorption des cellules* (Paris: Annales de l'Institut Pasteur, 1899).

8. R. Küss and P. Bourget, *An Illustrated History of Organ Transplantation* (Rueil-Malmaison, France: Laboratoires Sandoz, 1992), 53–54; C. F. Zukoski, D. A. Killen, et al., "Transplanted carcinoma in an immunosuppressed patient," *Transplantation* (1970), 9:71.

9. H. W. Muiznieks, J. W. Berg, et al., "Suitability of donor kidneys from patients with cancer," *Surgery* (1968), 64:871; S. D. Deodhor, A. G. Kuklinca, et al., "Development of reticulum cell sarcoma at the site of anti-lymphocyte globulin injection in a patient with renal transplant," *New England Journal of Medicine* (1969), 280:1104.

10. I. Penn, "The incidence of malignancies in transplant recipients," *Transplantation Proceedings* (1975), 7:325.

11. Quoted by F. M. Burnet, "Immunological aspects of malignant disease," *Lancet* (1967), i:1171.

12. A. Abbott and F. M. Burnet, "Immunological factors in the process of carcinogenesis," *British Medical Bulletin* (1964), 20:154.

13. C. S. Williamson, "Some observations on the length of survival and function of homogenetic kidney transplants: Preliminary report," *Journal of Urology* (1923), 10:275; R. E. Billingham, L. Brent, and P. B. Medawar, "Quantitative studies on tissue transplantation immunity. II. The origin, strength and duration of actively and adoptively acquired immunity," *Proceedings of the Royal Society B* (1954), 143:43.

14. P. I. Terasaki, "Histocompatibility," in Terasaki, *History of Transplantation*, 497–510.

15. Starzl, *Puzzle People*, 120.

16. M. R. Mickey, M. Kreisser, et al., "Analysis of HLA incompatibility in human renal transplants," *Tissue Antigens* (1971), 1:57.

17. Starzl, *Puzzle People*, 159.

18. Terasaki, "Histocompatibility," 527.

19. F. O. Belzer, "Organ preservation: A personal perspective," in Terasaki, *History of Transplantation*, 595–614; F. O. Belzer, B. S. Ashby, and J. E. Dunphy, "24-hour and 72-hour preservation of canine kidneys," *Lancet* (1967), 2:536.

20. F. O. Belzer, B. S. Ashby, et al., "Successful 17-hour preservation and transplantation of human cadaver kidney," *New England Journal of Medicine* (1968), 278:608.

21. G. M. Collins, M. Bravo-Shugarman, and P. I. Terasaki, "Kidney preservation for transplantation: Initial perfusion and 30 hours ice storage," *Lancet* (1969), 2:1219; G. M. Collins, M. Bravo-Shugarman, et al., "Kidney preservation for transplant. IV. Eight-thousand-mile international air transport," *Australian and New Zealand Journal of Surgery* (1970), 40:195.

Chapter 7. Prolongation of Life and Death

1. A. P. Lundin, "A personal experience with hemodialysis, 1966–1991," *Artificial Organs* (1996), 20:1332.

2. W. Drukker, "Hemodialysis—a historical review," in J. F. Maher, ed., *Replacement of Renal Function by Dialysis*, 4th ed. (Dordrecht, Netherlands: Kluwer

Academic Publishers, 1978); 20–86; J. J. Abel, L. C. Rowntree, and B. B. Turner, "On the removal of diffusable substances from the circulating blood by means of dialysis," *Transactions of the Association of American Physicians* (1913), 28:51.

3. G. Haas, "Ueber Versuche der Blutauswaschung am Lebenden mit Hilfe der Dialyse," *Naunyn-Schmiedeberg's Archives of Pharmacology* (1926), 116:158.

4. F. D. Moore, *Give and Take: The Development of Tissue Transplantation* (Philadelphia: W. B. Saunders, 1964), 54.

5. Cited in Drukker, "Hemodialysis," 35.

6. Ibid.

7. W. Quinton, D. Dillard, and B. H. Scribner, "Cannulation of blood vessels for prolonged hemodialysis," *Transactions of the American Society for Artificial Internal Organs* (1960), 6:104.

8. B. H. Scribner, cited in R. C. Fox and J. P. Swazey, *The Courage to Fail* (Chicago: University of Chicago Press, 1974), 240–279.

9. S. Alexander, "They decide who lives, who dies: Medical miracle puts a moral burden on a small committee," *Life* (November 9, 1962), 102.

10. T. E. Starzl, *The Puzzle People: Memoirs of a Transplant Surgeon* (Pittsburgh: University of Pittsburgh Press, 1993), 205.

11. Cited by G. Annas, "Organ transplants: Are we treating the modern miracle fairly?" in D. Cowan, J. Kantonowitz, et al., eds., *Human Organ Transplantation: Societal, Medical-legal, Regulatory and Reimbursement Issues* (Ann Arbor, Mich.: Health Administration Press, 1987), 166.

12. U.S. Renal Data System, *USRDS 2001 Annual Data Report: Atlas of Endstage Renal Disease in the United States* (Bethesda: National Institute of Diabetes, Digestive and Kidney Diseases, 2001).

13. R. D. Guttmann, "Technology, clinical studies, and control in the field of organ transplantation," *Journal of the History of Biology* (1997), 30:367.

14. Ibid., 371.

15. M. Sapperstein, "Dialysis: A poem," *NAPH [National Association of Public Hospitals] News* (1971), 2:8.

16. S. Aiken, *Remembrances: A Compilation of Thoughts and Tributes from Donor Families* (Boston: New England Organ Bank, 1998), 2–3.

17. M. Alexander, "The rigid embrace of the narrow house. Premature burial and signs of death," *Hastings Center Report* (1980), 10:25; M. A. DeVita, "The death watch: Certifying death using cardiac criteria," *Progress in Transplantation* (2001), 11:58.

18. A. Vesalius, *De Humani Corporis fabrica* (1543), cited in M. Lock, *Twice Dead: Organ Transplants and the Reinvention of Death* (Berkeley: University of California Press, 2002), 58; P. Drinker and C. F. McKhann, "The use of a new apparatus for the prolonged administration of artificial respiration: 1. A fatal case of poliomyelitis," *Journal of the American Medical Association* (1929), 92:1658.

19. J. Korein, "The problem of brain death: Development and history," *Annals of the New York Academy of Science* (1978), 315:19; F. D. Moore, *Transplant: The Give and Take of Tissue Transplantation* (New York: Simon and Schuster, 1972), 205.

20. "Pius XII: The prolongation of life," in *Pope Speaks* (1958), 4:393.

21. Cited in R. Küss and P. Bourget, *An Illustrated History of Organ Transplantation* (Rueil-Malmaison, France: Laboratoires Sandoz, 1992), 64; P. Mollaret and M. Goulon, "Coma dépassé et necroses nerveuses controles massives," *Revue Neurologique* (1959), 101:116.

22. Cited in Moore, *Transplant*, 207.

23. Lock, *Twice Dead*, 65; idem, "Death in technological time: Locating the end of meaningful life," *Medical Anthropology Quarterly* (1996), 10:575; *Newsweek*, December 18, 1967, 87.

24. "Report of the ad hoc committee of the Harvard Medical School to examine the definition of brain death. A definition of irreversible coma," *Journal of the American Medical Association* (1968), 205:337.

Chapter 8. New Departures

1. G. Majno, *The Healing Hand: Man and Wound in the Ancient World* (Cambridge, Mass.: Harvard University Press, 1975), 401; E. J. Trelawny, "Percy Bysshe Shelley (1792-1822)," in J. Sutherland, *Oxford Book of Literary Anecdotes* (Oxford: Clarendon Press, 1975), 192-196.

2. R. Warren, *Surgery* (Philadelphia: W. B. Saunders, 1963), 650.

3. T. Billroth, "Krankheiten der Brust," in M. Pitha and T. Billroth, eds., *Handbuch der Allgemeinen und Speziellen Chirurgie*, vol. 3 (Stuttgart: F. Ennke, 1882), 163-164.

4. A. Carrel and C. C. Guthrie, "The transplantation of veins and organs," *American Medicine* (1905), 10:1101.

5. J. J. C. LeGallois, *Experiments on the Principle of Life*, trans. N. C. Nancrede and J. C. Nancrede (Philadelphia: M. Thomas, 1813).

6. J. H. Gibbon, Jr., "Application of a mechanical heart and lung apparatus to cardiac surgery," *Minnesota Medicine* (1954), 37:171; quotation from F. D. Moore, *A Miracle, A Privilege* (Washington, D.C.: Joseph Henry Press, 1995), 224-225.

7. Carrel and Guthrie, "Transplantation"; F. C. Mann, J. T. Priestley, et al., "Transplantation of the intact mammalian heart," *Archives of Surgery* (1933), 26:219; V. P. Demikhov, "Experimental transplantation of vital organs," *Medgiz State Press for Medical Literature in Moscow* (Moscow, 1960); trans. B. Haigh (New York Consultants Bureau, 1962).

8. E. Dong, Jr., "A heart transplantation narrative: The earliest years," in P. I. Terasaki, ed., *History of Transplantation: Thirty-five Recollections* (Los Angeles: UCLA Tissue Typing Laboratory, 1991), 435.

9. N. E. Shumway, cited in R. Küss and P. Bourget, *An Illustrated History of Organ Transplantation* (Rueil-Malmaison, France: Laboratoires Sandoz, 1992), 113; E. Dong, Jr., E. J. Hurley, et al., "Performance of the heart two years after auto-transplantation," *Surgery* (1964), 56:270.

10. R. R. Lower, E. Dong, Jr., and N. E. Shumway, "Suppression of rejection crises in the cardiac homograft," *Annals of Thoracic Surgery* (1965), 1:645.

11. N. E. Shumway, W. W. Angell, and R. D. Wuerflein, "Heart replacement: The cardiac chimera versus mechanical man," *Lancet* (1968), ii:172.

12. J. D. Hardy, C. M. Chavez, et al., "Heart transplantation in man: Developmental studies and report of a case," *Journal of the American Medical Association* (1964), 188:1132; C. N. Barnard, "The first human-to-human heart transplant," in Terasaki, *History of Transplantation*, 565.

13. T. Stark, *Knife to the Heart: The Story of Transplant Surgery* (London: Macmillan, 1996), 79–105.

14. Moore, *A Miracle*, 201.

15. R. C. Fox and J. P. Swazey, *The Courage to Fail* (Chicago: University of Chicago Press, 1974), 135.

16. Ibid., 127.

17. R. Hoffenberg, "Christiaan Barnard: His first transplants and their impact on concepts of death," *British Medical Journal* (2001), 323:1478.

18. F. D. Moore, G. E. Birtch, et al., "Cardiac and other organ transplantation in the setting of transplant science," *Journal of the American Medical Association* (1968), 206:2489; D. E. Harken, "Transplantation," ibid., 2514.

19. *Times* (London), June 18, 1968; I. Page, "The ethics of heart transplantation," *Journal of the American Medical Association* (1969), 207:109.

20. "Transplants: Guarded outlook," *Newsweek*, July 21, 1969, 109–110.

21. R. Y. Calne and R. Williams, "Survival after orthotopic liver transplantation: A follow-up report of two patients," *British Medical Journal* (1970), 3:436.

22. J. D. Hardy, S. Eraslan, and M. L. Dalton, Jr., "Autotransplantation and homotransplantation of the lung: Further studies," *Journal of Thoracic and Cardiovascular Surgery* (1963), 46:606; V. P. Demikhov, "Some essential points of the techniques of transplantation of the heart, lungs and other organs," in Haigh, *Medgiz State Press*, 107–126, 129–135.

23. F. G. Veith, "Lung transplantation," *American Review of Respiratory Disease* (1968), 98:769.

24. Küss and Bourget, *Illustrated History*, 134.

25. J. D. Hardy, W. R. Webb, et al., "Lung homotransplantation in man," *Journal of the American Medical Association* (1963), 186:1065.

26. E. N. Meshalkin, V. S. Sergievskii, et al., "On the possibility of preserving the main function of the lung after surgical sections of all its neural connections (in autografting) under experimental conditions," *Experimental Surgery and Anesthesiology* (1964), 9:34.

27. F. Derom, F. Barbier, et al., "Ten month survival after lung transplantation in man," *Journal of Thoracic and Cardiovascular Surgery* (1971), 61:835.

28. J. M. Kriett and M. P. Kaye, "Registry of the International Society for Heart Transplantation, seventh official report—1990," *Journal of Heart Transplantation* (1990), 9:323.

29. C. W. Lillehei, in discussion of C. H. R. Wildevuur and J. R. Benfield, "A review of 23 human lung transplantations by 20 surgeons," *Annals of Thoracic Surgery* (1970), 9:489.

30. A. Carrel, "Surgery of blood vessels, etc.," *Bulletin of Johns Hopkins Hospital* (1907), 18:18; Demikhov in Haigh, *Medgiz State Press*, 29–48.

31. B. A. Reitz, N. A. Burton, et al., "Heart and lung transplantation: Auto and allotransplantation in primates with extended survival," *Journal of Thoracic and Cardiovascular Surgery* (1980), 80:360.

32. Küss and Bourget, *Illustrated History*, 141.

9. The Dracula of Modern Technology

1. R. C. Fox and J. P. Swazey, *The Courage to Fail* (Chicago: University of Chicago Press, 1974), 151.

2. H. H. Dale and E. A. Schuster, "A double perfusion pump," *Journal of Physiology* (1928), 64:356; A. Carrel and C. A. Lindbergh, "Culture of whole organs," *Science* (1935), 31:621; V. P. Demikhov, "Experimental transplantation of vital organs," *Medgiz State Press for Medical Literature in Moscow* (Moscow, 1960); trans. B. Haigh (New York Consultants Bureau, 1962), 129–135.

3. M. E. DeBakey, C. W. Hall, et al., "Orthotopic cardiac prosthesis: Preliminary experiments in animals with biventricular artificial heart," *Cardiovascular Research Center Bulletin* (1969), 7:127; Fox and Swazey, *Courage to Fail*, 149–214.

4. Fox and Swazey, *Courage to Fail*.

5. D. A. Cooley, D. Liotta, et al., "Orthotopic cardiac prosthesis for two-staged cardiac replacement," *American Journal of Cardiology* (1969), 24:723.

6. Ibid.; D. A. Cooley, "First implantation of cardiac prosthesis for staged total replacement of the heart," *Transactions of the American Society for Artificial Organs* (1969), 15:252; DeBakey, Hall, et al., "Orthotopic cardiac prosthesis."

7. DeBakey, Hall, et al., "Orthotopic cardiac prosthesis."

8. F. D. Moore, *Transplant: The Give and Take of Tissue Transplantation* (New York: Simon and Schuster, 1972), 275.

9. R. Bellah, "Civil religion in America," in *Beyond Belief: Essays in Religion in a Post-traditional World* (New York: Harper and Row, 1970), 168–189.

10. R. C. Fox and J. P. Swazey, *Spare Parts: Organ Replacement in American Society* (Oxford: Oxford University Press, 1982), 95–149.

11. J. Kolff, "Artificial heart substitution in the total or auxiliary artificial heart," *Transplantation Proceedings* (1984), 16:898.

12. "The forgotten man," *Boston Globe*, May 8, 2001; W. C. DeVries, J. L. Anderson, et al., "Clinical use of the total artificial heart," *New England Journal of Medicine* (1984), 310:273.

13. W. C. DeVries, "The permanent artificial heart in four case reports," *Journal of the American Medical Association* (1988), 259:849.

14. W. S. Pierce, "Permanent heart substitutions: Better solutions lie ahead," *Journal of the American Medical Association* (1988), 259:891.

15. "Dracula of modern technology," *New York Times*, May 12, 1988.

Chapter 10. The Abdominal Viscera

1. "A 'life' sentence for the justice," *American Liver Foundation, New England Chapter News*, (Summer/Fall 2000), 1.

2. T. Bartholin, in F. T. Fierichs, *A Clinical Treatise on the Liver*, trans. C. Murcheson (London: New Syndenham Society, 1860–1861).

3. W. Shakespeare, "Twelfth Night," act I, scene 3.

4. C. S. Welch, "A note on transplantation of the whole liver in dogs," *Transplantation Bulletin* (1955), 2:54.

5. F. D. Moore, H. B. Wheeler, et al., "Experimental whole-organ transplantation of the liver and of the spleen," *Annals of Surgery* (1960), 152:374; T. E. Starzl, H. A. Kaupp, Jr., et al., "Reconstructive problems in canine liver transplantation with special reference to the postoperative role of hepatic venous flow," *Surgery, Gynecology and Obstetrics* (1960), 122:733.

6. T. E. Starzl, K. A. Porter, et al., "Orthotopic liver transplantation in ninety-three patients," *Surgery, Gynecology and Obstetrics* (1976), 142:487.

7. T. E. Starzl, T. L. Marchioro, et al., "The use of heterologous anti-lymphoid agents in canine renal and liver transplantation, and in human renal homotransplantation," *Surgery, Gynecology and Obstetrics* (1967), 124:301; J. R. W. Ackerman and C. N. Barnard, "Successful storage of kidneys," *British Journal of Surgery* (1966), 53:525.

8. R. Y. Calne, "Liver transplantation," *Transplantation Reviews* (1969), 2:69.

9. S. H. Belle, K. C. Beringer, and K. M. Detre, "Recent findings concerning liver transplantation in the United States," in J. M. Cecka and P. I. Terasaki, eds., *Clinical Transplants* (Los Angeles: UCLA Tissue Typing Laboratory, 1996), 15–30.

10. E. P. Joslin, "Reminiscences of the discovery of insulin: A personal impression," *Diabetes* (1956), 5:67; M. Bliss, *The Discovery of Insulin* (Chicago: University of Chicago Press, 1982).

11. F. G. Banting and C. H. Best, "The internal secretions of the pancreas," *Journal of Laboratory and Clinical Medicine* (1922), 7:251; F. G. Banting, "The history of insulin," *Edinburgh Medical Journal* (1929), 36:1.

12. Banting, "History of insulin"; W. A. Selle, "Studies on pancreatic grafts made with new techniques," *American Journal of Physiology* (1935), 113:118; W. F. Ballinger

and P. E. Lacy, "Transplantation of intact pancreatic islets in rats," *Surgery* (1972), 72:175; R. Reckard, M. M. Ziegler, and C. F. Barker, "Physiological and immunological consequences of transplanting isolated human islets," *Surgery* (1973), 74:91.

13. D. E. R. Sutherland, "Pancreas and islet cell transplantation: Now and then," *Transplantation Proceedings* (1996), 28:2131.

14. A. M. Shapiro, J. R. Lakey, et al., "Islet transplantation in seven patients with type 1 diabetes mellitus using a glucocorticoid-free immunosuppressive regimen," *New England Journal of Medicine* (2000), 343:230.

15. Banting and Best, "Internal secretions."

16. W. D. Kelly, R. C. Lillehei, et al., "Allotransplantation of the pancreas and duodenum along with the kidney in diabetic nephropathy," *Surgery* (1967), 61:827; R. C. Lillehei, J. O. Ruiz, et al., "Transplantation of the pancreas," *Acta Endocrinologica* (1976), 83 (suppl. 205):303.

17. D. E. R. Sutherland, "International human pancreas and islet transplant registry," *Transplantation Proceedings* (1980), 12:229; J. S. Najarian, D. E. R. Sutherland, et al., "Kidney transplantation for the uremic diabetic patient," *Surgery, Gynecology and Obstetrics* (1977), 144:682.

18. J. M. Dubernard, J. Traeger, et al., "A new method of preparation of segmental pancreas grafts for transplantation: Trials in dogs and in man," *Surgery* (1978), 84:633.

19. Sutherland, "Pancreas and islet cell."

20. O. H. Wangensteen and S. D. Wangensteen, *The Rise of Surgery from Empiric Craft to Scientific Discipline* (Minneapolis: University of Minnesota Press, 1978), 106–111.

21. R. Margreiter, "The history of intestinal transplantation," *Transplantation Reviews* (1997), 11:9; E. Ullmann, "Offizielles Protokoll der K. K. Gesellschaft der Artze in Wien," *Wien Klinische Wochenschrift* (1901), 14:599; R. C. Lillehei, B. Goott, and F. A. Miller, "The physiological response of the small bowel of the dog to ischemia including prolonged in vitro preservation of the bowel with successful replacement and survival," *Annals of Surgery* (1959), 150:543.

22. W. G. Manax, G. W. Lyons, and R. C. Lillehei, "Transplantation of the small bowel and stomach," *Advances in Surgery* (1966), 2:371.

23. O. H. Wangensteen, in discussion of Lillehei, Goott, and Miller, "Physiological response."

24. R. C. Lillehei, Y. Idezuki, et al., "Transplantation of stomach, intestines and pancreas: Experimental and clinical observations," *Surgery* (1967), 62:721.

25. J. G. Fortner, G. Sichuk, et al., "Immunological responses to an intestinal allograft with HLA identical donor-recipient," *Transplantation* (1972), 14:53; E. Deltz, P. Schroeder, et al., "Successful clinical small bowel transplantation: Report of a case," *Transplantation Proceedings* (1990), 22:2501.

26. T. E. Starzl, *The Puzzle People: Memoirs of a Transplant Surgeon* (Pittsburgh: University of Pittsburgh Press, 1993), 78.

27. D. Grant, "Intestinal transplantation: 1997 report of the international registry," *Transplantation* (1999), 67:1061.

Chapter 11. A Modern Minotaur

1. L. Bailey, S. L. Nehlsen-Cannarella, et al., "Baboon to human cardiac xenotransplantation in a neonate," *Journal of the American Medical Association* (1985), 254:3321.

2. A. R. Shons, A. W. Moberg, and J. S. Najarian, "Xenotransplantation," in J. S. Najarian and R. L. Simmons, eds., *Transplantation* (Philadelphia: Lea and Febiger, 1972), 729–744.

3. L. Brent, *A History of Transplantation Immunology* (San Diego: Academic Press, 1997), 377; J. E. Canniday, "A simplification of the usual technique of skin grafting," *Journal of the American Medical Association* (1906), 46:1681.

4. D. N. H. Hamilton, "Kidney transplantation: A history," in P. J. Morris, ed., *Kidney Transplantation: Principles and Practice*, 5th ed. (Philadelphia: W. B. Saunders, 2001), 1–8; E. Ullmann, "Experimentelle Nierentransplantation," *Wiener Klinische Wochenschrift* (1902), 15:281.

5. E. Unger, "Nierentransplantation," *Wiener Klinische Wochenschrift* (1910), 47:573; Ullmann, "Nierentransplantation."

6. J. Ryzaard and C. O. Povlsen, "Heterotransplantation of a human malignant tumor to 'nude' mice," *Acta Pathologica, Microbiologica et Immunologica Scandinavica* (1969), 77:758.

7. H. Auchincloss, Jr., "Xenogeneic transplantation: A review," *Transplantation* (1988), 46:1.

8. C. R. Hitchcock, J. C. Kiser, et al., "Baboon renal grafts," *Journal of the American Medical Association* (1964), 189:934.

9. K. Reemstma, "Heterotransplantation," *Transplantation Proceedings* (1969), 1:251; T. E. Starzl, T. L. Marchioro, et al., "Renal heterotransplantation from baboon to man: Experience with six cases," *Transplantation* (1964), 2:752.

10. R. Y. Calne, "Observations on renal homotransplantation," *British Journal of Surgery* (1961), 48:384.

11. T. E. Starzl, J. Fung, et al., "Baboon-to-human liver transplantation," *Lancet* (1993), 341:65.

12. Cited by D. J. G. White, "Can the clinical application of xenotransplantation be justified?" *Graft* (1998), 1:55.

13. Brent, *History*, 384; A. C. Caplan, "Ethical issues raised by research involving xenografts," *Journal of the American Medical Association* (1985), 254:3339.

14. C. Patience, Y. Tekanchi, and R. A. Weiss, "Infection of human cells by an endogenous retrovirus of pigs," *Nature Medicine* (1997), 3:276.

15. "Animal-to-human transplants," in *The Ethics of Xenotransplantation* (Nuffield Council on Bioethics, U.K., 1996); "Animal tissue into humans" (Depart-

ment of Health, Advisory Group on the Ethics of Xenotransplantation, U.K., 1997); "Xenotransplantation, science, ethics and public policy" (Institute of Medicine, U.S., 1996).

16. H. Frankish, "Pig organ transplantation brought one step closer," *Lancet* (2002), 359:137.

Chapter 12. Coming of Age

1. "Thirteenth report of the Human Renal Transplant Society," *Transplantation Proceedings* (1977), 9:9.

2. N. L. Tilney, T. B. Strom, et al., "Factors contributing to the declining mortality rate in renal transplantation," *New England Journal of Medicine* (1978), 299:1321.

3. R. Y. Calne, D. J. G. White, et al., "Cyclosporin A in patients receiving renal allografts from cadaver donors," *Lancet* (1978), ii: 1323; R. C. Powles, A. J. Barrett, et al., "Cyclosporin A for the treatment of graft versus host disease in man," ibid., 1327; R. Y. Calne, K. Rolles, et al., "Cyclosporin A initially as the only immunosuppresant in 34 recipients of cadaveric organs: 32 kidneys, 2 pancreases, and 2 livers," *Lancet* (1979), ii: 1033 5.

4. J. F. Borel, "The history of Cyclosporin A and its significance," in D. J. G. White, ed., *Cyclosporin A: Proceedings of an International Symposium on Cyclosporin A* (Amsterdam: Elsevier, 1972), 5.

5. A. J. Kostakis, D. J. G. White, and R. Y. Calne, "Prolongation of the rat heart allograft survival by Cyclosporin A," *IRCS Journal of Medical Sciences* (1977), 5:280; D. C. Dunn, D. J. G. White, and J. Wade, "Survival of first and second kidney allografts after withdrawal of Cyclosporin A therapy," *IRCS Journal of Medical Sciences* (1978), 6:464.

6. R. Y. Calne and D. J. G. White, "The use of Cyclosporin A in clinical organ grafting," *Annals of Surgery* (1982), 196:330.

7. European Multi-centre Trial, "Cyclosporin in cadaveric renal transplantation: One year follow-up of a multi-center trial," *Lancet* (1983), ii:986; Canadian Multi-center Transplant Group, "A randomized clinical trial of Cyclosporin in cadaveric renal transplantation," *New England Journal of Medicine* (1983), 309:809; Borel, "History of Cyclosporin A."

8. Calne, White, et al., "Cyclosporin A in patients."

9. Calne, Rolles, et al., "Cyclosporin A initially."

10. T. Kino, H. Hatanaka, et al., "FK506, a novel immunosuppressant isolated from a streptomyces. I. Fermentation, isolation, and physiochemical and biological characteristics," *Journal of Antibiotics* (1987), 40:1249.

11. T. E. Starzl, S. Todo, et al., "FK506 for liver, kidney and pancreas transplantation," *Lancet* (1989), 2:1000.

12. L. K. Altman, "Drug shows stunning success in organ transplant operation," *New York Times*, October 18, 1989.

13. European FK506 Study Group, "A European multi-center randomized study to compare the efficacy and safety of FK506 with that of cyclosporine in patients undergoing primary liver transplantation: 6 month results," minutes of the 1993 annual meeting of the American Society for Transplant Surgery, 63; U.S. Multi-center FK506 Liver Study Group, "U.S. multi-center prospective randomized trial comparing FK506 to cyclosporine after liver transplantation: Primary outcome analysis," ibid., 33.

14. European Multi-centre Trial, "Cyclosporin"; Canadian Multi-center Transplant Group, "Randomized trial."

15. A. C. Allison, E. M. Eugui, and H. W. Sollinger, "Mycophenolate mofetil (RS-61442): Mechanisms of action and effects in transplantation," *Transplantation Reviews* (1993), 7:129; E. Cole, P. Keown, et al., "Safety and tolerability of cyclosporine and cyclosporine micromulsion during 18 months of follow-up in stable renal transplant recipients. A report of the Canadian Neoral Renal Study Group," *Transplantation* (1998), 65:505.

16. Avicinna, "Rules for testing new drugs," *Canon*, cited in H. Garrison, *An Introduction to the History of Medicine* (Philadelphia: W. B. Saunders, 1963), 130.

Chapter 13. The Industrialization of Transplantation

1. U.S. Department of Health and Human Services, *1996 Annual Report*.

2. N. Croft, "Supply of UK renal transplant surgeons dwindling," *Lancet* (1997), 349:708.

3. W. N. Hubbard, Jr., "The origins of medicinals," in J. E. Bowers and E. T. Purcell, *Advances in American Medicine: Essays at the Bicentennial* (Baltimore: Port City Press, 1976), 685–721.

4. T. Mahoney, *The Merchants of Life: An Account of the American Pharmaceutical Industry* (New York: Harper, 1959).

5. B. Werth, *The Billion Dollar Molecule: One Company's Quest for a Perfect Drug* (New York: Simon and Schuster, 1984), 268–271.

6. T. Bodenheimer, "Uneasy alliance—clinical investigators and the pharmaceutical industry," *New England Journal of Medicine* (2000), 342:1539.

7. M. Angell, "Is academic medicine for sale?" *New England Journal of Medicine* (2000), 342:1516.

8. M. E. Watanabe, "Not enough researchers in the clinic?" *The Scientist* (2001), 15:1; Angell, "Academic medicine."

9. "Yale spins off five biotech firms," *Yale Medicine* (Summer 1988), 4.

10. E. B. Chain, "Academic and industrial contributions to drug research," *Nature* (1963), 200:441.

11. R. D. Guttmann, "Technology, clinical studies, and control in the field of organ transplantation," *Journal of the History of Biology* (1997), 30:367.

12. K. Archer and F. McLellan, "Controversy surrounds proposed xenotransplant trial," *Lancet* (2001), 359:949.

13. N. L. Tilney, R. D. Guttmann, et al., "The new chimera: The industrialization of organ transplantation," *Transplantation* (2001), 71:591.

14. D. Weatherall, "Academia and industry: Increasingly uneasy bedfellows," *Lancet* (2000) 355:1574.

Chapter 14. Unexpected Specters

1. P. A. Ubel, R. M. Arnold, and A. L. Caplan, "Rationing failure: The ethical lessons of the retransplantation of scarce vital organs," *Journal of the American Medical Association* (1993), 270:2469.

2. C. O. Callender, "Kidney transplant allocation in America: An African American transplant surgeon's perspective," in J. M. Cecka and P. I. Terasaki, eds., *Clinical Transplants* (Los Angeles: UCLA Tissue Typing Laboratory, 1996), 355; R. H. Kerman, P. M. Kimball, et al., "Influence of race on cross-match outcome and recipient eligibility for transplantation," *Transplantation* (1992), 53:64; D. E. Butkus, "Primary renal cadaveric allograft survival in blacks: Is there still a significant difference?" *Transplantation Reviews* (1991), 5:91.

3. U.S. Renal Disease System, *USRDS 2001 Annual Data Report. Atlas of End-Stage Renal Disease in the United States* (Bethesda: National Institute of Diabetes, Digestive and Kidney Diseases, 2001).

4. U.S. organ procurement and transplantation network and scientific registry of transplant recipients, transplant data 1991–2000 (Washington, D.C.: U.S. Department of Health and Human Services, 2001).

5. K. C. Reddy, in W. Land and J. B. Dossiter, eds., *Organ Replacement Therapy: Ethics, Justice, Commerce* (New York: Springer-Verlag, 1990), 173.

6. M. Kauffman, W. K. Graham, et al., "UNOS donor data update," *Transplantation Proceedings* (1988–1999).

7. H. G. Welch and E. B. Larson, "Dealing with limited resources: The Oregon decision to curtail funding for organ transplantation," *New England Journal of Medicine* (1988), 318:171.

8. J. Rovner, "Anger at US transplant waiting times 'scare,'" *Lancet* (1998), 351: 1794.

9. A. S. Daar and R. A. Sells, "Living non-related donor renal transplantation—a reappraisal," *Transplantation Reviews* (1990), 4:128.

10. W. DeJone, J. Drachman, et al., "Options for increasing organ donation: The potential role of financial incentives, standardized hospital procedures, and public education to promote family discussion," *Milbank Quarterly* (1995), 73:463.

11. A. L. Caplan, C. T. Van Buren, and N. L. Tilney, "Financial compensation for cadaver organ donation: Good idea or anathema?" *Transplantation Proceedings* (1993), 25:2740.

12. J. H. Jones, *Bad Blood* (New York: Free Press, 1981).

13. R. Schwindt and A. R. Vining, "Proposal for a futures delivery market for transplant organs," *Journal of Health Politics, Policy and Law* (1986), 11:483.

14. D. Brahams, "Kidney for sale by live donor," *Lancet* (1989), i:285; D. J. Rothman, "The international organ trade," *New York Review*, March 26, 1998, 14–17.

15. M. Finkel, "This little kidney went to market," *New York Times*, May 27, 2001. Cited by permission.

16. Ibid.

17. The Council of the Transplantation Society, "Commercialization in transplantation: The problems and some guidelines for practice," *Transplantation* (1986), 41:1; World Medical Association resolution adopted at its 39th annual meeting, October 1987, Madrid.

18. F. D. Moore, "Three ethical revolutions: Ancient assumptions remodeled under pressure of transplantation," *Transplantation Proceedings* (1988), 20: suppl. 1, 1061; J. Radcliffe-Richards, A. S. Daar, et al., "The case for allowing kidney sales," *Lancet* (1988), 351:1950.

19. Brahams, "Kidney for sale."

20. P. A. Marshall and A. S. Daar, "Cultural and psychological dimensions of human organ transplantation," *Annals of Transplantation* (1998), 3:7; L. Cohen, "Where it hurts: Indian material for an ethics of organ transplantation," *Daedalus* (1999), 128.4:135.

21. K. S. Jarayaman, "Further fears of HIV in India," *Nature* (1989), 337:496; K. Banerjee, J. Rodrigues, et al., "Outbreak of HIV seropositivity among commercial plasma donors in Pune, India," *Lancet* (1989), 2:166; G. M. Abouna, M. S. A. Kumar, et al., "Commercialisation in human organs—A Middle East perspective," *Transplantation Proceedings* (1990), 22:918.

22. R. D. Guttmann, "On the use of organs from executed prisoners," *Transplantation Reviews* (1992), 6:189; C. Chelda, "China's human-organ trade highlighted by US arrest of 'salesman,'" *Lancet* (1998), 351:735; E. Rivera and M. Turner, "Body parts for sale," *Time*, March 9, 1995, 76.

23. R. Monroe, ed., "Human rights watch/Asia report," quoted in D. J. Rothman, E. Rose, et al., "The Bellagio task force report on transplantation, bodily integrity, and the international traffic in organs," *Transplantation Proceedings* (1997), 29:2739; R. Sheil, "Draft report: Use of organs from executed prisoners," *Transplantation Society Bulletin* (1996), 5:28.

24. Rothman, Rose, et al., "Bellagio task force report"; Council of the Transplantation Society, "Commercialization"; E. A. Santiago-Delpin, "Guidelines to assist authorities in each country with regard to transplantation," *Transplantation Society Bulletin* (1997), 6:9; Chelda, "China's trade"; Rivera and Turner, "Body parts"; quotation from E. Goodman, "The organ trade," *Boston Globe*, March 6, 1998.

25. Rothman, Rose, et al., "Bellagio task force report"; T. Leventhal, "The 'baby parts' myth: The anatomy of a rumor," United States Information Agency (Dec. 1994), 42; V. Muntarbhorn, "Sale of children," report of the special rapporteur to the UN Commission on Human Rights, January 12, 1993; Rothman, "International organ trade."

26. Monroe, "Human rights watch"; "Organ sales suggested in deaths of orphans," *Boston Globe*, March 18, 1999.

27. N. Scheper-Hughes, "Neo-cannibalism: The global trade in human organs," *Hedgehog Review* (Summer 2001), vol. 3; M. Lock, *Twice Dead: Organ Transplants and the Reinvention of Death* (Berkeley: University of California Press, 2002), 47.

28. Scheper-Hughes, "Neo-cannibalism."

29. J. Watson, "Harvesting," *New England Journal of Medicine* (2000), 343: 1499. Used by permission.

Chapter 15. Future Prospects

1. United Network for Organ Sharing, *2001 Annual Report*.

2. S. Westaby, A. P. Banning, et al., "First permanent implant of the Jarvik 2000 heart," *Lancet* (2000), 356:900.

3. D. Steinberg, "Stem cells tapped to replenish organs," *The Scientist* (2000), 14:20; G. R. Burgio and F. Locatelli, "Ethics of increasing programmed stem-cell donors," *Lancet* (2000), 356:1868.

4. M. McCarthy, "Bioengineers bring new start to stem-cell research," *Lancet* (2000), 356:1500.

5. L. Rosenberg, "Physician-scientists: Endangered and essential," *Science* (1999), 283:331.

6. W. M. Bennett, "American Society of Nephrology presidential address," *Journal of the American Society of Nephrology* (2000), 11:1548.

7. "Number of independent dialysis facilities climbed to 3065 in 1999," *Nephrology News and Issues* (September 2000), 10; P. P. Garg, K. D. Frick, et al., "Effect of ownership of dialysis facilities on patients' survival and referral for transplantation," *New England Journal of Medicine* (1999), 341:1653.

8. W. M. Bennett, presidential address in 2000 to the American Society of Nephrology.

Index

Pneumothorax, 180
Praxagoras of Cos, 213
Prednisone, 80, 169
Preservation, organ, 139–141, 174, 204
Prisoner donors, 48–49, 270–271
Public health measures, 84–85

Rabelais, François, 9–10
Radiation, total-body, 67–71, 72–73, 75
Ragosta, Vincent, 199–200
Raphael, 7
Reemstma, Keith, 222
Reitz, Bruce, 185
Rejection: circulating antibodies and, 137; of
    organ vs skin grafts, 110–112; pattern of,
    42–43, 83; second-set, 98; of skin grafts,
    17, 58, 97, 106, 110, 111–112, 136; tumor
    studies, 92–93; of xenogeneic organs, 223,
    225–226. See also Immunosuppression;
    Immunosuppressive drugs
Religion, transplantation motif in, 4–5, 7–9,
    8, 9
Renal transplants. See Kidney transplants
Renard, Marius, 49–50, 50
Research. See Medical research; Phar-
    maceutical research; Transplantation re-
    search
Rhinoplasty, 12–15, 13
Rich, Arnold, 93–94
Riteris, Andrew and John, 72–73, 74
Roentgen, Wilhelm, 165
Rowlandson, Thomas, 23, 24
Royal Colleges of Surgeons, 120
Russell, John, 182–183
Russell, Louis, 176
Russell, Paul, 102

Saliceto, William, 213
Salvarsan, 92
Sandoz company, 231–232, 241, 252–253
Sayers, Dorothy L., 29
Scaffolding, 280
Schwartz, Robert, 75, 76
Scientific fraud, 107
Scientific method, Medawar on, 117
Scola, James, 55
Scott, Helenus, 23
Semmelweis, Philipp, 25
Servelle, Marcel, 48–49
Sex glands, grafting of, 29–35, 43
Shaw, George Bernard, 92
Shroeder, William, 197
Shumway, Norman: on Barnard's heart
    transplant, 173; on heart donor/recipient

match, 169–170; heart-lung transplants of,
    185; heart transplant experiments of, 168–
    169; heart transplants of, 172, 178, 179; on
    xenografts, 228
Simonsen, Morten, 111
6–mercaptopurine (6–MP), 75–76, 77, 78,
    79, 169, 248
Sixty Minutes, 162, 258
Skin grafts: with artificial skin, 279; history
    of, 15–19, 16; radiation and, 68, 70; rejec-
    tion of, 17, 58, 97, 106, 110, 136; tolerance
    of, 114–115; xenografts, 218, 219
Smallpox epidemics, 84
Smallpox vaccination, 86–87
Snow, John, 84
Sophocles, 4
Sphinx, 4
Stanford University, 185
Stanley, Leo, 31
Starzl, Thomas, 126, 134, 138, 175, 202, 248;
    FK506 research of, 239, 240; kidney trans-
    plants of, 78, 80, 81, 134, 204, 205; liver
    transplants of, 201, 202, 224; multivisceral
    transplants of, 215–216; xenografts of, 222,
    224
Steinach, Eugen, 30
Stem cells, bioengineering of, 279–280
Stenburg, Lief, 197
Stevenson, Robert Louis, 23, 122
Streptomycin, 247
Summerlin, William, 106–108
Sushruta, 10–11, 11, 12, 38, 164, 213
Sutures, vascular, 36–37, 37, 39–40
Swine flu virus, 227

Tagliacozzi, Gasparo, 12–14, 13, 219
Tati, Moshe, 266–267
Teeth, transplantation of, 21–24, 24
Terasaki, Paul, 94, 96, 137, 137–139, 204
Testicular grafting, 31–35
Thomas, Dylan, 23
Thorn, George, 51–52, 54, 55, 62, 72, 79, 248
Thymus gland: removal of, 129–130; role in
    immunity, 96–97
Times, 178
Tissue matching/typing, 127, 136–139
Tolerance: clinical applications of, 76, 116–
    117; defined, 113; early research on, 113–
    115; Medawar's experiments on, 76, 113,
    115–116
Tolypocladium inflatium (Gans), 232
Total-body radiation, 67–71, 72–73, 75
Transplantation. See Transplantation, history
    of; Transplantation research; specific types